Psychological Adaptive Mechanisms

Psychological Adaptive Mechanisms

Ego Defense Recognition in Practice and Research

Thomas P. Beresford, MD

Professor of Psychiatry
Department of Veterans Affairs Medical Center
School of Medicine, University of Colorado-Denver

OXFORD
UNIVERSITY PRESS

OXFORD
UNIVERSITY PRESS

Oxford University Press, Inc., publishes works that further
Oxford University's objective of excellence
in research, scholarship, and education.

Oxford New York
Auckland Cape Town Dar es Salaam Hong Kong Karachi
Kuala Lumpur Madrid Melbourne Mexico City Nairobi
New Delhi Shanghai Taipei Toronto

With offices in
Argentina Austria Brazil Chile Czech Republic France Greece
Guatemala Hungary Italy Japan Poland Portugal Singapore
South Korea Switzerland Thailand Turkey Ukraine Vietnam

Published by Oxford University Press, Inc.
198 Madison Avenue, New York, New York 10016
www.oup.com

Library of Congress Cataloging-in-Publication Data
Beresford, Thomas P.
Psychological adaptive mechanisms : ego defense recognition
in practice and research / by Thomas P. Beresford.
p. ; cm.
Includes bibliographical references and index.
ISBN 978–0–19–979449–2 (hardcover : alk. paper)
I. Title.
[DNLM: 1. Defense Mechanisms. 2. Adaptation, Psychological.
3. Stress, Psychological. WM 193]
155.2—dc23
2012000399

"The best minds are those that are most various and most supple."

—Montaigne

For Ed, Hal, and Charlie
whose separate journeys from infancy to maturity
continue to give my life its wonder

CONTENTS

PREFACE

Were it not for the subject material itself, this book would have only its role as a training manual to recommend it to its readership. And, fundamentally, it remains an education tool designed to provide its readers with a practical method of recognizing the ways in which people adapt to the world around them. But the method does not exist in a vacuum or even in a laboratory. Its proper sphere of reference resides in everyday human life itself: how each of us comes to terms with the experiences of our lives, even at different times during our individual courses and through changing circumstances. As a result, the model of human psychological adaptation offered here and, more specifically, the stepwise algorithmic approach to recognizing observable human behaviors in the clinical and other practical settings offer, humbly, another window on the stuff of human life. Remembering Alexander Pope's famous comment three centuries ago, it is another episode in Man's proper study of Man.

This particular submission in that ceaseless project of human understanding represents the work of many years. It owes a large debt to the preceding scholars and observers, those whose science I discuss in Chapter 2, as well as those whose observations recorded either as fiction or as history that I have freely sprinkled in the body of the text throughout. More on those authors and their works shortly. But for now, I must thank formally those who have provided the truly practical inspiration for what I hope will readers will view as a practical book.

These comprise the members of generations following mine for whom I have been fortunate to serve as a teacher: the successive classes of psychiatry residents, medical students, and residents, fellows, and graduate students of other disciplines, whether medical or nonmedical. The psychiatry resident classes at the University of Colorado's School of Medicine from 1992 to the present deserve special mention as a group. When I began teaching about psychological adaptive mechanisms my offerings to them conveyed little more than an exposure to the work of George Vaillant. The classes found them, as I did, fascinating but repeatedly asked me a difficult question: How do we use this?

Talking about how people adapt wasn't good enough. My audience of clinicians demanded, in their gentle inquiry, a practical way of assimilating and then using the knowledge in *this* patient, that is, the one sitting in my office whom I must understand and assist. Over the next 19 years I began developing the systematic, practical use of Vaillant's concepts and glossary of ego defense mechanisms. I have worked daily for the majority of that time as a psychiatric consultant to internal medicine specialists and surgeons, seeing their hospitalized patients: the perfect classroom in which to see adaptive behaviors as people came to terms with illness, physical or mental or emotional. At the beginning, like the famous U.S. Supreme Court opinion on pornography, I knew human adaptation when I saw it but had to respond to putting that recognition in a systematic format that our residents could follow, apprehend, and then use consistently.

The hierarchical continuum of adaptive mechanisms that Vaillant reported empirically recommended itself as a natural algorithmic path with which to approach systematic recognition. I had previously had considerable success in applying a decision algorithm to the process of evaluating alcohol dependent candidates who requested liver transplantation (Beresford, 1990), a process too that entailed a clinical assessment method based in empirical knowledge. Applying the stepwise approach of a decision algorithm to the Domain hierarchy of the psychological adaptive mechanisms seemed to me a short step.

FROM EGO DEFENSES TO PSYCHOLOGICAL ADAPTATION MECHANISMS

But a stepwise approach alone did not suffice for my pedagogically demanding residents. They found the terms themselves confusing. Psychological adaptive mechanisms at the time were known as *ego defense mechanisms*, a term I used comfortably, having learned my specialty from a faculty who were known as the Young Turks of Boston psychoanalysis. While I am not now, and have never been, a member of any psychoanalytic society, I understood what the psychoanalytic model meant by the term *ego*, for example, and thought this common knowledge among psychiatric residency training programs. That too was insufficient: the students wanted to know what ego meant in *this* setting, what was it that the ego found itself defending against, and how was *defense* the same as *adaptation*. What did terms in common speech, like *acting out* and *repression*, mean when we used them clinically, and how did we define them with the precision needed to make them useful as medical specialists in taking care of our patients? These questions put me in their position—turned me back into a student rather than a professor—and made it clear to me that I had to come up with a model of greater clarity and greater simplicity in order to offer something that would be widely useful.

From this came the model of psychological adaptation and the observable behaviors, or mechanisms, presented in this volume. Ego defense mechanisms became psychological adaptive mechanisms, and the algorithm focused on the four Domains in the hierarchy, a much simpler clinical—and teaching—process than that of trying to pick one out of the eighteen specific styles impromptu. As this thought process continued, both in my conceptualizations and in the interactive discussions with questioning residents, the concept of adaptation itself came to the fore. The idea of human adaptation offered a much more dynamic and more positive formulation of the phenomenon that the residents found much easier to understand. Vaillant's work had included this all along, and the transition work of moving from empirical research into clinical usefulness served to actualize it. My role seemed to recall Michelangelo's conception of his artistic process: not creating a sculptured figure *de novo*, but finding the figure that already resided in the marble and bringing it out.

A MATTER OF MODELS

In locating the figure in the marble, my present goal, by analogy, is to present a simple, consistent, usable model and method in recognizing human psychological adaptive mechanisms. Science is always and everywhere a series of working hypotheses rather than a statement of absolute Truth. And that is certainly no less true in this instance. Human behaviors occur in such rich, varied, and emotionally moving, colors and textures that no one explanation suffices for all. Michelangelo found many figures residing in different blocks of marble, not just one. In order to serve the variety of human experience and the variety of observations we can make about it, I have freely—some might say shamelessly—borrowed from many different models in the course of this book.

These vary from models of experience as far disparate as early 20th-century psychoanalysis that originated the term *ego defense mechanisms* and the late 19th-century objective/descriptive psychiatry school that insisted on observable behaviors. Both of these function in our day, and I am happy to make use of any concepts that appear useful. Other models include mention of the formulation of the Unconscious that we owe first to the elder Freud and then to the more inclusive model of it that Jung saw as linked to the genetic and neural inheritance of the brain. Discussed first in Chapter 2, the concepts of both *mind* and *brain* take their turns in informing the discussion throughout. Words like *stress* and *anxiety* from other models form a particularly important part of the discussion as does the idea of an internal equilibrium that we owe to the early 20th-century biologists as they went about describing the inner workings of the cell.

Paradoxically, the goal of my borrowing freely from many sources resulted in establishing what I believe is greater simplicity in the systematic method of recognizing adaptive behaviors. Models, in my view, are not mutually exclusive, as compared to dogmatically stated "truths" that cannot be argued with or tested clinically. As a clinician I look for the most appropriate model from among several that may apply in day-to-day work. The adaptive model I offer in this volume is one of those, but is by no means intended as an exclusive one.

ABOUT UNDERSTANDING

Clinical recognition is always a process of detection. Proper recognition, whether viewed in one or in a series of models, leads to useful diagnosis. Diagnosis determines treatment, and treatment is measured in outcome, the most useful of all measures. As a result, my hope is to present, in sequence, (1) the phenomenon of human adaptation, (2) a simplified, coherent model of how it works, and (3) the systematic method for recognizing psychological adaptation mechanisms, followed by (4) continuing practice in applying the recognition method and (5) a brief description of where the use of recognizing psychological adaptation mechanisms may take us as we learn more.

While this work comes from my experience in the clinic and in teaching and in research, I believe the model proposed here, along with its recognition algorithm, can be used in any of a multiplicity of its settings from storytelling to international diplomacy. The prime object of his book is to make the knowledge it contains useful, practical, and available. Its ultimate goal is to add to our understanding of human experience and to aid in the effort of doing so. Paradoxically again, the more we understand human psychological adaptation, the better we will be in adapting to our circumstances both as individuals and as citizens of our planet.

WRITERS AS COLLEAGUES

As I have borrowed from many models, I have also added many colleagues whom the reader might not expect to show up in a book of this nature. Whether formulated as adaptive behaviors or not, how humans adapt to their own experiences has fascinated writers of many works in many eras. In my view writers were the first to record the observable behaviors that I formulate as psychological adaptive mechanisms. The heritage they gave us in doing so I regard as a rich source of information that frequently exemplifies psychological adaptation mechanisms and gives the recognition process a substance that readers and I can use.

Fiction writers in this volume do not turn up themselves as subject for "literary psychoanalysis" of the author or interpretations of their works according to the tenets of that model. Rather, I treat all of the authors I quote, fiction writers included, as colleagues and teachers. The best of them not only observe, but communicate what they see to us in ways that put us directly among their characters as observers. Where their work ends, ours starts. It is our responsibility to understand what they put before us, not as their interpreters, but as their students, standing beside them working hard to see what they see. Where I quote from history, I regard the writer in the same terms: as an observer whose words convey experience. Again, our responsibility involves trying our best to see what they see.

Even though, for practicality, I freely quote only small parts of longer fiction works, I realize that their authors have written them for other purposes. The work of a true artist serves on many different planes of consciousness and perception, by no means solely in a simple model of psychological adaptive mechanisms. By borrowing their words, I intend no detraction from these larger purposes or from the complex reactions of a reader to the whole of a writer's work. One small hope lies in my belief that some of the vignettes quoted here may lead readers to the originals, into the grand works of human imagination we can find in the best writers.

GRATITUDE

While this is a book about recognition and understanding, it is also one of gratitude. I had never heard of ego defense mechanisms until I learned that term from one of the faculty members at The Cambridge Hospital/Harvard Medical School program, where I trained in psychiatry between 1973 and 1976. George Vaillant had begun his landmark longitudinal research work on the subject, and I remember the lights going on, so to speak, as I read his seminal paper on the subject, as mentioned in

Chapter 2 and the first to offer a glossary of the mechanisms. It was my great good fortune to work with him as one of my supervisors during my year as chief resident, and my good fortune continues as I thank him here. George Vaillant was not alone in that magnificent cadre of clinical teachers in that place at that time. Another of them, Bennett Simon, one of the few psychoanalysts I have ever seen wearing a stethoscope, influences these pages by what he taught us from his studies of writers as observers, from the ancient Greeks to the present day. It is my great pleasure to thank him for his igniting the campfires and oil lamps: for turning on the lights for us to see the work of the gifted observers who guide us from their times to ours.

Three others of my teachers deserve special mention. The late John Pearce, who practiced psychiatry for many years in Cambridge, Massachusetts, taught me to think about adaptive behaviors and to begin to wonder about how they might apply to clinical situations. It took me many years to begin to see how adaptation ideas might be usefully applied in clinical psychiatry and how this might fit with George Vaillant's systematic studies. Were he with us now, it would be my very great pleasure to thank him, one of the most intelligent and perceptive physicians I have ever known. The second is Kenneth Fields, a professor of English and creative writing at Stanford, my teacher both as an undergraduate and later as a Stegner Fellow in poetry. It is my privilege to present two of his poems in Chapters 20 and 21 as exemplifying Sublimation and Humor, respectively. But my true debt goes back to his teaching the works of American poets from the point of view of "how poems get written." It was his scholarship that first taught me to consider what the poems meant, not just to a passing reader, but in lives of those who wrote them and who gave them to us so that we could stand at their shoulders and see what they saw. The present book, a far cry from the tentative essays of a struggling undergraduate, offers the thanks of all of us who learned from him and those of us who continue to do so. The third and last, if the reader will permit, is my late father. Just as I have never been a psychoanalyst so, too, I have never piloted a fighter plane. But the reader will notice that fighter pilots make several appearances in the ensuing chapters. My father served in World War II as a crew chief with the First Pursuit Group in what was then the Army Air Corps. He, along with his colleague Sgt. Gilbert Green, received the first two operational P-38s delivered to what is now known as the First Fighter Wing. Through the course of about three and a half years in the European theater of that conflict, he never lost a pilot. The boyhood interest I began in his shadow has transformed into an exploration of adaptive behaviors among those who flew those machines, as well as among those of us who see flight more in symbolic rather than concrete terms.

As the content of this book has taken shape over the past few years, mention of the topic in casual conversation with a number of others from professions besides psychiatry or medicine frequently brought forth their interest in it. This, I believe, attests to the aspects of human adaptive experiences that ring true in everyday life for most of us. More specifically, however, the diversity of discussions further informed my own thinking. Two instances especially deserve mention: conversations with one person on *Jane Eyre* that led to including a discussion of Charlotte Brontë's sharply drawn characters in the text, and comments and written criticisms from Elizabeth Karpinski Vonne that helped clarify the early chapters. I thank them both for their interest and their insights as educated readers not bound by technical jargon.

As this book began taking its final shape I was most fortunate to hire the editorial talents of two of my research associates, Jennifer Ratzlaff, M.A., and Chelsea Dize, Ph.D., who offered both revisions of content and of style in the manuscript, and did so during their off hours. Both are talented editors and writers of English prose and had no reservations whatsoever in pointing out instances in which my writing could be made simpler and clearer. I hope they see their work throughout this volume, and I know that readers will be grateful for the precision of language upon which they insisted. At the same time, it is appropriate to acknowledge the two institutions in which I work: the Department of Veterans Affairs (VA) that pays my salary in return for my clinical, research, and related efforts, and the School of Medicine of the University of Colorado Denver under whose auspices I carry my professorship and whose students and residents I teach in our VA medical center. For administrative clarity, let me state that this work is the product of evenings and weekends and was not pursued during normal working hours. Nonetheless, I consider myself doubly honored to work in our VA medical center, part of the national health system that is dedicated to the care of the veteran poor, and to serve on the faculty of the School of Medicine that is entrusted with the responsibility for continued development of the science and art of medicine. I hope that this continued form of inter-institutional cooperation will grow into even greater levels of effectiveness and that my work in this volume will reflect well on both entities.

My effort at furthering our ability to recognize the experiences of human adaptation would certainly not have seen the light of day without the interest and the effort of the Oxford University Press. Specifically, this project began as a proposal that Craig Panner first saw as valuable and then guided through the review and agreement stages. David D'Addona, who has served as the very patient editor of the manuscript itself, has done the heavy work needed to get this project off the ground, so to speak, and deserves special thanks along with his assistant, Kurt Roediger, as it tries a few banks and turns in the air. Emily Perry, Mary Anne Shahidi, J. Ramprasad, and their colleagues have provided irreplaceable contributions in copy editing and production. This is my second book with Oxford University Press (see Beresford and Gomberg, 1994), and it has confirmed my belief that any publishing house without a charter from Henry the Eighth is very likely a fly-by-night outfit. My heartfelt thanks go to all of them. I send special words of thanks to my son the architect who shares my family name and who turned my crude drawings into figures that clarify beyond words, as well as to Mr. Brian Beresford for his kind assistance with Chapter 3.

CONCLUSIONS: A BOOK OF LOVE

Through the course of writing this book, I have learned far more than I knew when I began it. Some specifics stand out. For one, I wonder about our understanding of human compassion. Psychological adaptation appears to be an active process that, in the model provided in Chapter 2, stress and anxiety call forth. But except in extreme circumstances, such as in the unrelenting stress observed in Major Edward

Mannock's case in Chapter 7, we are not necessarily engaged in overt adaptive behaviors during every hour of waking consciousness. When we do engage psychological adaptive mechanisms, however, the availability of compassion—that human attribute by which we share the feelings of others—now appears to me accessible to us only when active psychological adaptation occurs at the Mature Domain level. At the same time, it appears likely that we are capable of some level of compassion during times in which an active psychological adaptive response is not engaged, when waking consciousness enjoys relative calm. Is this true? Are we more capable of human compassion when we are not threatened? And when we are threatened, do only Mature Domain adaptive mechanisms allow us to share in the feelings of others?

In a related question, do the adaptive responses of the individual generalize into the adaptive responses of groups? For all of our history, human beings have adapted to the circumstances of their lives both as individuals and in groups. Formulated as group adaptations, some appear to have caused widespread destruction and loss of life: witness the totalitarian regimes of the 20th century that brought death on massive scales in different parts of the world. By contrast, other group adaptations have brought humanity its democratic forms of government, the world's best art and literature, and a setting in which the liberty of the human spirit has informed the education of generations of free people. How do psychological adaptive mechanisms apply to groups? What explains the wide variations in group adaptive behaviors? And what role do the Mature Domain mechanisms play in providing for compassion in groups of human beings, as contrasted to the three other Domains?

For another point of learning, I find it possible to conclude that the innate psychological makeup of human beings pushes each of us toward increasing maturity of psychological adaptive mechanisms rather than the reverse. This can be countered by the biological failure of the body's functions that mediate adaptation—including those of the brain. It can be slowed by the lack of the social and interpersonal environments needed to support natural psychological development toward Mature Domain adaptation mechanisms. It can be reversed, temporarily or perhaps permanently in some cases, when overwhelmed by acute or constant stresses that can drive psychological adaptation downward toward immaturity. How best can the basic psychological functions involved in work, play, and relationships with others maximize the individual human momentum toward Mature Domain adaptation styles? How does compassion make itself known in this process, and when and how can we maximize the human ability to connect with the thoughts and feelings of others?

From the point of view of the adaptation model offered here, I am less and less sure that we have sufficient systematic data that might answer these important questions. Questions that I believe have direct bearing on how we treat ourselves, each other, our children, and our planet. But a consideration of the processes and mechanisms of psychological adaptation makes it clear that we have the ability to adapt and, at our best, to do so with remarkable creativity and effectiveness. When Michel de Montaigne, writing in the 16th century, said that "our chief talent is the power of suiting ourselves to different ways of life" and that "to be tied and bound of necessity to one single way is not to live but to exist" (Montaigne, 1958, p. 250), he seemed to be asking us to pay attention to the flexibility of our adaptive natures. Some

300 years later, when Leo Tolstoy asserted in *War and Peace* that "to understand everything is to forgive everything" (Tolstoy, 1994, p. 111), he too appeared to be talking about human adaptation and human compassion. Ultimately, in following the paths of human adaptation described in these pages, human experience itself invites the reader to the understanding and to the shared feeling that unites us all.

Thomas P. Beresford, M.D.
March 2012

REFERENCES

Beresford, T. P., et al. (1990). "A rational approach to liver transplantation for the alcoholic patient." *Psychosomatics 31*(3):241–254.
Beresford, T. P., and E. S. L. Gomberg. (1994). *Alcohol and Aging*. New York, Oxford University Press.
de Montaigne, M. (1958). *Essays* (J. M. Cohen, Trans.). London, Penguin Books.
Tolstoy, L. (1994). *War and Peace* (C. Garnett, Trans.). New York, Random House.

Psychological Adaptive Mechanisms

CHAPTER 1

Humans Adapt

Psychological adaptation—the ability to come to terms with the stresses of one's environment, whether these come from sources internal or external to the individual person—remains a unique characteristic of the lives of human beings.

As an example, the earliest evidence of human burial ritual, ascribed to Neanderthal man, can be thought of as an internal adaptation to an external phenomenon, namely the death of another person. Where before the person was moving, breathing, and warm, now all three are absent. The living onlookers have before them a number of options, including simply ignoring the fact, moving away from it, or disposing of the remains as so much waste. Instead, they choose to bury both the deceased body and, along with it, objects that were important in life, such as carefully crafted stone tools. The living must come to terms with the event because, uniquely among animal, vegetable, and microbial beings, they have the ability to understand that the death of another prefigures their own passing. As an act of life, they engage in a ritual that draws them together and itself allows for a greater range of freedom in living their own lives. In this sense, although not negating the inevitability of demise, they come to terms with it in a way that allows them to function. As we shall note, the ultimate goal of successful psychological adaptation is to increase adaptive options to include the most flexible, creative, and therefore most effective actions available to any single person at any given point in time. Put another way, the highest forms of psychological adaptation promote the most effective human functioning. And at base, all forms of psychological adaptation, including the most psychologically primitive as we shall see, serve to make some form of action possible in response to a stress.

Observers from ancient times to the present have recorded their descriptions of humans coming to terms with their environment. This has taken many forms that can be communicated to others. As another example, one far down the millennia from the Neanderthal burial caves and taken from the visual arts, consider Rembrandt's painting *Bathsheba at Her Bath* (1654). In it the artist portrays the legendary biblical queen at the point of receiving the news of King David's interest in her. According to the biblical account, David has sent Bathsheba's husband Uriah, who is one of David's generals and a loyal soldier, to his certain death in a battle for territory. David has plotted to ensure that Uriah's soldiers desert him, leaving him to the enemy, who kill him.

In the painting, Bathsheba sits both physically and symbolically naked as she considers a written message from the king indicating his interest. A servant woman in the foreground prepares her bath. Bathsheba stands to gain from David's suit but, as Rembrandt portrays her, she has little actual power in a situation that could be considered a threat. But the Bathsheba of the painting is not stricken in a panic of anxiety or terror or even dread. Likewise, she is not celebrating or dancing for joy. Rembrandt's Bathsheba sits before us with a feeling of calm, an aspect of deliberation, and she exudes the sense that she will endure the circumstances that swirl about her and catch her up. It is a portrait of a woman in the process of adapting as best she can to a difficult situation, one that changes her life.

As onlookers, we glean all this from Rembrandt's painting because of the skill and invention with which he presents Bathsheba's pathos in having to respond to the change. We do not receive prior instructions, in the pedagogical sense, as to what he wants us to perceive in his painting, even though it assumes a passing acquaintance with the Bathsheba/David story. The artist, instead, expects us to work at seeing and understanding and feeling his work of art on its own terms. Rembrandt himself is nowhere to be found in the work and does not comment on it directly. This is both an advantage, as the work of art carries a life of its own, and a disadvantage, because the artist relies on our subjective perceptions. Communication comes about through the mechanisms that Carl Jung described in his groundbreaking model[1] of humans perceiving the world around them in patterns that are common to the biological/neural heritage of all human beings (Jung 1959). Without this ability, we would, in

1. *Model* serves as the operative word in this instance and in all those that follow when discussing conceptions of how the mind/brain works.

While I mention Jung here, the reader may find comfort in knowing that I do not consider myself a Jungian or any other *-ian* in this very complex setting about which we have much more to learn. As the reader will note, I freely and with no compunction borrow from any model that I believe has a positive contribution to make, including those of Sigmund Freud and Charles Darwin, of modern neurobiology, and of the great traditions of human myth, whether Western or Eastern, ancient, medieval or modern. The tapestry of human behavior is so rich that it seems to me important to consider many viewpoints and to avoid anointing any of them as the absolute truth.

As a clinician, however, my approach requires (1) collecting clinical data, (2) choosing one or more theoretical models in which to construe those data, and (3) providing treatment that best matches the data, with guidance from the most appropriate of the models available. As a result, in my view, clinicians require familiarity with a series of models, not just adherence to one at the exclusion of others. The approach in this book, as we shall see in Chapter 2 in detail, aims to provide a useful model, and in Chapter 3 its method for clinical use.

Carl Jung (1875–1961), a Swiss physician and psychiatrist, diagnosed and treated a variety of mental disorders, including those of considerable severity, before the discovery of effective medicines. His work with patients' mental productions led him to look for commonalities in perception that he could establish empirically. From this came his positing the existence of neural mechanisms by which humans perceive themselves and the world around them. In his model, because the forms of perception—what he called *archetypes*—appear common to all humans, he further posited that their basis exists in the biology of the organism. Modern neuroscience has much to learn from his observations and his empirically based model as that field of inquiry moves to understand how the brain works in its highest levels of complexity.

Jung's view, have to reinvent visual art each time we see a new painting, or indeed each time we receive any new perception not already stored in the brain. Rembrandt counts on our ability to perceive forms, and that is both the limit and the glory of visual art as a form of human observation.

Works of literature, in which words convey observations, offer by contrast much less visibly striking perceptions to the human eye than Rembrandt's artwork does. But they can deliver perceived details, and then the author's comments on them, in ways that allow for a wide range of perceptions. Those perceptions, at their best, include both the ideas and the feelings that describe human nature. Because of this, writers, from the earliest to the contemporary, have found human adaptive behaviors very fertile ground for using words to portray and comment upon human experience. They were probably among the first to discover that one ingredient in writing about human adaptive behaviors rests in the fact that those behaviors are observable. Consider, for example, these famous lines on the human emotion of anger that begin *The Iliad*:

> Sing, goddess, the anger of Peleus' son Achilleus
> and its devastation, which put pains thousand fold upon the Achaians,
> hurled in their multitudes to the house of Hades strong souls
> of heroes, but gave their bodies to be the delicate feasting
> of dogs, of all birds, and the will of Zeus was accomplished
> since that time when first there stood in the vision of conflict
> Atreus' son the lord of men and brilliant Achilleus.[2]
>
> (Homer, *The Iliad*, lines 1–7)

As we learn the story, Achilles' (Achilleus') anger occurs in response to a situation in which he feels himself insulted. He has just beaten the Trojans on a bloody Bronze Age battlefield where killing was done with broad sword and spear. He is the greatest, most effective of the Greek warriors laying siege to Troy, and he knows it. As the product of his human father and his mother, a minor goddess in the Greek ethos, he has a godlike strength in battle that is unparalleled by even the most worthy of his opponents. However, Agamemnon, the Greek king and leader of the forces invading Troy, has himself been denied a Trojan princess when the high priest Calchas tells him to return her to the Trojans or face the wrath of the gods. He complies with this but then claims for himself Achilles' prize: Briseus, another beautiful Trojan woman. This greatly perturbs Achilles, who perceives Agamemnon's action both as an injustice to his performance in the battle and as an insult to his status among the Greek warriors. Where before he was an effective fighter, now he is a very angry one.

---

2. Here, and in later quotations from both The Iliad and The Odyssey of Homer, I use the verse translations of Richmond Lattimore. Of Homer's translators in English, this author most closely approximates the structure of ancient Greek verse in the opinions of my learned colleagues in English literature and in classical Greek. More to the point, Lattimore's lines of six stressed syllables and varying unstressed syllables, each, make his work the most readable and pleasing to my ears of all the available translations.

The perturbation, or in present-day language used throughout this book, the stress, of the insult has called forth his fury. An obvious option lies before him—killing Agamemnon and stealing the woman—but Homer has the goddess Athena intervene, and Achilles chooses two other courses of action. First, he gives Agamemnon a verbal lashing in front of the other warriors, calling him a "wine sack, with a dog's eyes, with a deer's heart"—we might say a drunkard who follows a battle rather than leads it, and who runs away at the slightest provocation—among other things. And then Achilles retires from the battlefield, refusing to take any further part in the struggle. If the Greeks are to fight on, they must do so without him. This behavior, growing out of Achilles' reaction to what he perceives as a social disaster in being demeaned by his chief, in turn raises the anxiety of the other warriors who believe that without Achilles they are on their way to destruction and doom. And this indeed turns out to be the case.

We will make notice of this remarkable portrait of Homer's warrior in Chapter 8, but for now it is enough to recognize that Homer couches Achilles' behavior in adapting to the stress of the situation in the language of observation. He shows us what Achilles does, tells us what he says and what he thinks, and then provides his own commentary. Homer draws conclusions about Achilles from the data he gives us, for example, that Achilles is angry. And Homer shows his listeners and readers the effect of Achilles' emotion and how his method of adapting to it affects those around him. In this sense we "see" Achilles: that is, we *understand* his insult and we *feel* his anger. To Homer, and to us, human adaptation involves both cognition and emotion, both idea and feeling. Although the figure of Homer wrote this epic poem more than 3000 years ago, we perceive Homer's characters in their intellectual and emotional forms as though it were written yesterday.

Observable behaviors, then, make up the stuff of human adaptation. And if we consider the examples from the Neanderthal people, Rembrandt, and Homer reliable observations, that is, the kind of observations that can be repeated by other observers in other settings, then we may say that human adaptive behaviors abound in nature. That is, we can observe them as every day behavioral phenomena occurring out of human nature.

Their colorings and inflections, however, may come in very different forms, different languages, and even via different methods of observation. Like politics, that fine art of social adaptation, human adaptive behavior makes strange bedfellows. Consider these words of a man arriving at the house of a friend:

> I know not how it was—but, with the first glimpse of the building, a sense of insufferable gloom pervaded my spirit. I say insufferable; for the feeling was unrelieved by any of that half-pleasurable, because poetic, sentiment with which the mind usually receives even the sternest natural images of the desolate and terrible.
>
> (Poe 1998, p. 49)

The narrator goes on to describe the frightening aspect of the house in its horrid details. But for our purposes, in this passage he puts forth very clearly his inability to soften his perceptions at all: paraphrasing his words, he cannot see any poetry in it. In a very prescient and telling manner, far in advance of modern psychological theories of mind, the author describes the mental capacity to alter perceptions in a way that allows the perceiving human to take them in and adapt them for internal absorption. Although there is something horrible about this particular house that prevents the narrator from softening his perception of it, the author nonetheless acknowledges the capacity to do so, if only by its absence in this case. Edgar Allan Poe, in our day not always regarded as psychologically sophisticated, authors this observation as he begins his short story "The Fall of the House of Usher," published in 1839 (Poe 1998). And indeed it turns out to be a horror tale from this poet and writer known as the inventor of the modern detective story, and whose premature death itself remains a mystery.

If human psychological adaptive mechanisms are everywhere found in the varied colors that give us the rich textures of historical accounts, dramas, poems, novels, short stories, and journalistic reports—and we shall use all of these and more as sources of examples throughout the course of this book—our task is a much more technical one. The discussion that makes up this volume seeks to develop a clinical recognition tool that will allow us to make use of human adaptive behaviors in the dynamic processes of diagnosis and treatment, based in this psychiatric form of medicine and with potentially wider applicability. If this effort is successful, the reader will to learn to recognize human adaptive behaviors with clinical precision. This is not to say that we cannot see, and value, the individual shadings of these behavioral patterns. To do that would be to forgo much of the richness that clinical medicine brings to those who practice it and to limit much of our ability to be of use to other human beings. Rather, we look for the pattern that is common to adaptive styles because we want to use that pattern as it varies from the limiting simplicity of the most primitive methods of psychological adaptation through those that allow the enlightening and creative complexity of the most mature psychological adaptive styles.

Before proceeding to a method of recognition, the topic requires further definition of some of its keywords in the interest of clarity. These include some useful inklings of what we mean by *mind*, *brain*, *inside*, *outside*, *stress*, and *adaptation* and even technical words such as *ego*, *anxiety*, and *unconscious*. In providing these definitions, my purpose is not to create a comprehensive theory of the structure of either mind or brain; the result will not be a general field theory of the self or any of its components. Rather, I aim these definitions at the practical. I use them myself because I find them helpful in the psychiatric clinic or at the bedside on medical and surgical wards. For me, everyday usefulness is their ultimate test. For some readers, the definitions put forth here may seem too simple or simplistic, and for others they will seem arcane or at least too imaginary. This state of affairs calls to mind the words William Carlos Williams wrote near the end of "January Mornings," a poem to his wife Flossie:

> I wanted to write a poem
> that you would understand.
> For what good is it to me
> if you can't understand it?
> But you got to try hard—
>
> (Williams 1995, 103–104)

Dr. Williams, who returns in Chapter 19, practiced general medicine near Paterson, New Jersey, for all of his adult life. He understood very clearly the importance of perceiving the patterns in things around him. That function—the apprehension of patterns—often makes up the essence of what we refer to when we speak of the art of one thing or another, for example the art of medicine. It constitutes the diagnostic "feel" of sizing up a situation not only in medicine but in most human activities such as in business, parenting, creative arts, writing, and even in the performance of the best fighter pilots. In arriving at a diagnosis, in responding to the forces of the marketplace, in reacting to our children, in portraying human experience, and even in a split-second reaction in a high-performance flying machine, apprehending the patterns before us leads to the best understanding and most effective actions. The reader's task, as we proceed through the theory and many examples in recognizing psychological adaptation mechanisms and their uses, will be the same as Flossie's: to understand the patterns of the poetry[3] that human behavior puts before us. The complexity of human adaptation and our own responses to it require, for proper apprehension, that we all try hard. And, as in reading the best of Williams' poetry, learning the process should not occur without enjoyment.

MIND AND BRAIN

When we use the term *psychological adaptive mechanism* to describe specific responses to stress and anxiety in this discussion, the first word of that phrase implies the concept of mind. The first syllable in *psychological* derives from the ancient Greek word *psyche*, a word that can be narrowly defined as "conscious thought," or more specifically as "the experience of conscious thought"—what we notice in ourselves when we think. The original term meant far more than that: it included a much larger, more dynamic concept that is probably closest to what most of us mean when we speak of the human "spirit." That word usually connotes a dynamic and often systematic mingling of our thoughts, feelings, hopes, daytime dreams, affections, wants, needs, and more. No wonder that people before us from time to time separated out what they perceived as the various components of the *psyche* in order to understand it better.

The Romans coined the Latin noun *mens*, *mentis*, related to the verb *mentare* that meant "to think" and that contained the concepts of both the mind and the brain. Compare that to the Latin word *anima*, which more approached what we mean by spirit and what the Greeks meant by *psyche*. In medieval Christianity, the two functions were separated by what was seen—that is, the body, including the brain—and what was unseen, namely, "the soul." In Western civilization, most historians and scholars credit Plato in ancient Greece with the separation of the two concepts in respect to human experience: psyche, anima, spirit, soul—all having to do with the

3. The word *poetry* comes from the Greek *poesis*, meaning "create." The poetry of human behavior is that which humans create in their lives every day. Although it may not rise to the level of literature, it is nonetheless created. Everyday poetry itself offers an adaptive function viewed in the model discussed in this book.

aspects of human life that we cannot perceive directly with any of our five senses but which we nonetheless experience. In Eastern cultures, notably those of India and China, the division between spirit and matter is much less prominent, when it occurs at all. In those cultures, matter and spirit are traditionally regarded as one entity, creating a model in which the physical brain and the subjective experience of mind are one.

Late in the 18th century, Immanuel Kant took the Western idea a step further when he observed that the mind had its own innate capacity for what he called *a priori ideas*, that is, for the capacity of producing thoughts on its own that were not related to external perceptions. Psychiatrists in the early part of the 20th century developed these ideas even further in the concept of the Unconscious, which came into general awareness first with Freud's idea of a personal unconscious and then Jung's more complex observations about human thought processes as occurring in preset, biologically based forms in which the brain structures its perceptions. He referred to these innate forms that organize the influx of our perceptions as archetypes of the *collective*—or, we might say, "common to everyone"—unconscious. Jung's work circles us back to a reunion of the workings of the brain and the functions of the mind as referring to the same thing, that is, to a single process. Although perhaps much less cosmically related, the idea of mind-brain as a single entity more resembles the view in many Asian cultures than that of the Western bifurcation of the two. In the Eastern view, mind does not exist without brain nor brain without mind, something that those of us who do not care to risk one or the other would probably agree with.

How does this relate to the idea of psychological adaptation? Is a model of adaptive behaviors a model of the mind or a model of the brain? Is the character in Edgar Allan Poe's story looking for, and not finding, a way of adapting his thoughts to the horrors of his perceptions, or is this something he can alter only by altering his brain? Recalling Poe's own apparent alcoholism and opiate use, some might argue that he was interested in both.

The arguments continue to this day—and likely will for some time—in various circles as to whether mind and brain are separate or constitute a unity in creating thought. Most clinicians and a great share of the general public, for example, now consider that the unconscious mind is a fact of human life and, while theories exist, no one has specifically proven a specific locale in the human brain. On the other hand, we now know that the functions of judgment and social propriety have a reasonably specific locus in the medial orbital frontal cortexes, and that those functions we need in planning for and executing our conscious lives have to do with the dorsolateral prefrontal areas on both sides of our mirror-imaged, two-part frontal lobes in the upper brain (see Arciniegas and Beresford 2001). At the same time, research has shown that very basic human energies that we think of as basic drives for food, sex, territory, and so forth reside in the lower centers of the human central nervous system, popularly referred to as the "reptilian brain." That is most often the target of commercial advertising and the more lurid political campaign media bites. Referring to the terms of Freud's model of psychology, for example, we know that the *Superego*, that repository of things we ought to do, is best located in the orbital frontal cortex while the *Id*, that steaming cauldron of socially unacceptable things we want to do, is a function of the lower parts of the brain, those that we have in common with other animal species.

For the purposes of recognizing the various styles of psychological adaptation—viewing recognition as a specific skill and offering a stepwise algorithm whereby that can occur—my approach to the mind/brain dilemma will be all-inclusive. This will include a definition of *mind* as the subjective experiencing of conscious mental processes and the definition of *brain* as the physical organ that mediates those experiences. Rather than take sides, I will freely use the Monist view of mind and brain as a single phenomenon in which subjective experience and physiologic processes mirror one another, occur in specific association with each other, or require the physiologic process in order to create a subjective experience. This derives from the observation, discussed in detail below, that the most mature functions by which humans adapt to their experiences require the human brain to function at its best.

And I will just as freely use the Dualist view that the functions of the mind involve subjective experiences that themselves have no physical properties, and that the brain by definition is a physical object that can be measured both in its structure and its function if we have sufficient tools to do so. In this view, psychological adaptations have a subjective quality about them that can be perceived internally by those using them. At the same time, specific adaptive behaviors can be observed by others who note them in the actions of autonomous human beings whose behaviors occur under the neural control of the brain. Those who may be troubled by my license to use these, and any other reasonable formulations, despite their apparently obvious contradictions, may take comfort in their use as mere models of human functions rather than statements of necessarily enduring truths. An analogy in physics notes that, to human perception, light behaves both as an energy particle and as a wave. And the two models of light each offer their respective forms of understanding. I suspect that human thought can make use of more than one model of what we mean by mind and brain.

STRESS AS DISCOMFORT REQUIRING DESCRIPTIVE LANGUAGE

The word *stress* finds many usages in the languages of our time. Metals, such as steel, can be stressed, which is to say can lose tensile strength when a continuously applied force pushes the metal's molecular structure to the point of distortion at which it loses its integrity and breaks. Concrete, on the other hand, can be prestressed and thereby strengthened. People say that life is a stress, and often describe themselves and each other as stressed, stressed out, overly stressed, stressed to the point of exhaustion, or living in a stressful environment, to provide only a handful of uses of the word.

Psychologically, stress generally has a negative valence: stress is bad for you. Very few, if any, commentators today equate human stress as something good. Stress is no fun. This is overly simplistic, however, and doesn't do all stresses justice. When stress may be good, for example, we change its valence by using synonyms for stress, such as *challenge*. The situation is not *stressful*; it is *challenging*. Rather than overcome a stress, the person must instead overcome a challenge, and in so doing reach a new and positive plateau in human growth and development.

Common to both valences, however, is that the words we use to describe the phenomenon consistently imply a subjective sense of discomfort. Sometimes this is described as states of mind and at other times as sensations in the body, and frequently as both at the same time. Whether rising to a challenge or dealing with stress, the term also implies a sense of perturbation that is to be overcome or managed in one way or another. In this view, continuous, unrelieved challenge or stress is not the ideal state of existence for the human mind.

Biological studies over the last 40 years suggest that stress is not the ideal state of the human body either. Stress has been linked with heart attacks, alcohol and drug use disorders, and a host of other human maladies that, of themselves, do not make up the subject of this volume. Biologists who study the human brain have given the term *stress system* to certain nerve cell collections, neural tracks, and neuroendocrine capabilities of the brain, all of which connect to one another. These form networks of physical communication and appear to be especially active in animal models of stress-induced behaviors: that is, in models designed specifically to perturb the subject animals under study. Although it is interesting to note that no one has turned these same systems into "challenge systems," the stress systems work opposite the brain "reward systems" in order to find some way of managing the perturbation. One model, for example, of disordered brain physiology in drug and alcohol overuse postulates a dynamic balance between the stress and reward systems of the brain. Other biological models link social behavior in nonhuman primates to stress hormone (the glucocorticoids and others) production. In one line of research the highest concentration of stress hormones occurs among those lowest in the social order of an animal colony. In another, concentrations climb among those required to administer painful stimuli to other nonhuman primates. Some research suggests that continuously high circulating stress hormones have a damaging effect on the brain itself. Referring again to the negative connotation or valence of the word *stress*, more euphemistic "challenge hormones" and "challenge systems" also merit study. The effects of positive stress may elucidate a new layer of complexity in the models of brain functioning than exist at present.

The current models of brain functioning suggest that stress hormones heighten the activity of the sympathetic nervous system, that network of nerves and muscles that turns on when, in response to some discomfort, we choose to flee or to stand and fight. The first descriptions of the fight-or-flight reaction come from the work of biologists in the early part of the 20th century who observed that biological organisms that possess locomotion respond in one of these two ways when faced with a threatening or stressful situation. The combination of the sympathetic nervous system activity and the rapid dispersal of stress hormones has the effect, among other things, of raising the heart rate, increasing the blood pressure, increasing awareness of the surroundings, and sending glucose to the muscles for the work that requires this fuel be burned rapidly as needed. Subsequent biologists have noted that the same effects occur in humans who feel stressed or who report feeling *anxious*. We shall say more about that term later, but for now it is important to note the link between the mind, the brain, stress with either a positive or negative valence, and the systems in the body that ready us for action.

We can sum up briefly by saying that stress includes (1) a sense of discomfort, (2) the opposite of an ideally calm state of being, (3) brain activity that both indicates perturbation and seeks to manage it, and (4) changes in the body's physiological processes, in addition to those of the brain, that rise to meet the perturbation. At this point, however, it is important to recall that the objective of this book is to provide a reproducible mechanism of clinical recognition, not of stress itself but of the ways by which humans adapt to it. As a result, we must leave the studies of stress in its various aspects in the capable hands of other researchers. In the model presented in Chapter 2, we will continually make reference to stress. And in the examples that follow in subsequent chapters to which we will apply the recognition model, part of the work will be to identify each specific stress as it triggers an adaptive response.

STRESS PERCEIVED

Because the interest in this extended discussion lies in psychological adaptive mechanisms, it follows that we are interested in the psychological perceptions of stress. More specifically, in learning to recognize adaptive mechanisms we will focus on the subjective perturbation perceived by the mind, the brain, or both, depending on one's philosophical concepts as discussed above. In the recognition model, stress perturbs something else, and that something else notices it as a perturbation, an upset to its equilibrium or perceived sense of well-being.

What is that something else? First of all, we can characterize the perceiving mechanism as conscious and say unequivocally that we are describing a stress that perturbs us when we are awake. Because psychological adaptive mechanisms are observable, as we noted above, they are by definition productions of our waking hours no matter what may be going on in the mental processes during sleep. Put another way, both the perceptions of, and adaptations to, stresses occur during waking consciousness. Although no doubt deeper processes are likewise at work, and are mentioned further in this chapter, we must begin with the conscious sense of oneself, rather than the Self in more inclusive models, such as in Jung's Self or Harry Stack Sullivan's Person, concepts that will receive only passing mention in the quest to learn to recognize psychological adaptive mechanisms.

One term for a person's waking sense of his or her self is *Ego*. Here we have another commonly used word that may include many meanings, beginning with the Latin version of "I," as "et in Arcadia ego," roughly translated as "I am in Paradise," and including such things as personal narcissism, as in "He has a big ego." A host of other usages come and go, including examples like *egoist*, *egotist*, *false ego*, *alter ego*, *ego ideal*, *ego psychology*, and so forth. We owe use of the term *ego* in a psychological sense to the elder Freud, who used it to denote the conscious sense of one's self that, in his early model of the mind, lives uncomfortably between the pummeling's of the Id with its base and often consciously unwanted drives and the Superego, that repository of social rules and regulations. For the purposes of the present discussion, the definition of the conscious sense of itself as *ego* works perfectly well and links us to empirical research on adaptive mechanisms that grow from a model advanced by the younger Freud, Sigmund's daughter Anna.

For practical purposes, and in the interest of trying hard to acquire a new way of seeing in the great world, let us agree therefore that we will understand stress as perturbing the conscious sense of self: that is, the person we know ourselves when awake, to whom we say hello when we look in the mirror in the morning, and to whom we say goodnight as we close our eyes and drift into that other world of experience in which the conscious sense of oneself is not the primary actor. During wakefulness, the conscious sense of the self can be perturbed by stressful circumstances. In other words, stress bothers the ego, the conscious sense of oneself.

INSIDE AND OUTSIDE

The experience of stress as a perturbing discomfort to oneself during waking consciousness carries with it the implication that the stress has some kind of source. Following the traditional philosophical framework of human experience occurring within the bounds of space, time, and causality, we naturally look for some cause that we can pinpoint. Sometimes, causes are clear and obvious. In Rembrandt's depiction, for example, Queen Bathsheba holds the cause of her stress in her hand: a written note declaring King David's intentions. Similarly, Homer portrays for us the cause of Achilles' anger in response to Agamemnon's pulling rank and claiming Briseus, the beautiful Trojan woman, as his spoil of battle. From the points of view of both Bathsheba and Achilles, their respective stresses come from other persons, that is, from sources outside them. Outside stresses make up a significant share of those we experience every day in modern life. Pursuing work promotions, engaging in intimate relationships, or simply avoiding bad drivers on the highway all provide common examples. And outside or external stresses will make up a significant share of those exemplified for the purposes of our learning.

At the same time, stresses can come from within a person. As examples, we have only to consider the two kings, David and Agamemnon. Following the first story, David was overcome by his desire for Bathsheba sexually, what later generations would refer to as his lust, and what still later generations would call a primitive drive toward sexual pleasure emanating from the lower, "reptilian," centers of his brain. The desire is so strong that he is willing to arrange a murder of someone he trusts in his obedience to them. We could as easily say that the stress is so strong that David is willing to violate the prohibitions against murder and to do so in a premeditated manner, all in response to it. There is no mention of him balancing in a thoughtful way his desire for Bathsheba against other options that will observe the social sanctions against killing for personal gain.

Agamemnon provides a contrast to David, at least insofar as the nature of the stress he feels. As Homer implies, Agamemnon reacts not so much from lust as from envy, and that, in turn, appears to derive from a sense of insecurity in his social position. Against the best judgment of everyone involved, and with severe consequences, he vaunts his authority as the king and does it for all to see. Homer makes no description of anyone attempting to displace Agamemnon as the head of the Greek warriors besieging Troy. No political threat makes itself known. The only person who seems to be concerned about Agamemnon's authority is the Greek king himself. Achilles may be the greatest of all the Greek warriors, but Agamemnon must assert that he is the greatest of all Greek kings, even at the cost of violating the rules of war spoils and how they are distributed. Homer leads us to ponder whether this breach of custom among the warriors comes from the sources that Achilles cites when in his anger he calls Agamemnon a drunken, timid coward. For our purposes, Agamemnon reacts to a stress that he alone perceives, that is, to an internal cause based on internal perceptions.

Like external stresses, perturbations can grow in us from within. And we must adapt to them as we do to external stresses. From the point of view of adaptation, the origination point of the stress, whether from inside or from outside, is much less relevant than is the discomfort itself. Even if the stress is continuous over time, such as being held in a prison camp or living in a forbidden love relationship, it still requires adaptation to the discomfort even though some forms of psychological adaptive behaviors do not resolve the stress but provide only some measure of lessening of the discomfort. It is the lack of even this latter compromise that Poe's character decries in himself as he looks on the horror of the House of Usher.

In summary, the discussion thus far has provided the beginnings of a practical model for understanding the psychological adaptive behaviors of human beings. We posit that it involves a source of discomfort that we call a stress, and that the sense of discomfort reaches perception during the waking hours, in which we notice that it upsets our conscious selves. It is clear that this sense of being perturbed requires some kind of resolution: no one likes to continue in a sense of constant discomfort. Somehow or other, distress requires an adapting to, and how that occurs brings us to the model discussed in Chapter 2.

REFERENCES

Arciniegas, D. B., and T. P. Beresford (2001). *Neuropsychiatry: An Introductory Text*. Cambridge, Cambridge University Press.

Homer. (1951). *The Iliad of Homer* (R. Lattimore, Trans.). Chicago, University of Chicago.

Jung, C. G. (1959). *The Archetypes and the Collective Unconscious*. Princeton, Princeton University Press.

Poe, E. A. (1998). The Fall of the House of Usher. In *Selected Tales*. New York, Oxford University Press.

Williams, W. C. (1995). *The Collected Poems of William Carlos Williams, Volume 1, 1909–1939*. New York, New Directions.

CHAPTER 2

The Clinical Model

With the concept of psychological adaptation to stress in mind, we may now build a model that allows us to focus on psychological adaptive mechanisms with more detailed clinical specificity. For clarity, I have diagrammed the clinical model that will guide our method of recognizing observable adaptive mechanisms in a series of visual schemas, each with the aim of illustrating the descriptive text.

In Figure 2.1, the large, gray-shaded circle represents the concept of the Self, that is, the total composition of an individual human being. This includes everything subsumed by the word Self, whether physical or psychological, and, in the latter, whether conscious or unconscious. Within the diagram of the Self, a smaller oval represents the conscious sense of oneself that we know as the Ego, the same concept of the conscious self we discussed in Chapter 1. This refers to the conscious, subjective experience all of us have during our waking hours. Similarly, the arrow depicts the idea of a stress as impinging upon the Ego. As discussed in Chapter 1, the stress may come either from the outside environment or from inside the self, in the latter case emanating from its nonconscious parts. For simplicity of depiction, the arrow appears to come only from outside when, as we shall see with further examples, both may occur.

What happens next? We already know that stress, by definition, creates a subjective sense of discomfort. In human life most people notice not only a sense of psychological discomfort or upset, but a physiological reaction—for example, rapid heart rate, nausea, and sweating—as well. Both refer to what researchers in the 20th century began to describe as Anxiety. Viewed clinically, the most commonly used descriptors for the subjective feeling of anxiety include a sense either of impending *doom* or imminent *disaster*, or sometimes both. For purposes of clinical application in the chapters that follow, we will refer only to these two subjective aspects of anxiety. To differentiate them from each other, *doom* refers to an ongoing perception of hopelessness akin to Poe's description of his arrival at the Usher mansion in Chapter 1. In subsequent chapters, it presents in examples of chronic illness, unrequited love, and inappropriate career choice. It has a subjective connotation of eventual, lingering "death" of the spirit—a loss of subjective animation. By contrast, *disaster* refers to a sudden and permanent change near at hand. Examples of this will include airplane crashes, wartime combat, and the experience of falling in love. Doom—in the

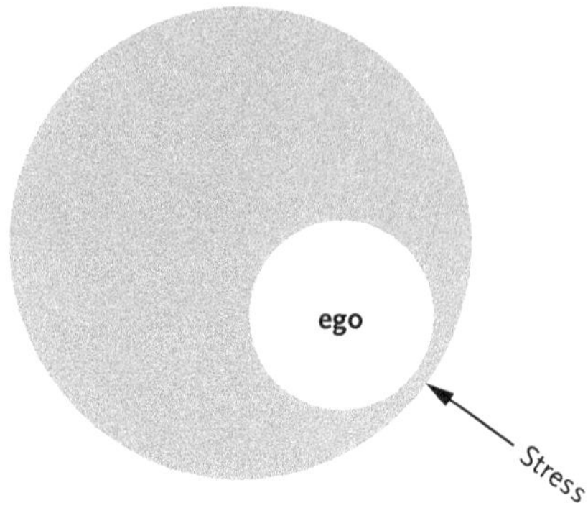

Figure 2.1
The circle with the gray shading represents the experience of Self, the subjective totality of one's personal being. The smaller circle, including the ego, represents subjective experiences that occur in waking consciousness. The gray shading itself refers to the unconscious parts of personal experience, including models of the Unconscious itself. The arrow attached to the word *stress* depicts a perturbation experienced in waking consciousness, that is, in the perceptions of the ego.

sense of hopelessness—usually results from a negative valence, while disaster—an indicator of sudden change—may occur irrespective of the stress's valence, either positive or negative, as we shall see.

Neither personal doom nor actual disaster need necessarily be present for this human response to occur. The subjective sensation alone alerts the human that some stress has moved into present consciousness. At the same time, however, a person may be aware of feeling significant stress without conscious awareness of the cognitive and/or emotional causes of their anxiety, For example, as recalled from Chapter 1, Homer portrays Agamemnon as one who does not appear to see his own behavior—in that case his treatment of his best warrior—as destructive, although everyone around him can appreciate that with perfect clarity.

Presented schematically in Figure 2.2, the adaptive recognition model posits that a stress perturbs the conscious sense of well-being—alternatively stated, it upsets the equilibrium of one's ego. The perturbation, or upset, of the stress causes an immediate effect in the person: it increases anxiety. That is, it results in the subjective sense of oncoming disaster or doom, both of which are uncomfortable. As we will learn in acquaintance with the algorithm presented in Chapter 3 and by repeating its use subsequently, identifying the stress and anxiety in each instance make up the first steps in recognizing psychological adaptive mechanisms clinically. In this chapter, we have the leisure to consider some thoughts on why humans have developed this biologic and subjective response to stress.

THE USEFULNESS OF DOOM AND DISASTER: PSYCHOLOGICAL ADAPTIVE MECHANISMS

One line of thought formulates anxiety in response to the stress as a signal to the organism that a threat is present. In this sense, some use the term *signal anxiety* to

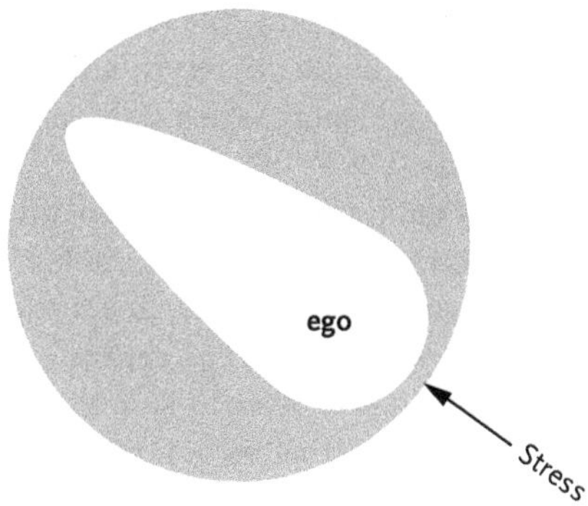

Figure 2.2
As stress perturbs the ego, it generates anxiety, defined as a sense of either impending disaster or oncoming doom.

describe this phenomenon. In a signaling model, the stress may be analogous to, and to some degree encompasses, what early 20th-century physiologists referred to as an alteration in the homeostasis of a cell. The French biologist Claude Bernard used the term *milieu interieur*, or internal state, to describe physiologic calm, or, put in more literary language, the sense of natural respite that any cell has in a resting or unperturbed setting. His American contemporary Walter Cannon used the term *homeostasis* to describe the same phenomenon in respect to the functioning of cells within organisms. Based on experimental evidence, both went on to describe the nature of the cell when perturbed as responding in such a way as to maintain its own internal equilibrium: its homeostasis or its own steady internal milieu. Cannon used the phrase "the wisdom of the body" to describe this internal ability of both cells and collections of cells to adapt in order to preserve its/their internal functioning. Their research, and that of others on the idea of biological flexibility in the interest of successful adaptation, opened new avenues of thought in 20th-century biology. They suggested that the adaptive responses that Charles Darwin described in his naturalistic studies of biological evolution were themselves mediated by mechanisms at the cellular level. Today, we would add molecular and micromolecular levels as well.

Considered further in terms of Darwin's survival-of-the-fittest observations, the physiologists of the early 20th century and after saw adaptations to immediate biological threats as carrying considerable importance. At their most basic, this includes the fight-or-flight reaction in which the organism either attacked the threat or ran from it. Because the functional goal of Darwinian evolution is to pass the biological heritage of one generation on to new generations of the same species, an individual's attacking or fleeing from a threat occurs in the service of continuing to live at least until passing on that individual's genetic material. For example, when out walking and encountering a snake, we may observe the snake either to flee from us or, in the case of some poisonous snakes, to attack. The fleeing snakes and the attacking snakes have each developed different adaptive responses to the presence of humans. From an evolutionary perspective, fleeing and attacking both represent behavioral means toward a biological end: to preserve the organism's health and well-being at least until it can reproduce itself biologically, and, for the luckier reptiles, through the course of the natural history of its life. However, although this may work with snakes, human beings have developed more varied and complex ways of adapting to physical and psychological threats.

For humans, anxiety—that subjective sense of either doom or disaster—can be considered the subjective human equivalent of the fight-or-flight discomfort that occurs in less neurally complex organisms. The subjective perception and the biological processes—whether described as separate in a mind/body Dualist model or as an integrated biological behavioral unit in a Monist formulation, as mentioned in Chapter 1—are nonetheless occurring at the same time, in the same place, and in a fashion that strongly suggests their exquisite, detailed integration with each other. When anxiety signals to consciousness that some discomfort is present, the body has its own set of signals that mediate anxiety and mediate adaptive behaviors. We referred to these in Chapter 1 in part as involving the stress systems of the brain. Some researchers have provided biological evidence suggesting that the brain's stress systems appear to function in a balance with the brain's reward systems—those neural networks in the brain that signal success and well-being as well as pleasure (Koob 2003). Although areas of knowledge involving the specific neural tracks and the details of their functioning lie outside the scope of this book, the fact of biological and psychological interactions informs both clinical knowledge and practical discussion.

Two cases of extremes—no capacity for anxiety on the one hand, and no capacity to moderate anxiety on the other—offer illustrative examples. Let us imagine that a person is walking through the woods on a pleasant day, when he or she encounters a grizzly bear. Were anxiety not at all present in the human walker as a part of his or her biological and psychological makeup, no physiological reaction or fear would attach itself to the presence of the bear in the human's perception. The bear, meantime, thinks only of satisfying his hunger and regards the human as something like dinner. In Darwinian terms, that human organism's existence ends and he or she may or may not have passed on their genetic material. Signal anxiety, in this sense, can be thought of as an adaptive mechanism that has itself evolved over the millennia of biological existence.

The opposite case, however, may also exist. In the same situation, immediately upon recognizing the presence of the bear, the human may experience an extreme, unrelieved, uncontrollable sense of anxiety in which he or she is paralyzed by an overactive nervous system and completely unable to respond to the bear's existence in even the most basic fight-or-flight manner. The bear, again concerned about its hunger, wins the adaptation contest between the two organisms at the expense of the human and the chances of the human species' preservation are fewer than before. From this scenario, we may reasonably conclude that it is in the best interest of the species for humans to have evolved some way of managing anxiety in order to serve both purposes: to be able to appreciate—that is to notice and put a value on-the signal of a threat to one's homeostasis and to be able to respond to that threat in the most adaptable way possible that preserves not only homeostasis but the life of the individual.

That way of managing anxiety calls forth the concept of psychological adaptation in the cause of maintaining an internal homeostasis in waking consciousness. The specific styles of adapting to anxiety we refer to here as *psychological adaptive mechanisms*. These mechanisms, classed below in four large groups, or *Domains*, occur in the present model in order to limit the subjective doom or disaster of anxiety immediately and to allow adaptations beyond the two basic fight-or-flight choices. Their engagement as adaptive response results in observable behaviors as discussed further below. Psychological adaptive mechanisms were originally termed *ego defense mechanisms* in the psychoanalytic model: a term coined by her father and developed more coherently by Anna Freud, as discussed below (Freud 1977).

CONTRAST WITH OTHER PROPOSED MODELS

To offer a present-day perspective, however, let us first contrast how another model than that proposed in this chapter has attempted to codify them for clinical use. The model is that of objective-descriptive psychiatry, originating with Emil Kraepelin, Eugen Bleuler (Carl Jung's teacher), and others in late 19th- and early 20th-century European psychiatry. The specific example comes from the modern-day edition of that model that focuses on collections of symptoms that associate with each other empirically and comprise syndromes, leading to syndromal diagnosis.

Although a useful method in many other clinical settings, the DSM-IV-TR (American Psychiatric Association 2000) descriptive approach to "defense mechanisms" suggests a one-dimensional phenomenological model of the psychological adaptive mechanisms, one that leaves out such variables as development and brain functioning. In contrast to the model advanced in this chapter, it portrays what appears to be a misunderstanding of the nature and purpose of the adaptive mechanisms themselves.

For example, the DSM-IV-TR discussion begins with the statement, "*Defense mechanisms* (or coping styles) are automatic psychological processes that protect the individual against anxiety and from the awareness of internal or external dangers or stressors." Taken in order, the term *automatic* brings the connotation of a machinelike, programmed response rather than a less predictable, if more complex, repertory of responses available to a human being. In describing the same attribute of the adaptive mechanisms, Vaillant himself has recently referred to the defense mechanisms as "involuntary."[1] This seems a likewise unfortunate term that appears to relate adaptive mechanisms to the involuntary functions of the body, such as involuntary extrapyramidal control of skeletal muscle tone and the involuntary innervation that controls the smooth muscle of the viscera, both functions that do not require conscious attention on a minute-by-minute basis. Both *automatic* and *involuntary* suggest attempts at mitigating the discussion or mention of the Unconscious, the home of defense mechanisms when not in use, according to a psychoanalytic model. Be that as it may, for purposes of general discussion and

1. See Vaillant (2011).

consideration of practical use, the word *spontaneous* appears far more appropriate. That is, the psychological adaptive mechanisms occur spontaneously in response to stress resulting in observable behaviors. While both psychodynamic and neural models may enlighten our understanding of this spontaneous response, the phenomena of psychological adaptive mechanisms appear far too complex to fit either *automatic* or *involuntary*.

The second part of the DSM-IV-TR statement suggests that anxiety is itself a threat against which humans deserve psychic protection, and that stress, whether internal or external, is best kept out of awareness. The implication seems to allow that *defense mechanisms* build walls against anxiety and stress rather than recognize and use them. Rather, as the adaptive model of this chapter presents, stress occasions adaptation and anxiety provides the human with an indication that adaptation must be accomplished to the best of the individual's ability. As a result, as noted in Table 2.1, psychological adaptive mechanisms cap, or moderate, anxiety rather than protecting against it as though it were itself some outside threat rather than a biologically and evolutionarily useful part of the human makeup. Likewise, resolution of the stress, best accomplished through the most flexible and creative Mature Domain psychological adaptive mechanisms as introduced in Chapter 3, remains the ultimate goal of human psychological adaptation and its mechanisms. In the present adaptive model, stresses are to be recognized in waking consciousness, rather than kept out of awareness.

As mentioned, the DSM-IV-TR text goes on to direct the clinician to observe and record up to 7 of the 31 specific mechanisms, and lists definitions of all of them, along with providing a form for noting them down. Although this approach avoids

Table 2.1 CLINICAL CHARACTERISTICS OF PSYCHOLOGICAL ADAPTIVE MECHANISMS

Psychological adaptive mechanisms:

- Occur spontaneously.
- Cap (moderate or limit) anxiety.
- Respond to perceived stress that threatens conscious psychological homeostasis.
- Allow time to deal with stress maximally.
- Exist on a hierarchy of Domains from Primitive to Immature to Neurotic to Mature.
- Develop along this Domain hierarchy from infancy through adulthood.
- Are normal by Domain at different life stages.
- May develop toward higher Domains at slower rates in socially vulnerable settings.
- Actively resolve stress at the level of the Mature Domain
- Vary over a spectrum of responses from rigid (Primitive) to flexible (Mature).
- Engage at the *most mature level available* in individual cases.
- Depend on optimal brain development and functioning for the greatest Maturity of response.
- Regress to lower, less mature Domains with impaired brain functioning.
- May regress to lower, less mature Domains with overwhelming or prolonged stress.
- Result in observable behaviors that can be measured.
- Empirically predict mental and physical health in relation to age appropriate maturity.

the clinical ease-of-use aimed at in this volume, it at least acknowledges that psychological adaptive mechanisms consist in observable behaviors. The present volume seeks to go beyond the DSM's approach by providing a systematic method for recognizing psychological adaptive mechanisms, namely, the stepwise recognition algorithm presented in Chapter 3.

The recognition algorithm itself proceeds from the more complex model described here. Table 2.1 lists for the reader a number of the aspects of the model that pertain to its clinical usefulness. Some of these, such as the hierarchical relationship of the psychological adaptive mechanism Domains, refer to existing empirical study data. Others, for example the assertion that individuals employ mechanisms from the highest Domain of adaptive styles available to them in response to the specific stress, find their usefulness as working hypotheses that the clinician is free to use or discard as he or she wishes. All of them may at some point be amenable to hypothesis-driven research that focuses on both the phenomena and causal relationships with such entities as human biology and the brain, evolutionary conservation of behaviors, and the mental or metaphysical considerations implied with the use of the word *mind*. In the meantime, the present approach aims at clinical usefulness when assessing and working with the patient sitting opposite the clinician in the consultation office or at the bedside. As writers of the last three millennia have made clear, human adaptation entails a very rich and creative tapestry of behaviors across cultures and over time. The approach offered here lives in the excitement of that complexity, in the adventure of the human spirit as it comes to terms with itself and the world around it.

WIDENING THE ADAPTIVE OPTIONS

In the model presented in Figure 2.3, the psychological adaptive mechanisms ideally fill both of the teleological roles in adaptation: assuring internal psychological homeostasis and adapting to stresses in order to preserve life and to function effectively in it. Stress engages them by raising anxiety and the adaptive mechanisms themselves in turn "cap" anxiety, that is, moderate it in order to harness its functions in the most successful ways available. Viewed in the context of the neural systems of the brain, this model suggests that both the stress and reward systems are involved, at the very least, and as we explore empirical examples of complex human psychological adaptation many other brain functions will make their contributions as well.

The present author is solely responsible for the schema that depicts the adaptive model in Figures 2.1, 2.2, and 2.3. In the setting of the current chapter, the reader may see the influence of Bernard, Cannon, and the other physiologists whose principles could be diagrammed in the same illustrations with some alteration of the various nouns to fit one or another biological system model. The original use of the psychological labels in the figures, however, belongs principally to Anna Freud. In her work *The Ego and the Mechanisms of Defense*, she both described the empirical phenomena of psychological adaptation and provided its first theoretical framework (Freud 1977). She published her book in 1936, well after Cannon and Bernard had

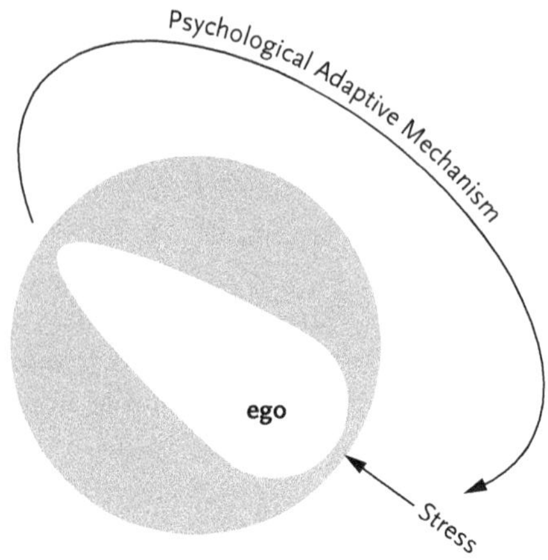

Figure 2.3
In response to the subjective anxiety generated by the stress, the Self activates psychological adaptive mechanisms with the object of coming to terms with the stress and reestablishing homeostasis in waking consciousness.

articulated their biological systems theories of adaptation and well into the acceleration of biological research in the 20th century. Whether consciously or unconsciously, in my view she incorporated those ideas in formulating her concept of the mechanisms that "defend" the ego against anxiety in order to maintain the ego's own homeostasis and therefore preserve adaptive functioning. Happily for us, she moved this line of thinking out of the more rigid models based in 19th-century physics that characterized much of the work of her father, Sigmund Freud. Happily as well, she developed her work to include empirically observable phenomena, namely human adaptive behaviors, that were not the particular interests of the scholars in early psychoanalytic efforts. Where the psychoanalysts of her father's and most subsequent generations sought only to study the unconscious processes of the Self, Miss Freud, as she was known, saw the value of empirical study of human adaptation. Based on her work, the attention of both the later researchers in the field, and the didactic effort in this book, focus on *observable behaviors*: what people actually *do* in deploying psychological adaptive mechanisms.

For practical purposes, Figure 2.4 offers another schematic version of the model that we will use repeatedly in going about the process of recognizing and characterizing human adaptive behaviors as they present before us. This model will take us from Anna Freud's conceptions into the work of George Vaillant as we develop a method of recognition aimed at clinical utility in everyday practice.

The interested reader can do no better than to explore the pioneering work that Vaillant has published from his prospective, longitudinal scientific studies (Vaillant 1992, 1998a, 1998b, 2003, 2008) of the observable phenomena we regard here as psychological adaptive mechanisms, to which he refers as "ego defense mechanisms," using Anna Freud's term for this class of human phenomena. Vaillant has carried out multidecade longitudinal, prospective studies of human adaptive behaviors that

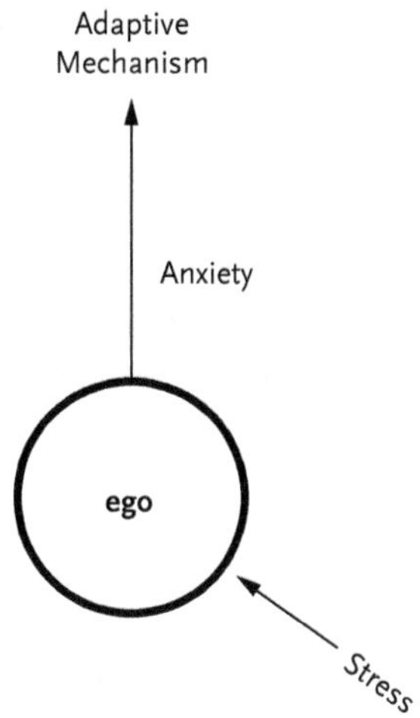

Figure 2.4
In a more schematized version that allows comparison of the adaptive strategy Domains, stress perturbs the ego, raising anxiety, which calls forth an adaptive response. See the variations on the schema in Chapters 4, 7, 12, and 17.

enrich our knowledge not only of those mechanisms but of the natural course of human life as well. In Chapter 22, we shall have more to learn from his methods of measuring empirical phenomenon in this area of study, one for which he quoted the term "the poetic science."[2]

For now, practical application requires that we denote some of Vaillant's many contributions to the field. For example, he was the first to describe that human psychological adaptive mechanisms, as found in Nature, belonged to a hierarchy (Vaillant 1971). These start from very primitive and inflexible adaptive mechanisms, and follow along an observable continuum of increasingly flexible adaptive responses to stress. They culminate in the most flexible adaptive mechanisms, those that characterize adult human functioning at its best.

Second, for our purposes, Vaillant assigned adaptive mechanisms to groups, according to their commonality of stress response strategies, that I shall refer to here as Domains. He named four of these: Primitive, Immature, Neurotic, and Mature. Vaillant's hierarchy refers to the rank ordering of these Domains as already noted (Vaillant, Bond, et al. 1986). Within each Domain, specific adaptive mechanisms occur that, although differing in style of adaptation, do not form a hierarchy within their respective Domains. Within its Domain, each specific adaptive style may be considered as equivalent to the others in that same grouping in respect to practical application, as we shall see.

As we progress through an algorithm of clinical recognition, presented in Chapter 3, our first and principal focus will be to differentiate each adaptive style Domain from the others as we approach our primary task. That task is to decide where the observable

2. See Vaillant (1998b, p. 27).

behaviors that we see in the unique individual before us fit best in the clinical definitions of the four respective adaptive-style Domains. Once reasonably assured from the clinical evidence of which Domain best fits the empirically observed behaviors in any given case, the observer will have constructed a working clinical hypothesis in respect to adaptive styles. He/she may then work to establish which of the specific psychological adaptive mechanisms within that Domain is at work and to engage continuously in the effort of monitoring the behavioral evidence that presents in a myriad of human experiences. For ease of use, the Domains and their respective adaptive mechanisms are listed in Table 2.2.

In this respect we encounter the third of Vaillant's contributions to our understanding of human adaptation, namely his glossary of ego defense mechanisms, or psychological adaptive mechanisms as we term them in this discussion. As noted in Table 2.2, his glossary defines three Primitive mechanisms, and five each in the Immature, Neurotic, and Mature Domains, respectively. Although he first published this glossary over 40 years before the writing of the present exercise (Vaillant 1971), it has remained a remarkably stable and useful glossary of psychological adaptive styles.

Other formulations, such as the Defenses list in the DSM series of the American Psychiatric Association, beginning with the third edition (1980), have been advanced but with only small increments, if any, in practical utility. As in most forms of human endeavor, the tendency to make things overly complicated provides a strong temptation to formulate and name as many possible styles of psychological adaptation as one can imagine based on the nuances of human words and actions. For example, in a section of its Appendix B, the DSM-IV-TR[3] lists the "Defensive Functioning Scale" under "Proposed Axes for Further Study." There follows a brief description and a list of seven "Levels," corresponding roughly to the concept of Domains in the present discussion, and within them a list of no less than thirty-one separate "defense mechanisms." Compared to the much simpler four Domains and 18 psychological adaptive mechanisms presented in this volume, the proposed DSM-IV-TR formulation presents an unnecessary complexity that renders this scale all but unusable clinically. And, as viewed in the temptation model of human behavior, unnecessary complication

Table 2.2 PSYCHOLOGICAL ADAPTIVE MECHANISM BY DOMAINS

Primitive	Immature	Neurotic	Mature
Denial (concrete)	Acting Out	Repression	Suppression
Avoidance/Distortion	Passive Aggression	Isolation of Affect	Anticipation
	Hypochondriasis	Dissociation[a]	Altruism
Projection (concrete)	Schizoid fantasy	Displacement	Sublimation
	Neurotic projection	Reaction Formation	Humor

[a] I list Dissociation as one of the Neurotic Domain psychological adaptive mechanisms, consistent with Vaillant's earlier formulation but not his later ones, as noted in Chapter 15. As I will discuss in detail there, I regard Dissociation as a very changeable mechanism and the only one that can appear in forms common to the definitions of the first three Domains.

3. American Psychiatric Association (2000, pp. 807–809).

is a good pitfall to avoid. For the purpose of providing clinical usefulness, the present discussion will follow both Henry David Thoreau[4] and Albert Einstein,[5] who enjoined us to keep formulations both simply stated and sufficient to cover the phenomena in question.

The principal advantage of a stable glossary lies in its usefulness in many different places at different points in time. The phenomena that the glossary describes can then be observed with confidence among different observers or through the behaviors of different cohorts of subjects even when those are viewed prospectively, serially, and over a long period. In my estimation, Vaillant's glossary is the most elegant and practical of the available guides to adaptive mechanisms, and the one that we will use in this discussion.

EMPIRICAL RESEARCH METHODS

One may reasonably ask—as our psychiatry residents, psychology interns, medical residents, and students of various stripes and disciplines often do—how does Vaillant ascertain whether a particular adaptive style is an operation? What is his scientific method? As he describes in his publications on the topic, his method begins with an interview of the patient or research subject, as the setting may indicate. In many respects, his research interview mirrors the clinical interview in that it focuses upon the patient's stress, or more specifically his or her sense of distress that brings them to the clinical encounter. In the standard format of clinical medicine, this would be the Chief Complaint and the History of the Present Illness. The object of the interview at the beginning is to identify and to formulate the stress to the person in as clear terms as possible. The person's related anxiety generally guides this aspect of the assessment process: ascertaining where, when, and how they notice that sense of doom or disaster and in relation to what possible source.

The interviewer then explores the various responses the person had to the stress in the interest of easing the anxiety. This is often open-ended and may involve different interview techniques ranging from the questioning of standard medical history taking through a more existential approach in which the interviewer explores the patient's subjective experiences, or, further, in an interpersonal style that may include a series of statements that the patient corrects in the conversation. The interviewer's object lies in establishing a clear understanding of the stress that creates the anxiety response and the various behaviors in adapting to and, in some styles, resolving the anxiety. Interviews of this kind often require considerable clinical latitude and flexibility because, as we shall see, any given subject or patient may employ more than one psychological adaptive mechanism.

Ideally, an interview with a second, outside person who knows the patient well, can focus on the details of the history the patient presents, although this is not always possible in every clinical setting. This kind of data gathering for convergent

4. Thoreau (1996).
5. Albert Einstein (1979, p. 73).

validity can be useful because all of us humans find ways of altering the tone, and sometimes the content, of what we say to one another, whether purposefully or not. The interview data from a significant other person by itself should not, however, constitute the primary data for adaptive mechanism recognition. Because the primary evidence for psychological adaptive mechanisms of one Domain or another rests on observable behaviors, what people *do* is far more important than what they say or what others say about them.

For research, the investigator abstracts specific interview vignettes in which the subject describes his/her response behavior to a stress. Two independent reviewers, blind to each other's assessments of the evidence and to the rest of the interview data, receive both specific individual vignettes and the glossary of mechanisms. Independently, the respective reviewers must sort each vignette by assigning it to a best-fit mechanism from the glossary list. From these data, one can calculate the statistical probability of agreement between the two or more raters: a rating of their statistical reliability. Other researchers have developed this method further and include group discussions when inter-rater reliability agreement is not present and proceed to establish a consensus of adaptive style recognition for the purposes of research clarity (Perry and Cooper 1989; Perry, Hoglend, et al. 1998).

This interview rating process also delivers cross-sectional validity with respect to recognizing the various adaptive mechanisms relative to their glossary definitions. It creates a picture of the psychological adaptive mechanisms in use at any given point in time. It is important to know, however, that this approach is always prone to possible distortions from several sources including the interview subject's memories, the interviewer's skills, and the abilities of the raters to understand the glossaries. But, as Vaillant himself points out, what people say may often be at odds with what they actually do. In this respect, true validity comes from two principal sources: (1) blind ratings of the same groups of people in a prospective fashion over long periods of time, and (2) comparisons of the adaptive mechanism ratings with independently gathered data that measures observable aspects of healthy human adult functioning. Longitudinal data, in particular, provides a functional measure of the consistency of the deployment of specific adaptive mechanisms over all or part of a life course.

It is from these longitudinal data, coupled with measures of adult functioning, that Vaillant gives us his fourth major contribution to understanding human adaptive behaviors and their consequences. He goes into considerable detail in showing the relationship between the hierarchy of psychological adaptive mechanisms and the relative success and failure of people in their lives in relation to them. Although a detailed discussion of that is not within the purview of this chapter—and is best left as an encouragement for the reader to explore Vaillant's published work—the prospective, longitudinal data from his studies point toward a consistent summary.

The Mature Domain of the psychological adaptive mechanisms of adult life is closely associated with successful function in living, such as in establishing and maintaining lasting intimate relationships, successful work progress, the ability to recreate in constructive ways that renew and revitalize, and parenting independent offspring. The list even includes continuing physical health. Conversely, persons who consistently deploy Primitive or Immature Domain styles as their primary psychological adaptive mechanisms in adult life live much less satisfying lives on these same independent measures when viewed in the aggregate over time. Those with access only to the Neurotic Domain of adaptive styles most frequently repeat behaviors that they find painful or unsatisfying, with attendant effects on the same measures. In very general terms, the relationship between successful psychological adaptation and lives lived with satisfaction expands on an old Roman saying, *mens sana in corpore sano* (a healthy mind in a healthy body). A healthy mind—in this instance referring to healthy adaptive styles—has a great deal to do not only with a healthy body but also with a healthy family and recreation life, and healthy adjustment to work functions. For the practical purposes of clinical recognition of the psychological adaptive mechanisms, it is sufficient for now to note that the terms with which we apply our recognition skills to those natural phenomena have received validation both from both cross-sectional and longitudinal, prospective research methodologies.

Other investigators have adapted the same concepts into a written scale form that may be used in research (Bond 2004). While this approach acquires much less data than the interview method, the scale survey approach offers brevity, requires fewer resources to administer, and adds the possibility of application to larger numbers of persons at a time. Though scholars, myself included (Beresford, Alfers, et al. 2006), have used this method of adaptive mechanism identification, the written scale method is not, at the time of this writing, available in a form useful for clinical recognition. Although it appears statistically valid for research analyses in aggregate samples, it does not now offer the empirically validated and reliable clinical cut points needed to recognize, with confidence, a specific mechanism in the single patient who fills it out and hands it to his or her doctor.

Offering a third way of going about the business of recognizing—and using the recognition of—psychological adaptive mechanisms constitutes the goal of this book. Author and reader aim to find a middle ground when interviewing patients that allows us to recognize, with clinical confidence, first the distinguishing Domains of the adaptive mechanisms and then styles of the specific mechanisms themselves. To achieve this, we will rely on a stepwise process that discussion of the recognition algorithm in Chapter 3 will provide; see Figure 3.1. It is an approach that I have developed and taught to successive psychiatry resident classes, and used with a great many patients in day-to-day consultations over the past 20 years.

As with Vaillant's interviews, the clinical method will begin by focusing on a specific stress. In the various examples and vignettes that follow, the first question we ask will be, what is the stress? In some cases it will be immediately obvious, as in a person having to react to sudden onset of physical illness. In others it will be much less so: for example in a person who was brought to the attention of the clinician by the local police and states that he has no idea why the police brought him in. In this respect, the clinical model for recognizing psychological adaptive mechanisms incorporates the various models of both psychological and adaptive functioning discussed so far. The final, practical outcome lies in the effort to create a stepwise, clinically driven examination of the stress and the adaptive responses in the person who sits immediately before us. How we begin to use this clinical method leads us to the subject of Chapter 3.

REFERENCES

American Psychiatric Association. (1980). *Diagnostic and Statistical Manual of Mental Disorders* (3rd ed.). Washington, DC, American Psychiatric Press.

American Psychiatric Association. (2000). *Diagnostic and Statistical Manual of Mental Disorders* (4th ed., Text Rev.). Washington, DC, American Psychiatric Press.

Beresford, T. P., J. Alfers, et al. (2006). "Cancer survival probability as a function of ego defense (adaptive) mechanisms versus depressive symptoms." *Psychosomatics* 47(3): 247–253.

Bond, M. (2004). "Empirical studies of defense style: relationships with psychopathology and change." *Harvard Review of Psychiatry 12*(5): 263–278.

Albert Einstein, *Autobiographical Notes*. Peru, IL, Open Court, 1979.

Freud, A. (1977). The Ego and the Mechanisms of Defense (1936). In *The Writings of Anna Freud* (Vol. 2). New York, International Universities Press.

Koob, G. F. (2003). "Alcoholism: allostasis and beyond." *Alcohol Clin Exp Res* 27(2): 232–243.

Perry, J. C., and S. H. Cooper (1989). "An empirical study of defense mechanisms. I. Clinical interview and life vignette ratings." *Archives of General Psychiatry* 46(5): 444–452.

Perry, J. C., P. Hoglend, et al. (1998). "Field trial of a diagnostic axis for defense mechanisms for DSM-IV." *J Pers Disord 12*(1): 56–68.

Thoreau, H. D. (1996). *Simplify, Simplify and Other Quotations from Henry David Thoreau* (Van Anglen, Ed.). New York, Columbia University Press.

Vaillant, G. E. (1971). "Theoretical hierarchy of adaptive ego mechanisms: a 30-year follow-up of 30 men selected for psychological health." *Archives of General Psychiatry 24*(2): 107–118.

Vaillant, G. E. (1992). *Ego Mechanisms of Defense, A Guide for Clinicians and Researchers*. Washington, DC, American Psychiatric Press.

Vaillant, G. E. (1998a). *Adaptation to Life*. Cambridge, Harvard University Press.

Vaillant, G. E. (1998b). *The Wisdom of the Ego*. Cambridge, Harvard University Press.

Vaillant, G. E. (2003). *Aging Well*. Boston, Little, Brown.

Vaillant, G. E. (2008). *Spiritual Evolution*. New York, Broadway Books.

Vaillant, G. E. (2011). "Involuntary coping mechanisms: a psychodynamic perspective." *Dialogues in Clinical Neuroscience 13*: 366–370.

Vaillant, G. E., M. Bond, et al. (1986). "An empirically validated hierarchy of defense mechanisms." *Archives of General Psychiatry 43*(8): 786–794.

CHAPTER 3

The Clinical Method

Before going into the specifics of the various discrete psychological adaptive mechanisms, the logic of clinical recognition requires first that we define as precisely as possible the large groups, or Domains, of psychological adaptive styles. Considered as Domains, the phenomena themselves lead forward in a stepwise progression, beginning with the most Primitive Domain adaptive strategies. These proceed by turns through what Vaillant first described as the hierarchy of Immature, Neurotic, and Mature Domain mechanisms.

At the same time, moving from the Model of psychological adaptive mechanisms in Chapter 2 to the Method of their clinical recognition in this, we will here begin use of a specific stepwise recognition approach that will apply in all of the subsequent chapters as a systematic method that we can repeat in identifying the Domains of the various adaptive styles. In each of the passages or vignettes provided in the subsequent chapters as examples for applied recognition we will invoke this approach in the form of the algorithm depicted in Figure 3.1. This serves two purposes: (1) it allows the observer to use the same recognition procedure over and over again in order to develop a consistency in the recognition process (reliability), and (2) it allows for a systematic delineation of the approaches common to each of the Domains themselves, providing consistent definition of the psychological adaptive mechanisms within those groups, and within the Model (validity). Observing the time-honored method of learning through repetition of use,[1] a third goal of the algorithm lies in its becoming second nature, if you will, as a tool at the disposal of the expert clinician/observer. Repetition always risks tedium, however, and the author hopes to avoid this in the variety of the vignettes and examples to which the algorithm may be applied.

The first step in applying the algorithm requires identification of the stress that disturbs the equilibrium of waking consciousness, which is to say perturbs the ego

1. Ambroise Paré and the other European barber surgeons of the 16th century provided this when they preferred learning from direct clinical experience as compared to the previous route to medical expertise that lay in reading ancient classics and writing a dissertation on some aspect of them.

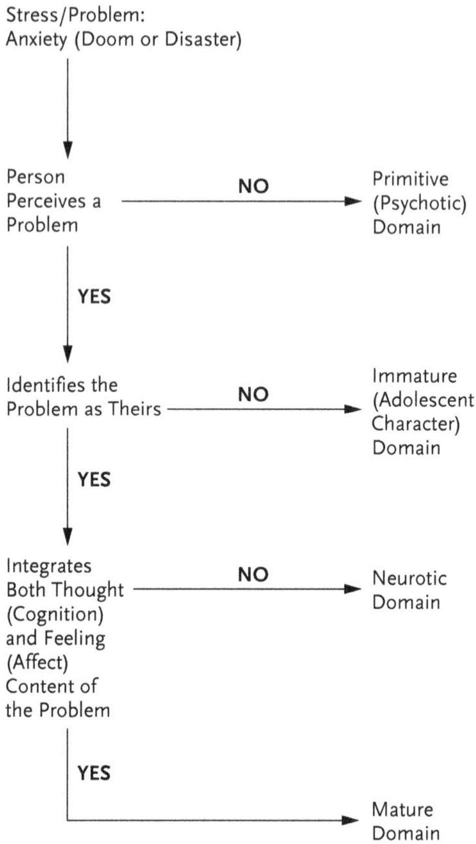

Figure 3.1
This diagram depicts the recognition algorithm for psychological adaptive mechanisms. It begins with clinical identification of the current stress and of the anxiety that the stress generates in waking consciousness. It then proceeds in a stepwise fashion. First, it assesses whether or not the patient recognizes the stress itself or ignores it in the style of the Primitive Domain adaptive mechanisms. If the patient recognizes the stress, it next asks whether he or she regards the stress as something within his or her range of responsibility or control, or locates it outside the Self. External location defines the adaptive strategy of the Immature Domain mechanisms. If the patient perceives the stress in waking consciousness and as within the purview of the self, the algorithm next asks whether the cognitive and emotional contents of the stress work together or whether they remain unintegrated. The lack of integrated thought and feeling characterize the Neurotic Domain strategies. Finally, if the person (1) recognizes the stress, (2) regards it as part of his or her life with its resolution belonging to him or her, and (3) integrates the thought and feeling contents of the stress, he or she functions in the Mature Domain of psychological adaptive mechanisms. Mature Domain mechanisms move to resolve the stress.

as defined in Chapter 2. The source of the stress, whether from within the person or from outside in the environment, carries less importance in the present model than the fact of the stress itself and its ability to raise anxiety in the conscious mental processes of a person. Anxiety—defined above and used consistently below as a sense of either doom or disaster—provides waking consciousness with a sense of discomfort.

The word *doom* carries with it a connotation of the ominous and the unavoidable, such as in misfortune or fate. *Disaster*, by contrast, brings to mind a more acute circumstance of immediate upsetting change of either positive or negative valence, such as falling in love or dying.

The observer's first task, therefore, in any situation in which the recognition algorithm can be applied, is to identify and to formulate in terms of the algorithm the specific stress or problem that raises anxiety as well as to verify the fact that anxiety itself does exist in relation to the stress. Because the advantage of a psychological adaptive mechanism to human life lies in its ability to manage anxiety in response to stress, the two go hand in hand and require simultaneous identification in order to use the algorithm as a recognition strategy. Let us illustrate this with the beginning example in the Primitive Domain of adaptive mechanisms, followed by further examples as the discussion proceeds up the hierarchy of Domains in psychological adaptation.

OH, *THOSE* PANTS! THE PRIMITIVE DOMAIN

Consider a young mother going about her work in her home, carrying an infant on one hip and her older child, a two-year-old toddler, running about at her feet. The mother notices a familiar although very unpleasant odor emanating from the toddler. She looks at the toddler in a kindly way and gently asks, "Did you poop in your pants?" The toddler looks back at her with a blank expression, straight in the eye, and then in an unemotional tone of voice states simply, "No."

What should the mother do? Is her child lying to her? Should she beat him or punish him in order to teach them to tell the truth? To view the situation in these terms—in the framework of a moral or ethical judgment—is to see the child not as a child but as an adult. It is to project the mother's own conception of adult behavior on to her toddler.

Rather, the mother recognizes the child as a child and understands that in the child's perception the dirty diaper simply doesn't exist. Perhaps because the experience itself is unpleasant, perhaps because the toddler has no idea how to change the diaper himself, or perhaps for no reason other than normal brain and psychological development at that stage of life, he does not recognize the stress as existing. And as a result, from his point of view, he provides a very honest "No." The mother accepts this difference in perception, takes the child in hand, changes his diaper, and sets him back at play as usual.

Notice how the algorithm applies in this everyday example taken from normal family life with small children. The stress, in this case the dirty diaper, comes into the child's conscious awareness when his mother asks him, "Did you poop in your pants?" Even asked in the gentlest of tones, this question nonetheless calls forth his anxiety, in this case perhaps the sense of some sort of unpleasant social "disaster" between child and mother at an age when the child's being depends on the mother and requires a response to avoid conflict in their relationship.

Those who might reasonably ask whether the concept of *anxiety* actually applies in very young children may consider the example of an extreme alternative. The mother begins yelling at her child, accusing him of lying to her, physically slapping him and then forcibly changing the diaper, all the while angrily shouting at the child. Is there any doubt that the child's reaction would be an upset in conscious equilibrium? Even if cognitively unformed at that age, the experience fits the definition of anxiety, if not terror. The child's response would be a continual crying that likely would exacerbate the situation. The much less frightening scenario of the child simply saying "No" and his mother acting appropriately involves the child's anxiety in a much milder form, considering the contrast with the more extreme example. With the knowledge and recognition of both stress and anxiety in hand, we can proceed to an understanding of the child's adaptation to the circumstance.

The algorithm next asks whether the two-year-old's perception of his mother's question about the status of his diaper registers as a conscious stress. In providing his mother with a straight-faced denial, he locates his response in the Primitive Domain: the problem simply is not there and therefore doesn't require being dealt with. According to the schema in Figure 3.1, the same "No" indicates the first right-hand-pointing arrow and identifies this in its proper Domain. In the vignette, his mother correctly reacts to his adaptive response as a Primitive one that does not deal directly with the cause of the stress itself, namely the diaper, but serves as an adaptive strategy designed to keep the equilibrium of the relationship between mother and toddler intact. Its purpose is to cap, or to limit, the anxiety the child feels and thereby preserve the economy of his conscious self in maintaining its equilibrium.

NORMAL VERSUS ABNORMAL: THE PRIMITIVE DOMAIN IN EARLY DEVELOPMENT

As mentioned in this example, the Primitive Domain mechanisms do not include pathology when humans exhibit them at an appropriate stage in psychological development. One practical view that Vaillant's longitudinal studies support holds that the progression of Domain mechanisms mirrors, or is a function of, normal human development, whether viewed as a continuing psychological phenomenon or as a dynamic process of brain development as that organ gains neural connections and myelinating capacity. In this respect, one useful question occurs that we may ask of all four of the Domains of adaptive mechanisms: When is this level of adaptation normal? That is, when is this group of adaptive styles commonly seen in the context of expected human development?

A corollary question follows: If specific behaviors are normal at one level of development, are they then pathological in subsequent stages of human psychological and brain development? If so, does the occurrence of early stage adaptive mechanisms—such as the Primitive or Immature groups—in adult life signal some compromise in the normal course of brain maturation and personality growth? We will consider these questions again in Chapter 22 after the extended discussion on recognizing the Domains and the specific strategies of each of the psychological adaptive mechanisms in the intervening chapters. But for now the beginning notion of the adaptive Domains as occurring normally, that is, in a nonpathologic fashion at appropriate stages of development, provides a useful context for understanding psychological adaptive maturity as its own developmental process.

Common to all of the Primitive Domain psychological adaptive mechanisms, the recognition algorithm in Figure 3.1 notes that, from the point of view of the person's state of waking consciousness that we call the ego, the stress is absent. That is to say, it is simply not perceived. It does not exist in conscious perception. Furthermore, the stress's lack of any perceived existence occurs in a very concrete manner. It is as though the reader of this book, holding it in his or her hands, does not perceive that it exists at all. At first, this may seem a very difficult point to grasp. We are all completely used to daily perceptions of what we consider to be real phenomena. Of course this book exists: I feel its weight in my hands, I see the written words on the page, when I speak the words I see I can hear them, and I can even smell the characteristic odors of the book's construction itself—of paper and glue or even the dust that may have collected sitting on the shelf. Were I so inclined—and most adults are not—I might even be able to characterize the taste sensation of the book. If these words come to the reader in an electronic version, the perception of the glare from the screen offers an analogous experience.

We owe the English empirical philosophers their due, however, when we recall that all of these "real" sensations are all mediated by our own perception mechanisms. Consider Bertrand Russell's brief description of a table:

> To the eye it is oblong, brown and shiny, to the touch it is smooth and cool and hard; when I tap it, it gives out a wooden sound. Anyone else who sees and feels and hears the table will agree with this description, so that it might seem as if no difficulty would arise; but as soon as we try to be more precise our troubles begin. Although I believe that the table is "really" of the same colour all over, the parts that reflect the light look much brighter than the other parts, and some parts look white because of reflected light. I know that, if I move, the parts that reflect the light will be different, so that the apparent distribution of colours on the table will change. It follows that if several people are looking at the table at the same moment, no two of them will see exactly the same distribution of colours, because no two can see it from exactly the same point of view, and any change in the point of view makes some change in the way the light is reflected.
>
> (Russell 1959, pp. 8–9)

The point is a simple one and yet one that is easy to forget: when dealing with the world around us, we are also dealing with our perceptions. Perceptions themselves are malleable and subject to all sorts of distortions. This is stated again in the uncertainty principle from 20th-century physics that holds that our ability to measure any natural phenomenon depends on the limits of instruments that we use to measure. The same phenomenon occurs in the Japanese tale of Rashomon and other examples of the reliability of human perception.

We may restate this in the case of psychological adaptive mechanisms in three ways. First, from the inside point of view of the adapting consciousness, the deployment of the highest available adaptive Domain response will depend on the ability of the ego in one model, and the brain in another model, to respond in the most flexible and mature way that either has at its disposal at the time. In some circumstances, whether developmental or pathological as we shall see, this may be only the Primitive Domain mechanisms. In others, the process may carry the person all the way to the Mature Domain adaptive mechanisms or to the two Domains that lie in between, the Immature and the Neurotic.

Second, from an observer's outside viewpoint in recognizing psychological adaptive mechanisms in the observable behaviors of others, the recognition itself will never be free of some element of clinical subjectivity. However, to a large extent this can be mitigated with careful use of the algorithm. Notice, for example, that practical use of the recognition algorithm asks the observer first to formulate as accurately as possible both the stress that perturbs waking consciousness and the anxiety that results from the stress. As we shall see, this is not always an obvious or easy process, but it is a necessary one for using the recognition approach with accuracy.

Once the stress and resultant anxiety have been identified, the next step in the recognition algorithm is to apply the criteria that define each of the four Domains and to do so in the sequenced manner by which each Domain succeeds that immediately previous as the adaptive strategies move along the hierarchy from Primitive to Mature, from limited options all the way along to creative flexibility. Practically speaking, it is less important to determine the specific adaptive mechanism employed than to establish the general Domain of the adaptive behavior in use. The Domains contain the respective overall adaptive strategies common to the *group* of mechanisms within each. The overall strategies define the success or the failure of the adaptive style as well as indicate the methods of specific interventions when these are needed.

The definitions of the mechanisms themselves that fall within the large Domains enhance the precision of both recognition and intervention. Consideration of the specific psychological adaptive mechanisms as variations on the theme that each shares with the cognate mechanisms of its Domain generally offers much greater usefulness than an approach that regards the respective adaptive mechanisms as operating independently and not related to each other in Domain patterns. Using the stepwise approach, therefore, the algorithm aims at improving recognition accuracy with its focus on Domains.

Third and last, the concept of accuracy requires an understanding that people may use more than one adaptive style—especially in the Mature Domain range—that the same person may use different adaptive mechanisms in different domains at different points in time or in response to different circumstances. In most of the examples provided in Chapters 4 through 21, for clarity and convenience of communication, the discussion will assume that a specific adaptive mechanism under consideration is the predominant, if not the only, adaptive style at hand. Although it is true that styles can change either for better or for worse, they can also be remarkably indurated and unresponsive to what would appear to be opportunities for further growth and development along the continuum to maturity. We will consider their malleability in Chapter 22 and for now warn the reader that this too requires a certain flexibility of observation in order to allow for the differences in time and circumstance. Like Mark

Twain's description of his experiences in learning to pilot a steamboat (Chapter 20), we too will have to get to know the river, so to speak, in recognizing which adaptive styles carry more hazard and which point toward health and well-being.

Summing up this section on the Primitive Domain adaptive mechanisms, therefore, advances the idea that *people adapt as best they can*, that is, by using the best options available to them, not the worst. According to the Model, always and everywhere, at any given point in time, people will respond to stresses with the most adaptive means possible at their command. When the clinician or other observer therefore finds Primitive Domain mechanisms at work, it is useful to consider that these may be the best that the person has at his or her disposal at the moment. In some cases, adaptive mechanisms will also fit models of the pathological conditions, or behaviors, or brain syndromes, as we will discuss in detail in subsequent chapters. In their proper developmental settings, as discussed in detail in subsequent chapters, these mechanisms are entirely normal and nonpathological, as in the following case.

THE BIRTH OF THE COOL, OR WITHER HOLLYWOOD? THE IMMATURE MECHANISMS IN ADOLESCENCE

Coming of age in the 1970s, a 20-year-old college student finds that his stylish appearance, in bell-bottom trousers, flowered shirt, long hair with a natural wave or two in it, accented by his Fu Manchu mustache, pleases himself and his friends. His father, a blue-collar worker and local union leader, tells him he looks silly in "that getup." But the student notes too that the women he talks with find him attractive and that the lines of his outfit accentuate the natural ability he has in interpreting disco music out on the dance floor. Some years go by, his "bells" go out of style, and he replaces them with the more conservative dress of the 1980s. He wears his hair shorter, and finds that jacket and tie gain him greater acceptance at work. He marries and begins a family. The only visible relict of his 1970s persona is his mustache, shortened now, reaching a little past the corners of his mouth and covering the lower part of his upper lip in a dark band more resembling Roman Novarro or Gilbert Roland in some of their movie roles than Mark Twain's leonine still portraits. Nevertheless, he feels it has become a part of him now and he cherishes it, as well as the look he sees in himself each morning in the mirror. He keeps it in good trim and comes to feel that it carries both an appearance of well-earned maturity as well as a secret sense of youth and rebellion.

Twenty-five years go by, and now, in his mid-50s, he has three daughters ranging from the mid-teens to early 20s, all living at home. One evening in late spring after dinner, his daughters ask if they can speak with him. They have convened and come to a unified decision. They ask him please to shave his mustache. They find it a social embarrassment because, as they say to him, it makes him look like "some kind of stalker or worse." They feel uncomfortable having their friends over to the house because some of them have commented on how "icky" mustaches look on boys their age. They find in this a natural extrapolation to their father's remnant of the facial hair they have seen in pictures of him taken in the 1970s when he looked even more "obtuse and uncool." He looks around for some age-appropriate support and sees his wife, her back to him and working with dishes in the kitchen sink, but clearly within earshot, shaking gently with unmistakable laughter. He tells his daughters that he will give it some thought, and they all go about their business in the evening. He looks at his mirror image thoughtfully that night before going to bed. The next morning, with a few deft strokes, he shaves off his companion of 40 years and finds, as he suspected he might, that his face more resembles his father's than he might have thought comfortable back when Fu Manchus were in style. Later that day at dinner, he asks whether his daughters approve of the new look. They compliment him, saying that he looks more distinguished, bears a resemblance to their grandfather, and that they now believe that he is presentable in public. In fact, they now want to have some of their friends over on the weekend. He sends them to their mother to arrange that, commenting, "I just work here. I'll help out if I'm needed."

In this vignette, most readers will find it easy to see two instances of adolescent "rebellion" from the preceding generation: first in the college student as he blends into his age group and then in his daughters for the same reason. Viewing both instances as forms of psychological adaptation in the model of Chapter 2, we can apply this chapter's recognition algorithm in the service of locating the proper Domain for their respective behaviors.

As in the previous example of the Primitive Domain styles, the first task is to locate the stress that serves to raise anxiety in waking consciousness, that is, that perturbs the ego with a sense of doom or disaster. At first glance, this stress might be attributed to (1) the college student belief of his father's low opinion of his cool outfit or (2) the three daughters' opinion of their socially unacceptable parent. Both reflect the true stress involved but do not make up its component parts. To understand the nature of the stress requires consideration of the phenomenon of adolescence itself, a process that entails pushing away from parents with the goal of standing independently on one's own. The natural process of development provides the stress: can I go from being a dependent child to being an independent adult, and, if so, how can I stand the frightfulness of standing on my own? Viewed in terms of the anxiety that flows from this quandary, to remain forever a child courts doom, while taking chances on independent adulthood risks disaster.

Having identified these two anxiety components of the stress of growing up, the algorithm next asks whether in each case the father or the daughters ignore the stressful situation or the anxiety it causes. Does the college student look his father in the eye and say, "What outfit?" Do the daughters avoid talking about the father's mustache? In either instance, do the protagonists regard (1) the disco uniform or (2) the unsightly mustache as put there by agents of the Devil or invading space creatures from Neptune? The answer of course in each case is *No*: the relevant stress and its anxiety in relation to normal adolescent development brings recognition of something relating to a sense of either doom—giving up the moustache—or disaster—a geeky Dad. Neither the college student nor his daughters in a later era ignore the concerns. In recognizing their respective dilemmas, they each clearly have progressed beyond Primitive Domain adaptive mechanisms.

Moving to the next level of the recognition algorithm, the observer's task requires an assessment of whether the protagonist/s in the vignette each locates the relevant anxiety and its stress as belonging to them for resolution or to someone else. In the first instance, from his point of view the college student's cool outfit provides him with friends and contact with interested females. If his old man hasn't got a sense of style, that's his problem. Similarly, the three daughters recognize their father's appearance as limiting their social acceptance. In their view, he clearly has no sense of style; otherwise he would recognize that the mustache makes him look like a dork. The fact that he doesn't is clearly his problem, not theirs. In each case, therefore, the sense of social disaster looming from a denied access to the respective peer social groups is somebody else's problem, namely one's parents'. In both cases, viewed as adolescents pushing away from their parents and finding their own identity, alarm at the parents' lack of good taste conforms to a normal and important developmental process.

The even greater stress in the developmental passage of adolescence—moving out of the childhood home and into an independent life of one's own—with an even greater sense of potential disaster, accounts for the necessity of relying on one's peer group to start with. It also accounts for the view of the parents' inadequacies from the point of view of the young people navigating the channel forward. From the adolescent's point of view, the psychological quandary could be paraphrased as "It's not that I'm inadequate. It's that my parents are clearly inadequate." This kind of projection of inner difficulties outward onto others makes up the subject of Chapter 11, and, as we shall see, it exists in pathological forms as well as in the normal developmental version described here. For the purposes of the present chapter, the instances of normal adolescent projection illustrate the Immature Domain of psychological adaptation strategies.

Reviewing the recognition algorithm schematic in Figure 3.1, therefore, adapting to a stress and its anxiety first involves acknowledgment of it, as opposed to ignoring the circumstance as in the formulation of the Primitive Domain mechanisms. Once acknowledged, the next level asks whether the stress and anxiety have to do with the person experiencing them or to locating them outside the person's waking consciousness, as in the formulation of the Immature Domain adaptive styles.

With the stress and its anxiety acknowledged and then "owned"—proceeding past the Primitive and Immature Domains, respectively—the recognition algorithm in Figure 3.1 next leads the observer to consider whether the Neurotic Domain adaptive mechanisms are at work. To illustrate this, we will now alter the fable of the mustache to focus on the college student now in middle age. And later, as we approach the Mature Domain through the algorithm, we will return to the original version.

MUSTACHE FOREVER! THE NEUROTIC DOMAIN IN ADULT LIFE

Recalling the scene in which the three daughters inform their father that his long-cherished mustache—in their view, a particularly unsavory facial characteristic—makes him look like a stalker or worse, the middle-aged hero of the story now responds with a very different behavioral reaction. He asserts, to the contrary, that the mustache provides a certain stylish dash. In fact, he decides to extend it by returning it to its original Fu Manchu configuration and begins growing the two vertical strips of whiskers that droop, one from either end of the mustache, down the creases of his chin. As this occurs, his daughters point out that he looks even dumber than before, now taking on the characteristics of the Old Coot from B Western movies as his mustache grows in with a two-toned appearance.

Meanwhile he has taken to pulling pictures out of the family photo album of himself in his younger days with the original monotone mustache, having them enlarged, printed and framed, and hanging them about the house. He orders a set of vanity license plates for the family sedan with MYSTASH printed on them and bolts them to the car, beaming with pride and saying only that he wished he had bought vanity plates 20 years earlier. His daughters find themselves even more appalled, telling him that the vanity plates advertise him as a drug dealer rather than a mustachioed movie hero. He, however, believes the contrary and begins to collect still photos of film swashbucklers from Douglas Fairbanks through Johnny Depp—including Ramon Novarro and Gilbert Roland—in their roles as movie characters with whom he believes he shares a certain panache, a savoir faire, and a zest for life that is rare for men his age who have largely lost touch with their adventuresome spirits. To his surprise, his daughters now refuse to bring any of their friends over to "New Dork City."

In applying the recognition algorithm of this chapter—warming up its use for all of the subsequent discussions—to this description of our middle-aged hero, the observer rightly focuses on the father's response to his daughters' criticism. Something about that criticism has created a stress. Something in it has perturbed his waking sense of the equilibrium of his conscious self. This in turn has raised his anxiety. The observer needn't look too far to find it: he or she learned earlier that the mustache originally encompassed a statement of individuality, recognition of social acceptance, and the last remnant of an age that the father experienced as characterized by personal adventure into the great world. At that time of life, the need for vanity license plates seemed as superfluous as the need for a family sedan. Now, however, his daughters tell him must look like everyone else and, worse yet, like everyone else in middle age. He hears in this his existential doom. He has become ordinary, adventureless, a physical mass against which rebellions occur rather than the rebel himself.

Having identified the stress and its anxiety, in stepwise fashion the recognition algorithm next asks whether the father's adaptation to them includes recognizing their existence or ignoring them altogether through use of a Primitive Domain adaptive style. The observer finds no evidence to suggest that the father denies any awareness of his daughters having made their statements about him, nor does he avoid the issue by talking about something else or claiming that his daughters have been bewitched and their spirits inhabited by the Devil. Far from ignoring their comments, he seems to have gone in the opposite direction and dwelt on them for some extended purpose. According to the algorithm, therefore, he has proceeded beyond the Primitive Domain.

Following Figure 3.1 in its stepwise fashion, the recognition algorithm next asks whether one of the Immature Domain mechanisms might be at work: does the father acknowledge the stress of ordinariness/middle age and its associated sense of doom as having something to do with himself, or does he perceive it as entirely someone else's fault? His behavioral crusade on the Importance of the Mustache provides evidence of perceiving the perturbation as within himself rather than locating it in some external place where he can do nothing about it. He has not blamed it on his daughters, calling them stupid, for example, which would reflect an Immature Domain response. Neither has he retreated into a fantasy world of adventure and excitement to which only he has access, nor has he passively promised his daughters that he would remove the mustache, knowing that he will never do so in order to spite them. The mustache and all it symbolizes belongs to him in his waking consciousness and requires him to adapt directly. There is no evidence of an Immature Domain adaptive style at work here.

Bearing in mind his having acknowledged the stress and its anxiety, and having taken responsibility for adapting to them, the recognition algorithm now directs the observer to the next step: consideration of the Neurotic Domain of adaptive mechanisms. The term *neurotic* implies the nature of the psychological adaptive styles that form this group: each stress—each perturbation to waking consciousness—contains two component parts best characterized independently as an idea and a feeling. Respective synonyms include cognitive and affective contents, or a thought and an emotion. In this discussion and all subsequent in this volume, *cognition*, *idea*, and *thought* mean the same thing: each is an equivalent description of conceptual content in the absence of emotion. At same time, the words *affect*, *emotion*, and *feeling* all equivalently refer to emotional content in the absence of any concept. To illustrate, we refer to the earlier example of the man walking in the woods who meets a bear. "Here comes a bear," states the cognition, the idea, the thought content of the experience. "I am frightened of the bear!" gives voice to the affect, the emotion, the feeling content of the experience, in this case, one of terror.

The observer's next task then, following the algorithm, requires identification of both the cognitive content and the affective content, respectively, of the stress that causes his anxiety, that raises the sense of doom. In the case of the father and his mustache in the more recent version of the vignette as stated above, the observer may formulate the cognitive content of the stressful circumstance as "I am ordinary and old," in the middle-aged hero's perception. Its affective content finds voice as "I am sad and not a little terrified."

Having identified idea and feeling, in order to establish the presence of a Neurotic Domain adaptive mechanism, the observer must judge the evidence for thought and feeling as integrated and working together, or as uncoupled and not at all working together toward a constructive purpose. The latter defines the Neurotic Domain in which idea and emotion never settle in each other's company.

In the case at hand, the father's crusade on behalf of his mustache indicates that it carries more psychological weight for him than simply decorative facial hair. Rather than setting his daughters' criticism of his looks in the context of their adolescent passage, and finding usefulness in a sense of parental distance and objectivity in the process, his response calls forth his own concerns instead. He defines the mustache and all that it symbolizes for him as good and makes it a cause célèbre in his household. Fueled by the fear of losing, or having lost, or never having gained a sense of his own unique human individuality, he chooses to attack the painful emotion with behavior based in the idea content of being unique. He will preserve his mustache despite the family opprobrium, extend it, publicize it, and turn it into a hobby. But this does not address the emotional issue. It merely repeats it. Repetitive restatements[2] of how important mustaches are—an insistence on his own sense of uniqueness—does not resolve the underlying fear that this may not be true.

In this regard, the cognitive content of his worry about being ordinary and the emotional content of his fear that he is unhappy with himself have not reached a resolution between them. Instead they are disjoined: the fear triggers the idea of being ordinary that in turn triggers the behavior meant to exemplify individuality that in turn worsens the fear. The lack of integration of idea and feeling defines the Neurotic Domain psychological adaptive mechanisms, in this case an adaptive style of Reaction Formation, which will be discussed in greater detail in Chapter 16.

A useful clue that the Neurotic Domain mechanisms may be at work often makes itself known when the observer notices repetitive, unsatisfying, and sometimes painful behaviors that carry with them a sense of being locked into a pattern with no other choices. A true resolution, by contrast, requires the father's own careful recognition of his anxiety, and it sources in the painful ideas and feelings he carries with him. To move from the Neurotic Domain adaptive mechanisms, however, may require patient assistance from another person with professional training. To paraphrase Robert Burns' formulation[3] of the phenomenon, in one or another circumstance—and especially in the setting of difficult thoughts and feelings—all of us have difficulty seeing ourselves as others see us. And from time to time we may need help from them to do so.

IT'S JUST ONE OF THOSE THINGS: THE MATURE DOMAIN MECHANISMS IN ADULT LIFE

To illustrate the Neurotic Domain mechanisms, this chapter's discussion took an imaginative side trip. But with a bow to our middle-aged protagonist and his vanity plates, we can return him to the original description in which we find the Mature Domain psychological adaptive mechanisms at work. The progression of the recognition algorithm, however, will not take our word for it and requires application of its stepwise process to the facts that the vignette provides. Fortunately we have already done most of the hard work. We have established in respect to the father in the story that his daughters' request for him to remove his mustache perturbs him as

2. Other models have described this repetitive process as counterphobic behavior or as repetition compulsions.

3. Burns, "To a Louse, on Seeing One on a Lady's Bonnet at Church" (1955, pp. 137–138). In current vernacular, *louse* refers to a ne'er-do-well or scoundrel. Burns here writes about the actual bug, a louse crawling on the woman's bonnet.

a stress to his waking consciousness, what we have defined as his ego that we refer to as his conscious sense of himself. This in turn raises his anxiety, which takes on the characteristic of a sense of doom. As we have seen, he does not ignore the circumstance, nor does he ascribe it as a problem for others outside himself to solve: he does not engage the Primitive Domain or Immature Domain psychological adaptive mechanisms. In examining the Neurotic Domain mechanisms in the last section, we find that the stress entails the cognitive content of the father's believing that he is ordinary/middle-aged without the mustache and the concurrent emotional content of fearfulness or disappointment related to the sense of doom. In that circumstance, he attacks the painful idea and feelings with an opposite reaction that his daughters regard as absurd. He does this in a way that does not allow affect and cognition to work together but keeps them both separate and at arm's length.

Contrast this to the first version of the episode, in which the father responds very differently to his daughters' request that he alter the appearance, his greeting card to the world. Both the idea and feeling contents remain in his awareness. The first relates to a subjective sense of ordinariness/aging and the second to fearfulness that his fate is to be ordinary, old, and resembling his father. He clearly regards the issue as something he must settle for himself when he tells his daughters that he will think about it. Unlike one of the Immature Domain defenses—that of Acting Out, as discussed in Chapter 7—he does not behave impulsively in an attempt to rid himself of the painful feeling and thought. Instead, he tolerates the anxiety and its associated idea and emotion by capping his sense of doom—putting a lid on it, so to speak—and then coming to terms with it over the next day. He revisits it that night before bed as he looks at his mustache one more time, and again in the morning when he shaves it off. At that point, with a recognition that one might call poetic, he sees his resemblance to his father that the mustache partly obscured. And 24 hours after the first conversation, he and his daughters have another one on the issue. They thank him for his having removed it and invite him to join in their plans with their friends. He politely refuses, leaving their generation to their own social devices in much the same manner as his did, and claims his ordinariness by saying that he just works there.

In this vignette, he adapts by combining the painful thought of being ordinary and the feeling of fearfulness that he is like everyone else—especially his father—in a way that allows him to navigate through a step in adult development. It requires him to give up a cherished remnant of his personal past that, as the Cole Porter song has it, was "great fun but just one of those things." Notice here that he does not keep idea and feeling at bay in some repeating pattern of behavior that aims to do just that. Instead, his adaptation includes experiencing them, looking at them serially in waking consciousness, and then coming to a resolution of them in giving up the mustache and then making a joke about it. We shall see both processes again in the exploration of Mature Domain adaptive styles. The first of them noted here, that of working through the perturbation with its difficult thoughts and feelings in manageable increments over time, describes Suppression, the subject of Chapter 17. The second, in which the father makes a small but significant joke as both the subject and the object of his own lightheartedness in embracing the ordinary, describing himself

Table 3.1 A COMPARISON OF THE DOMAINS OF PSYCHOLOGICAL ADAPTIVE MECHANISMS

	Primitive	Immature	Neurotic	Mature
Recognition of the stress	0	X	X	X
Stress ownership	0	0	X	X
Integrated thought/feeling	0	0	0	X
Resolution of the stress	0	0	0	X

as one who simply works there, exemplifies true Humor, another of the Mature Domain mechanisms. It rounds out the discussion of the specific mechanisms as the subject of Chapter 21.

For the purpose of the present chapter, namely introducing the systematic use of the recognition algorithm, Table 3.1 offers a comparison of the Domains. The Mature Domain mechanisms, in contrast to the other three groups, offer (1) an integration of affect and cognition, and (2) a true resolution of both the stress that perturbs waking consciousness and its associated anxiety. In this way, by definition, the Mature Domain mechanisms are never pathological. As Vaillant has pointed out, they represent healthy human psychological functioning at its best. Because of this, and again unlike the other three groups, the Mature Domain psychological adaptive mechanisms link people in adult life together rather than push them apart. The psychotic unreality of the Primitive Domain mechanisms, the Immature Domain styles' characterological blaming of inner upset on outer people and things, and the repetitive behaviors of the Neurotic Domain mechanisms that render human compassion impossible, each respectively restate the systematic steps of the algorithm in Figure 3.1 as it assesses the attributes of the observable human behaviors before us. The recognition algorithm will guide us in assigning the respective Domains of adaptation behaviors in the same progressive pattern from Primitive to Mature as these occur in nature. With this approach in hand, our next immediate task entails using it in recognizing specific psychological adaptive mechanisms within the Domains. To do this, we will apply it in each of subsequent chapters, devoting one chapter to each of the specific psychological adaptive styles.

REFERENCES

Burns, R. (1955). "To a Louse, on Seeing One on a Lady's Bonnet at Church." In James Barke (Ed.), *Poems and Songs of Robert Burns*. London and Glasgow, Collins.

Russell, B. (1959). *Problems of Philosophy*. Oxford, Oxford University Press.

CHAPTER 4
Denial

In differentiating the Primitive adaptive mechanisms from those of the other three Domains, the first task is to view them in very concrete terms. For example, as I set my coffee cup on the table in front of me, I observe that it is a fresh cup with steam rising off of it, and I smell a delicious fresh ground aroma. If, however, for some reason, such as a malfunctioning in my adult brain or the overwhelming weight of an intolerable stress or series of them, I am using Primitive Denial, in my perception the cup of coffee does not exist. In this sense, what may seem completely obvious to someone else does not occur in my range of perceptions. The term *denial*, therefore, we use here in a very specific sense with respect simply to nonexistence in the perception of the person using that psychological adaptive mechanism. The schematic diagram in Figure 4.1 represents this. Where in Figure 2.4 in Chapter 2, a stress perturbed the ego—the conscious sense of oneself—and that in turn raised anxiety resulting in the activation of an adaptive mechanism, we see in this instance that the adaptive mechanisms of the Primitive Domain strategies in one way or another eliminate recognition of the stress itself. Pictorially, the word *stress* at best appears with a question mark in Figure 4.1, as if to say "What stress?" And the person does not perceive it as having anything to do with anxiety that, itself, may not be recognized.

For the most part, cups of coffee contain very little in the way of emotional meaning, and we can consider this example a trivial one. However, the example is useful in illustrating the concrete nature of both this Primitive Domain adaptive mechanism and the other two Primitive styles so as to recognize them in the persons immediately before us, whether in clinical or other relevant situations. To illustrate further, consider the following case.

IT MAY GO AWAY: PRIMITIVE DENIAL AS REACTION TO ILLNESS

An outlying hospital transfers a woman in her mid-50s to an urban medical center where more definitive tests can be run in an effort to explain why she is having difficulty swallowing. She has carried a diagnosis of paranoid schizophrenia since her late teenage years, a condition that has been very well controlled with specific medicines

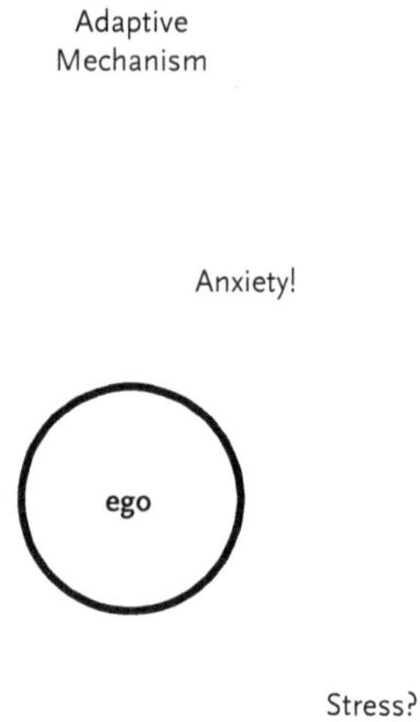

Figure 4.1
As compared to the template in Figure 2.4, the Primitive Domain mechanisms demonstrate no conscious recognition or acknowledgment of the stress. In this schema of the Primitive Domain strategy, therefore, no arrows connect among the components of stress, ego, anxiety, and adaptive mechanism. This Domain's mechanisms deny, avoid or distort, or project out the stress, all in a very concrete manner as if the stress were a physical object.

for that disorder. Although she has never married and has difficulty maintaining a regular job, her treatment has allowed her to live with her siblings and her extended family, wherein she is regarded as an amiable, if somewhat dotty, aunt. Her swallowing disorder, thought to be a side effect of her psychopharmacological treatment, requires two technical procedures to sort out a diagnosis. First, she must undergo a magnetic resonance imaging (MRI) study in which she has to lie motionless in a large, donut-shaped magnet, and then, possibly, an upper endoscopy procedure in which, while sedated, her doctor introduces the tube that can follow the track of her throat and esophagus down to her stomach. Although the patient's schizophrenia is generally well controlled, the medical staff is careful to explain each procedure clearly and in detail, as she has occasional difficulties—usually when she has stopped taking her psychiatric medications—with worries that the government is trying to harm her. After each explanation, she says simply, "Fine." And she completes each procedure without any difficulties. Unfortunately, however, both procedures reveal the presence of cancer in her esophagus, one that carries a poor prognosis. Uncertain as to how to go about telling her the news, the medical team invites the hospital psychiatrist into the conversation to discuss the findings with her. With the group assembled, the team presents a careful and very clear explanation of the problem, and the possible treatment options, including their recommendations. When they ask her which of the treatment possibilities she would prefer, she states that she trusts the judgment of the doctors and would go along with their first choice. Then, in perfect seriousness, she turns to the psychiatrist and in an even tone of voice says, "Or, it might just all go away."

To apply the recognition algorithm in its stepwise order, the observer first identifies the stress to the conscious equilibrium. In this case, it is the diagnosis of cancer. In most persons, that word alone raises a sense of doom or disaster—the subjective experiences that the recognition model identifies as manifesting anxiety. The algorithm next asks whether the person perceives the stress in their conscious state or whether he or she regards it as not there. In this case, the woman listens politely and then adds that the cancer might go away on its own, despite no indication of this from her doctors who recommend treatment. In the adaptation model, her response exemplifies the mechanism of Primitive Domain Denial. As an adaptation, it eases her sense of doom. To some, this vignette may simply illustrate an example of wishful thinking, and who among us wouldn't want some of that in the face of a difficult medical diagnosis? But in our model of psychological adaptive mechanisms, this patient's last statement demonstrates the concrete Primitive Denial that often characterizes persons who have schizophrenia. Without benefit of her medicines, she may well have become delusional about the diagnosis, believing that the government had caused her cancer. But as it was, faced with a stress that entails the emotional impact of life and death, her principal relief lay in her view that her cancer would simply not exist.

Establishing whether or not the person in question recognizes the stress, referring to our ongoing model for clinical observation, makes up the observer's first decision point in assessing which of the adaptive Domains the person uses. By definition the adaptive Domains are progressive: if a person has not first come to recognize the stress to which they respond with anxiety, there is no assignment to any of the other three adaptive Domains, each of which requires recognizing the stress itself as a condition of defining less primitive ways with which to adapt.

THE SLEEPY INTERN: PRIMITIVE DENIAL IN ADULTHOOD

As one way to characterize the differences among the Domains and adaptive mechanisms themselves across the boundaries of the chapters of this book, we will refer in each case to an overworked, sleep deprived, medical intern who finds himself (or herself, as the character will vary in different chapters) working at three o'clock in the morning on an extended shift, when most human beings are engaged in a restful sleep. As if this weren't difficult enough, in each chapter our intern will face an additional stress that perturbs his waking consciousness. And in each chapter our valiant—if not always well adapted—intern will deploy a response to illustrate the psychological adaptive mechanism for that chapter.

In the present chapter, we find our intern working hard with four very ill patients in the intensive care unit (ICU) and six more out on the hospital ward in various stages of medical health who are serious enough to require hospitalization. Despite this, and despite the lateness of the hour, our intern receives a phone call from the emergency room (ER) team notifying him that they are sending up another patient who is critically ill and must be admitted to the ICU. The intern politely hangs up the phone and goes about his work. But when the new patient arrives, the intern does not respond to the nursing staff's efforts to page him. They contact the hospital ward staff and the ER team, neither of which knows where he is. Becoming concerned, the ICU staff call the hospital security officers, who search the building. They find our intern sitting in an on-call room, staring at a blank computer screen and repeating over and over again, "I have no patients. They've all gotten better and gone home." The intern is relieved of duties the next day and sent on a leave of absence for health reasons.

Applying the clinical recognition algorithm, we first identify the stress that perturbs the intern's conscious well-being in this situation—in this case, it is the admission of yet another critically ill patient. As often occurs with the Primitive Domain mechanisms, an observer can only infer the person's anxiety, in this case a sense of imminent disaster, by his response to it rather than necessarily perceive it directly. Both the stress and anxiety it calls forth can be shut out of conscious thought in Primitive Domain adaptive mechanisms. His behavior provides an example of Denial in the very concrete form in which we use it in this volume. Common to the other Primitive Domain adaptive mechanisms, the behavioral response ignores the stress and anxiety. In the case of Denial, they simply do not exist.

Needless to say, however, the nursing and ER staff require a fully functioning physician who can recognize the need to care for the medically critical patient they bring to the ICU. They move on to some other arrangement with a covering physician until permanent help can arrive in the daytime. The next day, the intern's faculty supervisors recognize that his response is well short of acceptable adaptation to the stress of a very difficult job. They identify his Primitive Domain response as a psychotic reaction and refer him for mental health treatment.

PSYCHOSIS AND PRIMITIVE DENIAL

Viewed clinically, when Primitive Denial of this nature is a primary mechanism—that is, a first choice adaptive mechanism for anyone in adult or young adult life—we class it as a psychotic defense. The term *psychosis* has traditionally meant a state of mind in which a person has lost contact with the immediate reality around him or her. While this can be defined in many forms with many nuances in other theoretical frameworks, our current model of psychological adaptive functioning would define it simply as a nonrecognition of the stress presented to the person. Our sleepy intern serves us well in this context. Owing in this case to the overwhelming nature of the stresses relative to the intern's own psychological resources, he has responded by simply not recognizing his difficulty in the situation. To the intern, the last patient "isn't there" in a very concrete sense, and this expands to the perception that none of his patients are there because he has cured them all. It is in this sense, therefore, that the Primitive Domain adaptive mechanisms, when seen in a context that is not age appropriate, we term as Psychotic adaptive mechanisms.

Psychotic denial may occur in other clinical settings in which patients suffer a major mental illness—such as schizophrenia, severe forms of major depression, or bipolar disorder—as listed in the diagnostic and statistical manuals (DSMs)[1] of our era. In DSM syndrome models, diagnoses occur when a sufficient number of observable symptoms present themselves at the same time in the same patient. The model of psychological adaptive mechanisms—the focus of this book—contributes another view of the process. It suggests that humans adapt through deployment of the best psychological strategies available to the individual at the time, no matter how inflexible or primitive they may be. In the case of Psychotic Denial, the patient's best adaptive option is to ignore the anxiety and deal with the stress in the same manner. Impairment syndromes of brain functions in such cases limit the available choices of adaptation mechanism and may do so very severely.

In order to increase the number of options—that is, to move to a less rigid, more flexible adaptive style—the patient's neuropsychiatric function must improve. The great preponderance of scientific evidence identifies pathological or pathophysiological brain functioning as the basis for the three classically described psychotic disorders mentioned in the previous paragraph. In each case, schizophrenia, major depression, and bipolar disorder can be improved with specific medications that assist the return to normal brain functioning. The same Primitive Domain adaptive strategy of Denial can also be seen in other conditions in which the brain functions suboptimally, as in this case.

BRAIN FAILURE AND PRIMITIVE DENIAL

A 55-year-old male comes to the hospital with a police escort. They found him wandering about the streets in a confused state. On examination, when asked to describe why he has come to the hospital, he says, "I'm all right, Mac," repeating this phrase over and over. Hospital records show that he has had a long history of alcohol use. His physical examination also reveals nystagmus on lateral gaze—that is, an inability to fix his ipsilateral eye to the right or left depending on the direction of his gaze—along with signs of cerebellar incoordination. A further examination of his cognitive capacities finds that he is able to repeat words immediately but is unable to retain them in his memory when asked to repeat them five minutes later. His clinicians diagnose alcohol amnestic syndrome, also known as Wernicke-Korsakoff's disease.

Delirium states impair brain functioning and limit the range of adaptive styles available. The alcoholic patient in this case suffers a brain impairment that most regard as due to insufficient nutrition and too much alcohol. The perseverated phrase "I'm all right, Mac" reflects the same Primitive/Psychotic adaptive strategy of Denial: there is no problem. The same is true of the dementing illnesses and any other conditions that may lessen optimal brain functioning. In this respect, therefore, seeing the Primitive/Psychotic defenses in adult life should occasion a careful differential diagnosis in the search for specific, treatable causes of what we may call adaptive

1. At the time of this writing, the DSM-IV-TR (American Psychiatric Association 2000) is the current version of this manual. DSM-V is forecast to appear in 2013.

failure: a regression from Mature Domain to Primitive Domain psychological adaptive mechanisms. We will have more to say about regression in Chapter 22.

NORMAL PRIMITIVE DENIAL

However, recall Chapter 3's example of the two-year-old who answers "No" when his mother, overtaken by the unmistakable odor, asks him, "Did you poop in your pants?" We noted there that Denial is a normal Primitive Domain adaptive style in early childhood. The anxiety resulting from the mother's implied judgment, the physical discomfort, or some combination of both, calls forth an unconscious response that says "Let's ignore the problem." At that age, we call forth Denial in the context of our brains' early stage of development. And a caring environment, in this case a loving mother, regards this adaptive strategy as "cute kid" behavior, and she tends to the problem herself.

NORMAL PRIMITIVE DENIAL IN A PATHOLOGICAL ENVIRONMENT

The adaptive mechanism of Primitive Denial in early childhood will function irrespective of the environment in which a young child might find him- or herself. But we have much to learn about how Primitive Domain adaptation to a pathological environment at an early age can surface at a later age in ways that trouble patients subjectively and result in impaired psychological or social functions as a result. Consider this case.

At age four, a young girl and her older sister girl encountered regular abuse from a parent who was later sent to prison when the abuse was discovered. The child herself did not receive any treatment at that time. Twenty years later she came to treatment complaining of "nervousness," and her husband was concerned that she was frequently using barbiturate tranquilizing medicines to quell the anxiety she experienced after the birth of her own child. In the course of an evaluation, the psychiatrist noted that she exhibited far more symptoms of anxiety than could be accounted for on the basis of her recent parenthood, having given birth to a healthy, normal infant and with a caring and supportive husband. She began referring to the anxiety as being a sense of impending disaster that was "down in the basement." Working with a therapist over a number of weeks, she slowly began to notice that there was a connection between her ongoing sense of disaster and the childhood recollection of her older sister's loud cries in the next room. Over several months, both the fear associated with her own abusive experience at the hands of the offending parent and the cognitive recollection of it came into her consciousness. She had known for many years that her parent had gone to prison for mistreating her sister. But the cognitive memory and the anxiety of her own trauma had remained consciously unavailable until she became responsible for the care of her own infant. As her psychotherapy unfolded, the availability of her own traumatic memories and anxiety allowed her to work to a resolution that included a much less anxious relationship with her own child.

Applying the recognition algorithm from Chapter 3 to this case offers a particular challenge. In the first step—that of identifying the stress to waking consciousness—observers will quickly recognize it as the abuse the woman suffered at a very early age. But that abuse and the original stress it caused, as formulated in the current model of psychological adaptive mechanisms, occurred many years before. Did it include a sense of anxiety, the second ingredient that the algorithm seeks to characterize in recognizing psychological adaptation? We note her anxiety's presence when it flowed forth some 20 years later: the patient describes it as a feeling of impending disaster, and her family becomes concerned about her overuse of medication to calm that feeling. Until that time, however, neither the stress itself nor the associated anxiety existed in the woman's conscious recollections. Present knowledge suggests that only the Primitive Domain psychological adaptive mechanisms are available to four-year-olds. Brain development in early childhood simply has not reached the more sophisticated capacities for perception and judgment that characterize adult life. For this reason, children require supervision by adults and the special protection of the laws. The woman in this case, as a child of four, could make use of Primitive Denial, and the unavailable personal data of her own trauma fits most consistently with this. Following the recognition algorithm, her original adaptive option was that of a very concrete form of denying that the trauma ever existed.

Although one could argue reasonably that this patient presented a repression of her early experiences—an adaptive style that we will examine in Chapter 12—an important distinction lies in *both* the emotional content and the cognitive memories of her experience being unavailable to her conscious self for many years. That suggests the much more likely occurrence of an age-appropriate Denial of the trauma that she suffered when it occurred at age four, and that Primitive Domain mechanism remaining intact until the birth of her own child. Although normally young children grow out of Primitive Denial in favor of much more effective adaptive styles, cases such as this one suggest that Primitive Domain adaptive styles in response to specific conditions in a pathological environment may be much more specific and more indurated. In this case, the Primitive Domain Denial appropriate to the four-year-old remained intact until many years later. In her 20s, the same patient did not characteristically use Primitive Denial in any other part of her life. It is as though this process had become loculated and unavailable for resolution until some other occurrence triggers its sense of doom or disaster. Taking this idea one step further, the original anxiety does not appear until the original adaptive mechanism begins to fall apart, losing its property of managing or capping the sense of disaster.

VANKA: PRIMITIVE DENIAL IN MIDDLE CHILDHOOD

For another example, consider this description from a famous story of Anton Chekhov's, himself a physician and a keen observer of human behavior. The scene is very late Christmas Eve in Russia in the latter half of the 19th century. Little Vanka, a nine-year-old boy apprenticed to a shoemaker, writes a letter to his grandfather, a night watchman in another town who drinks heavily during the day.

"Dear Grandad Konstantin Makarich," he wrote. "I am writing a letter to you. I send you Christmas greetings and hope God will send you his blessings. I have no Father and no Mummie and you are all I have left." . . . .

"Come to me dear Grandad," continued Vanka. "I beg you for Christ's sake take me away from here. Pity me unhappy orphan they beat me all the time and I am always hungry and I am so miserable here I can tell you I cry all the time. And one day the master hit me over the head with a last and I fell down and thought I would never get up again. I have such a miserable life worse than a dogs. And I send my love to Alyona one-eyed Yegor and the coachman and don't give my concertina to anyone. I remain your grandson Ivan Zhukov dear Grandad do come."

Vanka folded the sheet of paper in four and put it into an envelope which he had bought the day before for a kopeck. . . . Then he paused to think, dipped his pen into the ink-pot, wrote: "GRANDAD," scratched his head, thought again, and added: "KONSTANTIN MAKARICH IN THE VILLAGE"

Pleased that no one had prevented him from writing, he put on his cap and ran out into the street without putting his coat on over his shirt.

The men at the butcher's told him, when he asked them the day before, that letters are put into letter-boxes, and from these boxes sent all over the world on mail coaches with three horses and drunken drivers and jingling bells. Vanka ran as far as the nearest letter-box and dropped his precious letter into the slit.

(Chekhov 1886, p. 52)

Following our clinical algorithm, we first ask whether Vanka perceives a stressful occurrence, one that gives him a sense of anxious doom. On the surface, it seems obvious: he lives in an abusive situation in which he is treated as a slave and exploited merely for his labor. Does he deny that this situation exists? The answer is obviously *No*, since his response is to write a letter asking his grandfather for help. But Chekhov gives us a more subtle and, at the same time, more terrifying stress that threatens Vanka and one that affects us deeply as readers. Chekhov makes it clear that there is no help for the boy and no hope of any. As if to underline Vanka's desperation in the face of his beatings and abuse, the boy does not have a working address for his letter and no real way of contacting his last hope, his grandfather who is likely too drunk to respond. It is the absence of hope that truly threatens Vanka. And it is this that he cannot recognize, even though Chekhov leaves the reader both in no doubt and with profound feelings of terror and sadness. It is in this way, therefore, that Vanka depends on primitive Denial as his best adaptive option, no matter how inadequate that may appear to the reader and certainly to Chekhov.

As will occur with several other terms used in this volume to denote the various psychological adaptive mechanisms themselves, we have here defined that ubiquitous and often overused term—Denial—in a very specific way. The specificity of definition allows precise characterization from observable human behaviors. Use of the stepwise recognition algorithm allows the observer first, and most important, to follow behaviors into their proper Domains, as it has in this chapter in respect to the Primitive Domain. Once clarified, the definitions of specific styles will differentiate the various psychological adaptive strategies within their respective Domains.

REFERENCES

American Psychiatric Association. (2000). *Diagnostic and Statistical Manual of Mental Disorders, Fourth Edition—Text Revision*. Washington, DC, American Psychiatric Press.

Chekhov, A. (1886). "Vanka." In *Anton Chekhov's Short Stories*. New York, Norton.

CHAPTER 5

Avoidance/Distortion

In one of his most famous tragedies, William Shakespeare draws the character of King Lear, a man used to giving orders and requiring obeisance, who completely misjudges the characters of his three daughters among whom he divides his kingdom. Contrary to his perception, two of his daughters, Regan and Goneril, mean him no good, while the third, Cordelia, extends to him the saintly love of unambivalent and unconditional acceptance. Continuing in his misperception, the King banishes Cordelia for her refusal to take a share of his kingdom, something he interprets as a lack of loyalty. He splits his kingdom, therefore, between the two remaining daughters, and they proceed to shear him of all his wealth and power. In the third act of the play, the audience finds King Lear wandering about the fields in a thunderstorm, wearing rags, with no shelter of his own, and accompanied by the Duke of Kent and others of his few remaining true friends. He complains loudly as if shouting to the sky.

> *Lear*: Filial ingratitude!
> Is it not as this mouth should tear this hand
> For lifting food to 't? But I will punish home:
> No, I will weep no more. In such a night
> To shut me out! Pour on; I will endure
> In such a night as this! O Regan, Goneril!
> Your old kind father, whose frank heart gave all,—
> O! That way madness lies; let me shun that;
> No more of that.
> *Kent*: Good, my lord, enter here.
> *Lear*: Prithee, go in thyself; seek thine own ease:
> This tempest will not give me leave to ponder
> On things would hurt me more.
>
> (Shakespeare, *King Lear*, Act III, Scene 4, lines 14–25)

What adaptive mechanism does King Lear use in this example? Following the recognition algorithm for psychological adaptive mechanisms, we first assure ourselves that Lear is reacting to a stress that threatens his conscious sense of himself or, in other words, his ego. In his case, two concurrent stresses add to each other's painful impact. The first is the loss of all his regal trappings and resources that he had thought to keep to himself when giving over his kingdom to his daughters. And the second, one that is more subtle and probably much more devastating, is his complete misjudgment of his daughters, thinking that the two to whom he has given his kingdom would love him as a person more than they love his wealth and power. They do not love him, and they do not show him even the lesser virtue of gratitude.

Second, in the recognition algorithm, does this double stress raise his anxiety and cause emotional pain? As he says in the quotation above, it drives him not only to pain but even to the point of what he considers to be madness. And third, how does he deal with anxiety that is so extreme as to be considered madness? As he says, he will "shun" madness. His method is simply to avoid it or, as he says, "no more of that." He has, in effect, said that he will refuse to allow either his thoughts about the stress—about his ungrateful daughters—or the painful anxiety from his situation into his conscious thought. He will "weep no more" and urges the storm to distract him from his painful thoughts and feelings by its violence upon him: "Pour on; I will endure / In such a night as this."

Although this last statement at first gives us a picture of a man standing up to the elements of thunder and lightning in the tempest storm, Shakespeare portrays him in yet another dimension. The Duke of Kent, the king's loyal and longtime friend who has been with him through his banishment, offers to come with him into a nearby hut to take refuge from the driving rain. But Lear refuses him, saying that he finds use in the storm because it helps him avoid his madness. So long as he has to fight with the storm, he does not have to face the pain and anxiety of deceitful daughters and the loss of his kingdom. We can conclude that Lear uses the adaptive mechanism of Primitive Domain Avoidance at this point in the play. Like Primitive Denial, its use in an adult asks us to consider the possibility of a psychotic adaptation, one that is not fully coming to terms with the details of a reality.

At the same time, Shakespeare offers us the insight that in King Lear's case Primitive Avoidance is not a passive process: he does not stop at merely ignoring his madness in a simpleminded fashion, but actively makes use of the storm as a way to continue to distract him from his own pain. He does this at least at the price of his own discomfort, and perhaps physical illness, as well as the concern of his friends. And, as with any avoidance, indeed any of the Primitive adaptive mechanisms, King Lear has not solved the problem. He has only temporized, put off a resolution of, his madness for some short while, or perhaps forever.

PRIMITIVE DISTORTION WITHOUT PSYCHOSIS

If King Lear avoids what we term *anxiety* and what he calls his *madness*, Ignatius J. Reilly manages his by distorting the circumstances around him. Using the recognition algorithm, consider this passage from John Kennedy Toole's famous comic novel, *A Confederacy of Dunces*. The setting is New Orleans, and we hear a mother talking with her grown son: an overweight, overeducated, and underachieving man somewhere in his 30s who records his thoughts on life in copious notes written in pencil on wide-ruled Big Chief tablets. His mother worries about him.

> "Ignatius, don't you think maybe you'd be happy if you went and took you a little rest at Charity?"
>
> "Are you referring to the psychiatric ward by any chance?" Ignatius demanded in a rage. "Do you think I am insane? Do you suppose that some stupid psychiatrist could even attempt to fathom the workings of my psyche?"
>
> "You could just rest, honey. You could write some stuff in your little copybooks."
>
> "They would try to make me into a moron who liked television and new cars and frozen food. Don't you understand? Psychiatry is worse than communism. I refuse to be brainwashed. I won't be a robot!"
>
> "But, Ignatius, they help out a lot of people got problems."
>
> "Do you think I have a problem?" Ignatius bellowed. "The only problem that those people have anyway is that they don't like new cars and hair sprays. That's why they are put away. They make the other members of society fearful. Every asylum in this nation is filled with poor souls who simply cannot stand lanolin, cellophane, plastic, television, and subdivisions."
>
> "Ignatius, that ain't true. You remember old Mr. Becnel used to live down the block? They locked him up because he was running down the street naked."
>
> "Of course he was running down the street naked. His skin could not bear any more of that dacron and nylon clothing that was clogging his pores. I've always considered Mr. Becnel one of the martyrs of our age. The poor man was badly victimized. Now run along to the front door and see if my taxi has arrived."
>
> (Toole 1980, pp. 468–470)

Let us beg the reader's patience in allowing application of the recognition algorithm to the portrayal in this vignette, something that Ignatius himself, and very likely his late author, would never allow us to do unless we did so with no intended solemnity, whatsoever. Seriousness, yes, but solemnity, no.

First let us locate the stress to Ignatius in this description, which in this case is obvious: Ignatius's own mother thinks he should admit himself to the mental ward of the local public hospital. He is indeed a Charity Hospital case because he has no other medical resources of his own and, as we learn elsewhere, his fortunes and those of his mother are in decline. She nonetheless cares about him and thinks he should get help. Does this stress, viewed in these terms, raise Ignatius's anxiety? We can reasonably say that something is perturbing him because he flies into an immediate rage. But he is not a violent sort and his mother knows him very well. So they continue to talk.

Does Ignatius see anything in himself that might indicate a need for him to seek admission to a mental ward? This too is a resounding, or should we say a bellowing, *No!* He proceeds into a riff on how wrong the world is, how right he is, and concludes with a brass band heroic portrait of poor Mr. Becnel, all of it completely serious from his point of view—and completely comic from ours. Following one of his great comic strengths as a literary character, Ignatius has distorted the facts around him entirely to his own advantage to stave off the anxiety of acknowledging his mother's concerns—and perhaps his own—about his mental health. Although his response is clearly in the Primitive domain, in which one behaves as though the stress did not exist, it serves to put his own anxiety in check, and he quietly asks his mother to look out the window to see if his taxi has arrived.

In so distorting the facts about him, Ignatius completely avoids having to face either them or, indeed, his anxiety—his sense of personal doom or disaster as someone who is unable to function in the real world—that we can imagine is well hidden below his rage. Distortion, then, in the model of adaptive behaviors can be considered the equivalent of, or a form of, Primitive Domain Avoidance. Among many other things in the novel, this is what Ignatius J. Reilly has to teach us, and for it we thank him profusely. We then send him our apologies, beg his author's pardon, and quietly tuck him back into his literary context in one of the great comic novels of our time. But we do so with a sense of the ominous, however: in day-to-day life, distortion as a form of Avoidance/Distortion can be much more destructive than its comic portrayal might suggest.[1]

PRIMITIVE AVOIDANCE/DISTORTION: A CLINICAL EXAMPLE

A woman in her early 30s arrives at the ER of a hospital, brought there by family members, who sign her in and then promptly depart. The ER staff quickly triage her to the psychiatrist on call. When the doctor—a woman in her mid-40s—arrives, she asks the patient how she might be of help. In response, the patient screeches at the top of her lungs: "MURDER!" "MURDER, MURDER, MURDER, MURDER, MURDER!" She grabs the nearest object she can find—a partially filled plastic water pitcher—and hurls it as hard she can at the psychiatrist, barely missing the doctor's head. ER staff respond with a show of force, gathering half a dozen people around her and helping her onto a hospital gurney, where they put her in soft restraints, both for her own safety and for the safety of those around her. The psychiatrist, using an even tone of voice and a businesslike manner, states, "Perhaps you could be more specific." The patient continues to speak in a loud voice and, with intermittent tearfulness, voices more phrases that sound like newspaper headlines. These include examples such as "THIS UNDESERVING PERSON THROWN OUT," "EMPLOYERS ARE ALL THIEVES," and "MEN ARE ONLY BEASTS." Despite her patient probing, the psychiatrist does not elicit any further information and elects to make a phone call to the family. In that conversation, she learns that the patient's boyfriend had broken off their relationship two days before. The family spokesman, the patient's brother, described the boyfriend as a very tolerant, unemotional sort—a "saint" in the family's consensus view—a man whom the patient herself had herself described as "the most perfect human being on earth" prior to their parting. In the two days following their breakup, she had first fallen into a rage at one of her fellow department store

---

1. John Kennedy Toole committed suicide at a young age before *A Confederacy of Dunces* was published, allegedly because he felt that no one valued his work.

employees, threatened that person and then destroyed store property, for which she was fired, and then continuously treated the family with anger and abusive language including throwing objects about the house and breaking two windows. They decided to bring her to the ER when they became fearful that she might inadvertently hurt the young children in the house.

Reviewing this vignette, we first find only a very rageful person who acts violently and for whom other human beings either appear perfect or, as now, completely worthless if not hurtful. But we can structure our understanding of the situation by referring to the clinical algorithm for recognizing adaptive mechanisms. The first task is to gain some understanding of the stress to the patient's psychological equilibrium that resulted in the rageful behavior. This takes some investigating, aided perhaps by the clue that emotional reactions of this violence very often involve relationships with other people. In this case, the boyfriend's departure triggered the course of events that resulted in the patient being extruded from her normal family setting and into the ER for psychiatric care.

Did the stress of the patient's breakup result in an increase in her anxiety, that is, in her sense of impending disaster? Listening to the word *murder*, one that she repeats with considerable emotional force, not only connotes the feeling of impending disaster but also denotes a sense of death. Viewed symbolically, it is easy on the surface to sense her murderous wishes toward someone else and perhaps much more difficult, in the face of an emotional torrent, to understand that she herself may be the victim of a murder, that is, symbolically the death of her relationship with her boyfriend and the horror of feeling unloved. Faced with this level of extreme anxiety resulting in uncontrolled behavior, the psychiatrist appropriately adopts a very calming, unemotional approach and uses soft restraints to provide the patient with the control that, for the time being, she cannot provide for herself.

Having identified the stress and her anxiety reaction to it, does the patient herself address either of these? She is unable to give the psychiatrist any but the most emotionally laden, nonspecific, clichéd responses by which she tries to put her emotions into words. The psychiatrist gains the needed information only through conversation with the patient's more rational family member. The patient herself uses her rage, much like Lear uses the storm, as a way of distracting herself from the anxiety. And, like Lear, she avoids having to deal directly with the situation or her emotions simply because she is unable to do so. Her adaptive mechanism is Distortion, which, as we have seen, is a form of Avoidance and a Primitive Domain psychological adaptive mechanism. By setting limits, the psychiatrist and ER staff provide a structured environment to stabilize the patient emotionally until she can move beyond the Primitive Domain mechanisms.

PRIMITIVE AVOIDANCE: NORMAL USE

In a volatile and emotionally laden clinical incident such as this one, it seems difficult to conceive of Primitive Avoidance as ever possibly having any function an adaptive mechanism, let alone a normal one. Although it is true that, in the above vignette, the patient's adaptive behavior is not pleasant or particularly constructive, it is important to remember that the adaptation she presents is the best of which is capable at time. And Primitive Avoidance/Distortion is not imported from Mars. As with Primitive Denial, Avoidance/Distortion appears most commonly as a normal adaptive mechanism among very young children. When the young mother, for example, asks her toddler, "Did you poop in your pants?" and the toddler runs to the other end of the house, we chuckle and see him avoiding the issue.

For most adults, use of a Primitive Domain adaptive mechanism involves a regression: a downward movement from less primitive, more mature adaptations previously reached through the normal progression that the recognition algorithm describes. Some very dysfunctional adults, however, use Primitive Domain mechanisms as their primary adaptive measures in adult life because, in those cases, appropriate psychological development requires very long periods of time to mature into more flexible adaptive maneuvers. In DSM models, for example, the terms *borderline* or *severe personality disorder* describe these clinical syndromes.[2]

But there is something of Ignatius J. Reilly's consternation in all of us. And this common experience, in turn, allows us to see even the Primitive Domain adaptive mechanisms as belonging to the human race. This is not to say that we shouldn't respond to Primitive Domain adaptive mechanisms with appropriate external structure when it is needed—the rageful patient requires restraint in the ER and the mother will need to change the toddler's diaper. Appropriate action, however, depends on the most accurate recognition we can bring to the observation of adaptive processes. Recognition accuracy in those who remind us most of ourselves often brings the most difficult challenges, as in the following case.

THE SLEEPY INTERN DISAPPEARS

We find our intern again at three in the morning bustling about the hospital in a sleep-deprived state. He is standing at the desk in the intensive care unit busily entering orders for his last admission: a man with a probable heart attack who was admitted a half-hour before. The phone rings a few feet away; the nurse on duty answers it and then calls to the intern to tell him that the senior ER resident wants to speak to him. The intern thanks the nurse, listens politely on the phone, and then, with more thanks, hangs up. He tells the nurse that the ER has another patient with chest pain and that they may send that person to the ICU if they feel it's needed. He finishes his orders and then leaves the hospital, turning off his pager and mobile phone. He takes himself to an all-night pancake house and buys breakfast. After eating, he falls asleep in his car for a few hours, wakes, and drives back to the hospital in time for seven o'clock rounds. He finds the nursing and medical personnel in an uproar, and he finds this puzzling. The chief resident takes him into his office and informs him that the second patient arrived at the intensive care ward a few minutes after the intern left and then suffered a cardiac arrest shortly after. A team from the

2. American Psychiatric Association (2000); see also World Health Organization (2012).

ER had to be called up to intensive care for this purpose, and one of their residents remained to take care of the patient as well as cover the others in the ICU. The intern stares blankly at the chief resident and says there was no actual second patient and that the ER resident had never said there was. The chief resident looks down at his notes and comments that the ER resident said, "I told him there is a patient down here that is coming to intensive care," and he asks the intern for an explanation. "Well," our intern tells the chief resident, "that depends on what your definition of 'is' is." The chief resident relieves him of his duties and refers him to a disciplinary evaluation in their department.

Applying the recognition algorithm, the second admission appears to tip the balance toward an intolerable stress level for our intern. Whether sleep deprivation is the cause for his subsequent behavior is not clear, but it is likely that it does not help the situation. He then avoids any sense of anxiety and proceeds to avoid the situation itself by physically leaving the location. He then returns as if nothing happened and, when called to account, provides a distorted explanation reminiscent of a public official caught in an embarrassing situation. Neither the stress nor the anxiety reach any relief or resolution because of his behavior. We conclude that he is in the Primitive adaptive Domain and that his behavior reflects the mechanism of Avoidance/Distortion, in this instance including some of both styles. And in response to these, the chief resident sets an appropriate limit. The vignette underscores the nature of Primitive Domain psychological adaptive mechanisms: common to all of them, the stress itself doesn't reach the level of conscious recognition. Like T. S. Eliot's mystery cat, Macavity, it simply isn't there.[3]

REFERENCES

American Psychiatric Association. (2000). *Diagnostic and Statistical Manual of Mental Disorders, Fourth Edition—Text Revision*. Washington, DC, American Psychiatric Press.

Eliot, T. S. (1982). *Old Possum's Book of Practical Cats*. New York, Harcourt, Brace.

Shakespeare, W. (1955). *King Lear*. In W. J. Craig (Ed.), *The Complete Works of Shakespeare*. New York, Oxford University Press.

Toole, J. K. (1980). *A Confederacy of Dunces*. Baton Rouge, LSU Press.

World Health Organization. (2012). *ICD9-CM* (9th ed.). Philadelphia, Saunders.

3. See Eliot (1982, p. 37).

CHAPTER 6

Psychotic Projection

King Lear is not done with us, nor are we with him. A few lines after those quoted in Chapter 5, Lear, Kent, and the King's Fool encounter Edgar who, like them, wanders about the heath in the thunderstorm. Edgar is the displaced son of another of Lear's vassals. He enters the scene disguised as a partially naked madman who wears only a blanket and calls himself Tom O' Bedlam, or "poor Tom." He speaks, as if to a hallucination:

> *Edgar*: Away! The foul fiend follows me!
> Through the sharp hawthorn blow the winds.
> Hum! go to thy cold bed and warm thee.

And Lear, who has not seen him before, responds:

> *Lear*: Didst thou give all to thy two daughters?
> And art thou come to this?...
> What! Have his daughters brought him to this pass?
> Couldst thou save nothing? Didst thou give them all?
> *Fool*: Nay, he reserved a blanket, else we had been all shamed.
> *Lear*: Now all the plagues that in the pendulous air
> Hang fated o'er men's faults light on thy daughters!
> *Kent*: He hath no daughters, sir.
> *Lear*: Death, traitor! Nothing could have subdu'd nature
> To such a lowness, but his unkind daughters.
> Is it the fashion that discarded fathers
> Should have thus little mercy on their flesh?
> Judicious punishment! 'twas this flesh begot
> Those pelican daughters.
>
> (Shakespeare, *King Lear*, III, 4, 44–73)

Note how, in this scene, Lear's reaction on meeting the madman is to ask whether the man's own daughters have created poor Tom's madness. When Kent tries to correct him by pointing out that poor Tom has no daughters, Lear misinterprets the correction by saying that he is glad the madman's daughters are dead and that they got what they deserved.

Viewed in the stepwise progression of the recognition algorithm, we first ask what perturbs Lear. The answer is the same as in Chapter 5: he has suffered the loss of his rank, power, and resources—all due to his own poor judgment of his daughters' characters; that is, from the impact of his own actions. The second question asks whether this generates an impending sense of disaster—the definition of anxiety—in Lear. Shakespeare leaves little doubt when he describes the storms both outside Lear and, metaphorically, inside him: in Lear's perception the thunderstorm outside on the heath is the far less painful of the two.

The algorithm then directs the observer to ask, as earlier in the scene, whether Lear recognizes the stress in a way that allows him to adapt to it. Where before he invoked Primitive Domain response of Avoidance, now he attributes his perceived "madness" to poor Tom and to poor Tom's battering at the hands of his imaginary daughters. Lear will not admit correction of his belief, what the present era would call reality testing. He will have no part in recognizing the reality of his own situation even when he sees his own attributes as belonging to another human being when they do not actually do so.

We conclude that we are once again in the Primitive Domain of adaptive mechanisms in respect to Lear. The stress and its madness are simply not recognized. In this case, however, Lear has taken on a different adaptive strategy within the Primitive Domain: he projects the stress and its pain outward, onto another human being in attributing his own predicament to poor Tom. Shakespeare's King Lear provides us with a clear example of Psychotic Projection. Recall once again that all of the adaptive strategies in this Domain have to do with *concrete* perceptions of the stress, the anxiety, and the adaptation, taken altogether. Lear does not speak symbolically when he ascribes poor Tom's madness to Tom's disloyal daughters; instead, he is speaking of them very concretely in his perception as actual daughters. When Kent challenges this rigid and invalid view, Lear has no room in which to consider an alternative perception. In Lear's view, poor Tom's daughters have driven him to this madness, and that's that.

WHAT PSYCHOSIS PROJECTS

In the Primitive Domain of psychological adaptive mechanisms wherein we have already considered Denial and Avoidance/Distortion, Psychotic Projection offers us something extra. Although all three have in common the strategy that stress and anxiety simply do not exist, psychotic projection is the only adaptive strategy of the three that casts something outward, outside the person so to speak. Shakespeare portrays Lear as casting his own dilemma with respect to his daughters outward and onto the person of poor Tom. The character ascribes to poor Tom his own anger, torment, and revengeful fury, perceiving them as Tom's own and caused by Tom's disloyal daughters. In establishing the recognition of the specific psychological adaptive mechanism, and indeed in understanding the specific person in more depth, clinicians and others do well to look for the content of the Projection itself. The projected material will contain two perceptible components: one a cognition and the other an emotion. Said slightly differently, the projected contents will contain an idea and a feeling, at least, and oftentimes complexities of both ideas and feelings. Simplifying Lear's case, the idea he projects onto poor Tom is the fact of Lear's own daughters' disloyalty, while the emotion is best described with words such as betrayal, fury, and ultimately a very deep sadness that has shaken Lear's own view of himself as a competent human being.

THE SOUTH SEA WARRIOR: PRIMITIVE PROJECTION VERSUS THE SELF DESTROYED

For another example in which to exercise both the recognition algorithm for adaptive mechanisms and an assessment of the content of projected material, let us consider the following vignette from a very different writer. At its surface, Joseph Conrad provides a romantically remote locale, the sea trading world off Southeast Asia in the late 19th century. In the following passage, taken from one of his short stories, Karain, a Malay warrior chieftain, recalls his youth when he and his "only friend" went on a mission to kill the friend's disgraced sister who has run away from their village with a Dutch trader. During the several years of hardship they encounter as they pursue their target, Karain himself begins seeing his friend's sister, first in his nighttime dreams and then in his daydreams. He talks with her vision affectionately and promises her image that he will not kill her. At last, the two pursuers find the sister and her husband; Karain waits in the foliage with a rifle as the brother steals up to his unwitting sister. Just as he raises his knife to kill his sister, Karain shoots his friend dead. He escapes by saying that he is simply a passerby. But the farther he gets from the scene, and the closer to his home village, the more he hears the voice of his dead friend. The voice torments him for a long time until an old man gives him a charm and the voice goes away. The old man remains as his bodyguard as Karain—free of his hallucination with the old man around—rises in stature to become the chief of the village. Many years later, when the old man dies, Karain once again leaves the village and swims to a ship anchored off his land. There he talks with three of the traders whom he knows. One of them narrates:

> The sound of my voice seemed to steady him into a sudden rigidity, but otherwise he took no notice. He seemed to listen, to expect something for a moment, then went on—
> "He cannot come here—therefore I sought you. You men with white faces who despise the invisible voices. He cannot abide your unbelief and your strength."
> He was silent for a while and then exclaimed softly—
> "Oh! the strength of unbelievers!"
> "There's no one here but you—and we three," said Hollis quietly. He reclined with his head supported on elbow and did not budge.
> "I know," said Karain. "He has never followed me here. Was not the wise man ever by my side? But since the old wise man, who knew of my trouble, has died I have heard the voice every night...."

> "Where is the danger?"
>
> "Everywhere outside this place," he answered mournfully. "In every place where I am. He waits for me on the paths, under the trees, in the place where I sleep—everywhere but here."
>
> (Conrad 1977, pp. 30–31)

To begin applying the algorithm, we first ask whether there is some perceived stress that Conrad puts in his character, Karain. The hallucinated voice of the friend he murdered pursues him to the point of Karain leaving his home and his position of great social dignity, in favor of what he perceives as a safe harbor, so to speak, on the trading ship. His behavior, as Conrad describes it, reflects the stress of what the character perceives as life-threatening danger. Its life-threatening quality, in Karain's perception, makes an excellent description of his anxiety, a sense of impending disaster in our Model. Both Karain's stress and his sense of disaster occur in the vignette.

Next the algorithm asks whether the character can identify the stress in such a way as to allow him to resolve it. In Conrad's description of his character, the answer is a clear *No*. The perturbation in consciousness from the hallucination's sense of threat has been checked for many years by the presence of the old wise man, and at his death, the specter is now unleashed. In Karain's perception, it is the avenging voice of the man he killed many years ago and the voice is the harbinger of Karain's destruction. Conrad's warrior does not recognize the hallucination as part of himself—any more than Lear did his delusion about poor Tom's daughters—but sees it as a real threat to him from his environment. Because of this, Karain's first response is to run from the danger to a place where he can successfully avoid it according to his own beliefs. That is on the ship with the Western traders who do not believe in hallucinations. In this respect, Conrad portrays an element of Primitive avoidance.

But he also gives us much more in his portrait of the Malay chieftain. His hero finds himself incapable of the murder that he and his friend set out to commit and in fact falls in love with the sister whom his friend and he have sworn to kill. He saves the life of the sister who has violated the cultural mores that he and his friend observe, and then does the exact same thing when he fires the rifle and ends his friend's life. Unlike the sister, however, Karain returns to a place deep within the cultural context whose highest rules he has violated. There, his hallucination finds relief only by the old man's presence, as something of a truce. Add to this the reaction of having shot the best friend from his youth, and we find in Conrad's character a man seized with his own guilt. When we ask, therefore, whether in reality his dead friend pursues him, either in his own person or as a symbol of Karain's violating their culture, the clear answer is that he does not—the friend is dead. Instead, the hallucinated voice that threatens and condemns Karain comes from Karain himself even though Conrad's character does not perceive that. The voice is always external and always goes where Karain goes, with the exception of the trading ship. According to our recognition algorithm, therefore, Conrad very clearly describes Karain as adapting through the Primitive mechanism of Psychotic Projection.

The projected material in this case is Karain's own guilt in the form of the friend's voice as an ever-continuing hallucination that follows him "in every place that I am." Can the voice of his friend kill him? In the direct sense, the answer is of course that it cannot. But in Conrad's story, we meet only one actual killer, and that is Karain. The true danger to Karain, we come to understand, is Karain's own violence. If he could kill his best friend, he could kill himself. His only adaptation, and a fragile one at that, requires him to project his lethality into the ever-tormenting voice. The story affords a strange irony: the adaptive mechanism in the form of the friend's threatening voice is Karain's last alternative mechanism in adapting to the guilt. By so doing, his friend's voice serves the purpose of keeping Karain alive. Although all this refers only to the fiction that Conrad sets before his readers, clinically the inflexibility of the Primitive Domain psychological adaptive mechanisms can occur in adult life as the last line of defense against potentially lethal emotional forces. The standoff can manifest itself in suicidal behavior, with special attention to those who, like Lear and Karain, see projected fury or guilt, respectively, as actual, outward threats coming from somewhere else, rather than the inward emotional states they truly are.

NORMAL PRIMITIVE DOMAIN PROJECTION

A delusional medieval British king and a hallucinating Malay chieftain: how can we ever consider such a very concrete form of projected anxiety as a normal human phenomenon? For the answer, we must look to some of the most creative, and also the most concretely thinking, of all human beings: toddlers. These small ones, of about age two or so, we can think of as being completely swept up in the brain and neural development processes that reach their completion in early adulthood, to the best of our present knowledge. At the toddler age, however, the dendritic connections among the nerve cells and populations of nerve cells, the myelinating processes that insulate the neural connections as they reach toward each other, and the intricate dances between the brain, the rest of the body, and the outside world all take place in a rapid, formative state of transition.

The casual outside observer may see a cute little kid running about the house, getting into mischief, and spending long periods of time in imaginative play wherein any object becomes a toy. But the toddler's mother knows better. Recall the situation mentioned previously in which she notes a pungent and unpleasant odor rising from the child that prompts her to ask the anxiety-laden question, "Did you poop in your pants?" Where in the previous example the child simply said *No* or tried to avoid the issue by running to the other end of the house, in this case his mother is completely taken off guard by a remarkable burst of youthful creativity. Pointing straight at his younger brother, an infant that his mother holds her arms, the toddler says with a prosecutorial air, "Jimmy did it!" The mother replies, "Jimmy pooped in his pants?" "No!" the two-year-old argues in rebuttal. "He pooped in *my* pants." His mother says, "Let's change yours anyway," and goes about the process with the budding conviction that her child is a creative genius.

Using the algorithm, the unwelcome excrement and the mother's inquiry, provides the stress and the anxiety, respectively, from the little one's point of view. This, however, has nothing to do with him and is clearly all his little brother's doing: that interloper who has upset a previously tranquil home with mother. Notice, for example, that the toddler didn't blame the whole occurrence on the family dog, a gentle and generally unobtrusive beast. It is far better to blame the little brother toward whom one harbors at least ambivalent, if not antagonistic, feelings. When we ask the question we asked of the Malay warrior—What is projected out?—one answer is a certain amount of rage at the prospect of one's little brother. Although this example may seem facetious, and is certainly intended in a lighthearted manner, projected rages of this kind are very common in childhood. Often they involve ascribing fearful concerns to inanimate or otherwise nonthreatening objects. Examples include frightening machines, such as vacuum cleaners or lawnmowers, animals, or imaginary characters such as robbers or statues. These serve as worthy depositories of painful emotions that will gradually be taken back in again and integrated usefully as the child and the personality develop. In this respect, they not only occur normally as phenomena, but they serve useful developmental functions in allowing the child to work through the difficult challenges that emotions bring.

One need only think about what the experience of childhood would be like if there were no relief from overwhelming emotions, nowhere to put them for a while before bringing them back in again. Little by little, in manageable doses, psychological development makes peace with them and goes on to use them as energy sources for the competent adult when dealing with the outside world or with oneself. In the absence of a temporary respite like Primitive Projection, the early childhood personality would be beleaguered 24 hours a day, seven days a week, every week by unceasing emotional upset, tossed about in the storms of an ever unsettled violent and rolling sea. In that context, Primitive Domain mechanisms including Primitive Projection serve as the young child's life preserver and source of emotional relief. And Vaillant has noted this as one model of adult sociopathy in which Primitive Domain mechanisms are adaptive even though, to the outside observer, the sociopathic person may appear to have no emotions whatsoever.[1] But let us leave our toddler to his play and consider Primitive Projection further, this time as an adaptive mechanism in a normally developed adult facing overwhelmingly anxiety.

STRESSED OUT: THE INTERN FROM MARS

Our overburdened intern is again hard at work trying his best to manage five very ill patients in the intensive care unit along with six others on the general medical ward. It is three o'clock in the morning, and he has had no sleep. An ER resident phones to say that there is another patient coming up to the ICU who is suffering from what appears to be advanced pneumonia, and will require careful monitoring and very likely a breathing tube followed by mechanically assisted ventilation. Very politely

1. Vaillant (1975).

and with no emotion whatsoever, the intern says, "Thank you," and hangs up the phone. The night nurse notices him stand up from the computer desk where he has been entering medical orders, take a stethoscope out of his pocket and insert the earpieces properly into his ears, and then walk across the room. Stopping at a nearby wall, he places the end of the stethoscope flat on it and begins glaring intently at the wall. When the nurse comes up behind him and says, "Doctor are you all right?" he glances at her sternly and then waves her aside with the words, "Hush. I have to hear all this. Please don't interrupt."

When, inevitably, she asks, "Hear what?" he states, "The latest instructions on the new admit, of course. This patient is in the throes of some artificially constructed virus that was originally produced from germ warfare and now threatens all of mankind. This is top secret, of course, and the only way to learn about it is to listen carefully at this spot. I've been given special security clearance to do so because my excellent record in medical school and my graduation at the top of my class. Germ warfare is very dangerous for everyone involved. I've got to get the directions exactly right or someone may die this evening. It's a great privilege to have been chosen to do this. And I don't mean to sound condescending when I tell you how important this is and that I must be left alone to do it. Please leave."

The wide-eyed nurse backs away slowly, picks up the phone, and alerts hospital security. Two uniformed officers come to the unit and gently lead the intern away. He expresses a certain amount of consternation, but they tell him that the transmissions for the day are over and won't resume until tomorrow evening. They take him to a seclusion room on the psychiatry unit, where he is committed and bedded down for the night with the door locked behind him. The next morning the psychiatry team diagnoses his delusional disorder as a psychosis and begins treatment. The chief medical resident visits his intern to let him know that all will be well and that his patients will be taken good care of without him. The intern eyes him suspiciously and says that he has diagnosed that the chief resident has himself been exposed to the virus. The chief resident thanks him for the information and departs.

The adaptive style recognition algorithm asks us to identify the stress in this situation. In this case, the admission of yet another very ill patient provides the straw that broke the camel's back. Frederick Nietzsche described early adulthood symbolically as that time of life in which we emulate the camel who asks his master to give him as much burden as possible—work to do.[2] It is a time of proving oneself, and, therefore, the greater the burden, the greater the proof. And although it is true that that stage of life is one of high-energy, hard work, and long endurance, one can get too much of a good thing. The intense experience of a good residency training program has stood the test of time as the best way to bring beginning doctors into a maturity of clinical wisdom and discretion. But one individual is never the same as the next, and some who take on a residency may not be particularly well-suited for it. As an example, the person who has grown up in the troubled home environment in which trusting relationships were inconsistent may find it difficult to trust

2. Nietzsche (2005, p. 25).

him/herself in high demand situations. When this occurs, the expectation of performance in a high-stress environment can be overwhelming.

According to the recognition algorithm, the stress manifests itself in an overwhelming anxiety that limits functioning. In this case there is clearly an anxiety present in the intern's mind, but in his perception it is not anxiety about his own performance. Rather, he is extremely anxious, worried, and perhaps somewhat fearful of the viral infestation that he believes he can understand by listening through his stethoscope clapped on the wall. He did not identify any anxiety in himself, nor does he identify the stress of yet another seriously ill patient coming to him for treatment and critical care. He is therefore functioning in the Primitive domain of ego adaptive mechanisms.

The fact that he locates a substitute object of his anxiety outside himself tells us that he is using a Psychotic Projection rather than Denial or Avoidance/Distortion. Akin to Lear, his situation has inundated him, and his best adaptive strategy involves distraction by the storm of unreal viruses rather than recognizing the pain of feeling inadequate and overwhelmed. His treatment team may postulate that the situation has in some way injured his own narcissism, his ability to think well of himself, and that this is intolerable. Thinking of it in the same way as the toddler who is afraid of the vacuum cleaner, our intern may, perhaps, locate this difficult pain outside himself before he can find a way to recognize it in incremental doses that may allow him to engage higher level adaptive mechanisms to integrate it and then grow beyond it. The same process can be seen in some of the most severe cases of posttraumatic stress disorder (PTSD), although overwhelming stress is by no means the only process that can result in the use of Primitive Domain adaptive strategies in adult life. At the same time, we assume from our intern's history that his biology is intact, which is to say that his brain is working properly and, in the absence of the overwhelming stress, would allow for higher level adaptive mechanisms. Although, let us say, this is true in his case, it may not always be so.

ADAPTATION IN DELIRIUM: A CLINICAL EXAMPLE

The police bring a man in his 50s into the hospital ER, where he is found to have an infection in one lower leg from a wound that looks to be several days old and not properly dressed. He is admitted to the medicine ward, where he receives an intravenous line and his medical team begins treatment with antibiotics to clear the infection. A few hours later the medical student on the team notices that he is pointing at the ceiling with the index finger of his right hand and making occasional whirring and buzzing noises. When the medical student asks what's wrong, the man stops the behavior completely and turns his face into a flat expression, closing his eyes as if in sleep. The medical student asks if he is all right, and the man nods but does not open his eyes. The student alerts his resident, who then calls for a psychiatric consultation.

A senior psychiatry resident arrives in the hospital room, where the man is still lying on his bed with a very blank expression and his eyes partially open in a squint through which he appears to be looking again at the ceiling. The psychiatrist notices the man's squinting behavior and his suspicious glances at the ceiling. Sensing a likely psychosis, the psychiatry resident states, "Perhaps it is not inconceivable that all may not be well with the ceiling."[3] The patient waits for a moment, and then opens his eyes wide and looks at the psychiatrist. He begins pointing again at the ceiling. As he does so, his eyes begin filling with tears. The psychiatry resident comments, "It would not be seen as unhelpful were you to put into words what appears to be so upsetting." The patient, in a barely audible whisper, says, "The spaceship. Up there." Over the course of the next few minutes, in an interview that takes careful account of gently creating an atmosphere in which the patient can tell of his concerns, the psychiatry resident learns that the patient is convinced that a spaceship from another galaxy hovers just above the hospital. It is a very large spaceship carrying a "death ray" that will allow it to incinerate the hospital and all the people in it within a matter of a few seconds. Further, the psychiatry resident learns that the patient's leg wound occurred from a fall in his backyard in which he cut his leg on a low metal fence in his garden. The patient says that the spaceship knocked him over with a "Taser ray" as a demonstration of what it would do were the patient not to cooperate. He divulges further that the spaceship has been following his every move for the previous eight months, since the death of his wife in an auto accident. The patient has become acutely aware that if he displeases the aliens who control the spaceship, a mass incineration will follow, beginning with the hospital. The spaceship is only one of a fleet of ships that can destroy "humanity as we know it."

At this point the psychiatry resident conducts a careful examination of the man's cognitive functions and finds that he has lost the ability to remember new words over a five-minute span, to add numbers with a carryover accurately, and to manage standard tasks that involve judgment and planning. Examining the man physically, he notes that the patient's eye movements, when looking to one side or the other, are abnormal and that his reflexes are abnormally brisk. The resident establishes a working diagnosis of delirium in this patient and alerts the medical team that this may be the first stage of incipient crisis relating to the man's infection. Approximately an hour later, the patient develops a high fever, fast pulse rate, and greater confusion in which he is now no longer sure of where he is or what day it is. The team transfers him to the ICU, where they treat him vigorously with intravenous fluids and more antibiotics, as well as very low dose medicines that the psychiatry resident suggests to clear the man's perception difficulties. The next day, his fever is down, he is awake and alert, and his thinking has cleared dramatically. He is no longer concerned about a spaceship hovering above the hospital.

Although in this case, the medical team's patient clearly suffers from a delusion about the spaceship, his case demonstrates one limit—and one strength—of the recognition algorithm. As to the limit, if we look for a stress in this case in regard to a specific perturbation of the conscious self, we will not find one. There is no doubt, however, that the patient is very anxious and frightened of enemy spaceships and immediate disaster. The difficulty in applying the algorithm in this case has to do with the definition of "the conscious self" that, to this point, we have assumed is in

3. This psychiatric resident has learned Sullivan's interpersonal style of interviewing from his teachers, a style particularly useful in conversation with very disturbed patients. See Sullivan (1970).

good order. In this case, however, it is not: the patient suffers from a physical impairment, namely his infection that has resulted in the loss of his normal ability to think properly. This includes his ability to sort his perceptions of what is real and what is not. As a result, he is frightened of the spaceships. Although it is true therefore, in the psychological adaptation model discussed in Chapter 2, that stress can perturb waking consciousness, that same conscious functioning of the self that we refer to as the ego depends on healthy brain functioning.

This points up a remarkable property of the recognition algorithm as a clinical tool. The recognition process when, as in this case, it identifies a Psychotic Projection in the clear absence of any identifiable psychological stress, immediately raises concern about the state of conscious functioning. This in turn triggers a differential diagnostic process with the target of establishing why the brain has lost its ability to function and how that can be returned. The list of illnesses and conditions that can cause a loss of normal brain function—and therefore an impairment in its conscious functions, whether perceived subjectively by oneself or objectively by others—is a long one. Because of this, the process of diagnosis and treatment requires careful, and yet aggressive, pursuit. From the point of view of our task in this volume, however, a shift to Primitive Domain adaptive mechanisms, especially in respect to Psychotic Projection, in an otherwise healthy functioning adult may make up one of the earliest, and most subtle, indications of an oncoming, or worsening, medical illness. We will visit this common clinical phenomenon again in Chapter 22.

Whether in response to the psychological stresses of Lear's misjudgment of his daughters or Karain's inability to tolerate the guilt within himself, whether in the neurodevelopmental staging of the two-year-old's concerns, the life-or-death stresses that pile up to crush the sleepy intern's conscious well-being, or the impaired brain that harbors delusional beliefs about spaceships, Psychotic Projection, and all of the Primitive Domain adaptive strategies, afford a final common pathway of basic psychological adaptation. Their presence early in life is a sign of normal consciousness and adaptation. Their evidence in adult life in settings when the Primitive Domain adaptive mechanisms constitute the best methods of adaptation at an individual's disposal at that moment, calls forth a wide consideration of possible causes and treatments. As subsequent chapters will elucidate, many more flexible adaptation styles make up the options humans have in maintaining their conscious sense of equilibrium. They always exist, however, against the background of the Primitive Domain styles.

REFERENCES

Conrad, J. (1977). Karain: A Memory. In *Tales of Unrest*. London, Penguin.

Nietzsche, F. (2005). *Thus Spoke Zarathustra*. New York: Barnes and Noble Classics.

Shakespeare, W. (1955). *King Lear*. In *The Complete Works of Shakespeare* (W. J. Craig, Ed.). New York, Oxford University Press.

Sullivan, H. S. (1970). *The Psychiatric Interview*. New York, Norton.

Vaillant, G. E. (1975). "Sociopathy as a human process. A viewpoint." *Arch Gen Psychiatry 32*(2): 178–183.

Primitive
Immature

CHAPTER 7

Acting Out

For most adults, to discuss the Immature Domain of adaptive mechanisms is to recall adolescence. For a small minority of adults, it may be a constant struggle to grasp one's own responsibility in working through the painful feelings and thoughts of everyday life. For others, driven down from higher Domain adaptive mechanisms by overwhelming or unrelenting stress, a return to the Immature Domain styles may signal both the beginning of psychological reconstruction and the likelihood of increased behavioral risk.

Occurring normally in the teens and early 20s, adolescence is both empirically and by definition a time of cognitive and emotional immaturity. For this reason, civilized legal systems limit the young person's ability to enter into binding contracts, or to make decisions on irreversible courses of medical care, without the consent of an adult guardian.

At the same time, adolescence itself is one of the most intensely creative periods of life and one that sets the flooring for the creative structures we build around the poetry of our individual experiences. Where before, during that period of childhood from about six through about 12 years, in which daily experiences appear linked to inevitable cause and effect, now all of life seems experimental. What we have learned from elders, parents, history books, churches, and even from Sir Isaac Newton now requires proof, as shown in the following example.

FAST FORWARD: ENERGY INTO ACTION IN NORMAL ACTING OUT

The sun shines on a spring day, warming the crest of a hill where stands a 15-year-old tenth-grader who has recently mastered the balance and thrust of the skateboard. His eyes follow the long downward slope of the sidewalk before him. He imagines the cooling breeze and the cool sense of accomplishment waiting on the flat ground at the bottom to which he can all but fly to the accompanying scream of the wheels on the concrete. He thinks to himself an emphatic *Yes!*

He kicks the board forward, standing on it at a right angle to its motion and aimed down the hill. He balances to and fro like a surfer who has just caught a wave to ride at a constant speed all the way to the beach. But there is no constant speed here. Gravity propels him, and the board accelerates as it goes downhill. The drop seems somehow steeper than it did only a few yards back. And the board hurtles down the hill faster and faster. A few yards ahead, a curve in the sidewalk bends to the left, away from the street and the hard, stubby curb that lines it. Automobiles come and go on the street to the right of the walk. The board aims squarely at them now, and if the board rider hits the curb he will fly into the street and into oncoming traffic. He digs the board hard to the left and crosses the pavement left into the grass of the park lawn. The board catches, and its rider tumbles forward, first landing on his belly, then his chest, and finally upon his elbows, his arms instinctively protecting his face from the ground. A bounce knocks the breath out of him as his momentum ceases. For a minute or two he crawls around on his hands and knees waiting for his breath to return, and then lies back looking at the sky with the crook of one elbow over his forehead. We can imagine that our intrepid skateboarder is now considering that perhaps there is something to be accounted for beyond imagination of moving like the wind.

To some, this vignette suggests that the magical thinking of childhood has yet to be replaced by the rational thought of adulthood. To others, the seeking after experience is a creative process that requires the leavening that only experience itself can provide. And to others still, that *Yes* forms the basis for the adventures of a lifetime. What, however, in the present context, does this vignette of misjudged momentum—the product of mass × velocity—have to do with psychological adaptation?

Referring again to our standard algorithm, is there any stress to be appreciated here? Of course, losing control of the skateboard in the face of oncoming traffic and at a high rate of speed provides its own threat. But that is not the focus of our discussion. Rather, what perturbs, or in this case entices, the conscious sense of the rider's self before the skateboard has started its motion? We may characterize that as the thrill of racing downhill with little effort on the rider's part—the thrill of something for nothing—the thrill of the experience itself.

Stresses, if we define them as such, can carry both positive and negative valences depending on the experience involved. The anxieties generated from *positive stresses* can themselves take on positive forms: they may be thrilling, or exciting, or enticing. And in that context they often entail the subjective sense of impending disaster along with the activities of both the sympathetic nervous system, which quickens the pulse and the breathing and elevates the blood pressure, and those of the glucocorticoid system, which shifts glucose stores into the bloodstream for availability in the muscles. This phenomenon not only characterizes riding a skateboard downhill but many other human experiences, including that of falling in love. Here, for example, is a modern translation of a stanza from a love poem written by Sappho around the sixth century BC in ancient Greece.

> I am in a cold sweat, and trembling
> Seizes me all over, and, pallid
> As range grass, I think I am almost
> On the point of death.
>
> (Cunningham 1997, p. 106)

If, as we apply the recognition algorithm to the board rider's vignette, the stress is the positive thrill of the downhill, effortless ride and it results in an exciting form of anxiety, what is the rider's reaction to it? More specifically, does he think through the circumstances of gravity, proximity to the road, and speed at the turn in the sidewalk? Or does he simply act? Purposefully in this portrayal, the rider jumps on the board with no consideration other than for the thrill of it.

In the present model of psychological adaptation, the movement from anxiety directly into action with no time for, or interest in, recognizing the anxiety as a signal to be sorted and thought through, defines the adaptive mechanism of Acting Out. That term has found its way into common speech and can carry a number of different meanings, both denotative and connotative. For our uses in the interest of recognizing specific adaptive behaviors, however, we define Acting Out as an immediate translation of anxiety directly into action aimed at dispelling the anxiety itself. The skateboard rider at the top of the hill wishes to live in the moment and experience the thrill of kicking the board into motion, not dwell on it before moving into it. He will race through the thrill that will disperse itself when the experience is over. The positive anxiety will have disappeared.

Why, one may reasonably ask, is this regarded as an Immature psychological adaptive mechanism? The answer lies in understanding that in Acting Out, the anxiety is to be gotten rid of. It is to be cast outward so as no longer to be troubling, either as a thrill or as a pain. When it is cast outward, it has "no more to do with me." In this way, the anxiety is "not me" in a subjective sense and therefore: "I no longer have to deal with it." Had this been Sappho's adaptive mechanism in response to the thrilling pain of falling in love, we would never have read her poem. She never would have written it. Rather, her experience would have dissipated quickly and we may never have heard of her. Fortunately for all involved, she adapted by using the Mature psychological adaptive mechanism discussed in detail in Chapter 20, and her poem comes down to us in a way that allows us to share her experience with our own.

THE MODEL AND THE IMMATURE ADAPTIVE MECHANISMS

Acting Out presents a first example of the Immature Domain adaptive mechanisms, and we will discuss the others in Chapters 8 through 11. At this point, however, it is important to understand the adaptive stance common to all of the mechanisms in the Immature Domain. Clinically, they provide the observer with different attributes than do the Primitive Domain adaptive mechanisms. Where in the Primitive Domain the person struggles to see any kind of problem or stress as in any way perturbing them, in the Immature Domain the stressful threat to psychological equilibrium presents itself clearly. Because of this, our algorithm has moved one rung up the hierarchical ladder from Primitive to Mature. Recognition of a problem, the barest sort of recognition in this case, provides a greater measure of flexibility in dealing with it than does denying its existence, avoiding it altogether, or ascribing it to Martians. The stress, at least to some degree, occurs. That is, it exists in the perception of the person who must find a way to adapt.

Although this is a step in the right adaptive direction, the Immature Domain mechanisms, by definition, all locate the perturbing problem where it cannot be addressed, namely, for someone else to solve. Any causes, and therefore remedies, lie outside, not inside, the person. "Yes, there is a problem," the person using an Immature Domain psychological adaptive mechanism tells us, "but it is not my problem." He or she simply does not see it as his or her responsibility in any immediate sense. Figure 7.1 presents this concept schematically. In the psychological adaptive mechanism model, the stress perturbs the conscious sense of oneself and this raises anxiety—the sense of impending doom of disaster. The Immature Domain adaptive strategy, however, does not recognize the stress as related to the person whom it perturbs. The person does not "own" it, so to speak, in subjective consciousness. The stress is "not me," as diagrammed.

For the person experiencing the threat to their psychological homeostatic stability that the stress provides, being able to accept their own role in adapting to the situation requires a giant step. He or she has to tolerate the anxiety that the threat engenders, and that anxiety is uncomfortable. In some instances, especially in the setting of stress with a negative valence, that anxiety not only threatens adaptive stability but can shake the foundations of the personality itself. Consider, for example, the following study in adaptation, recorded in *The Iliad of Homer* over 3000 years ago.

THE TROJAN MEN: ACTING OUT TO RELEASE ANXIETY

The setting is near the end of the tale: Achilles (or Achilleus in the translation below), the mightiest of the Greek warriors during the siege of Troy, has taken himself out

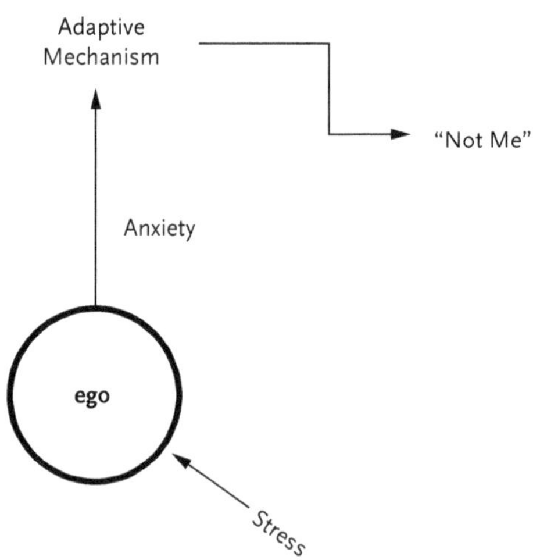

Figure 7.1
In this schematic version of the Immature Domain strategies, the person recognizes the existence of the stress. This raises anxiety and engages Immature Domain psychological adaptive mechanisms. Those mechanisms define the stress as outside the control of the conscious ego. That is, the stress is "not me."

of the game, as it were, in a fit of pique and benched himself on the sidelines of this very bloody contest. This has occurred for reasons that we mentioned in Chapter 1 and will discuss further in Chapter 8. As a result, the Trojans, led by King Priam's son Hektor, have staved off the Greek army's breaching the walls of their city: they have fought the Greeks to a draw on the bloody battle plains before Troy. Things have changed, however. Achilleus, fired by revenge for the death of his comrade, Patroklos, has once again taken the field. His return has caught the attention of the Trojan warriors, who know they must respond to it in some way. One of them, Poulydamas, makes an argument to which we will also refer in Chapter 17. But for now we will focus on the description of Hektor in relation to the algorithm for recognizing psychological adaptive mechanisms in those immediately before us.

In respect to the recognition algorithm's first question, the source of the stress to Hektor's conscious sense of himself, Homer tells us clearly as the Trojan warriors gather together:

> They stood on their feet in assembly, nor did any man have the patience
> to sit down, but the terror was on them all, seeing that Achilleus
> had appeared, after he had stayed so long from the difficult fighting.
>
> (Homer, *The Iliad*, lines 246–248)

They are not merely apprehensive; they are terrified. In Homer's description, they all suffer the one emotion that is the least consistent with the identity of the warrior. For all of us, terror remains the most emotionally intolerable of all the moods that human beings can experience. It is that against which we are most fiercely defended, a point commonly used in teaching residents and others to pay attention, rather than to ignore, their fearful feelings in a clinical situation: feeling terrified is often an indication that the situation itself is unsafe and is one in which we require assistance from others. Returning to Homer's portrayal of Hektor, we find a different reaction:

> Then looking darkly at him Hektor of the shining helm spoke:
> "Poulydamas, these things that you argue please me no longer
> when you tell us to go back again and be cooped up in our city....
> If it is true that brilliant Achilleus is risen beside their
> ships, then the worse for him if he tries it, since I for my part
> will not run from him out of the sorrowful battle, but rather
> stand fast, to see if he wins the great glory, or if I can win it.
> The war god is impartial. Before now he has killed the killer."
> So spoke Hektor, and the Trojans thundered to hear him;
>
> (Homer, *The Iliad*, lines 284–286, 305–310)

Homer makes it clear that tolerating the affect—the emotional content, in this case the terror—does not lie within the capabilities of the majority of the warriors who applaud Hektor's plan. Hektor and the others have a clear choice before them: withdraw into the city and devise a battle plan as Poulydamas suggests, or go out onto the battle plain now and face Achilleus impromptu. The first course requires that they tolerate the terror. In the second, they must act now to dispel it, and with it the threat to their warrior-ness no matter the cost. Homer gives us his judgment when he calls them:

> fools, since Pallas Athene had taken away the wits from them.
> They gave their applause to Hektor in his counsel of evil,
> but none to Poulydamas, who had spoken good sense before them.
>
> (Homer, *The Iliad*, lines 311–313)

Notice that Hektor ascribes any problem in the situation to Achilleus, not to himself or to the war god[1]—whom we can read symbolically as a projection of himself and whom he regards as neutral in a fair fight. He makes no calculation that Achilles may actually be the better warrior or that Hektor who himself has more often been the killer, may now himself be killed.

In this careful description, Homer gives us a very clear portrayal of Acting Out. The stress perturbs Hektor and most of the other Trojan warriors' conscious sense of themselves, creating an upsetting anxiety. They show themselves unable to tolerate this impending sense of disaster and must act to dispel the anxiety as quickly as possible. Characteristic of the Acting Out adaptive mechanism, no thought occurs between anxiety and action. In Acting Out, anxiety results immediately in action aimed not at resolving the stress, but at relieving the anxiety as instantaneously as possible. In concert with the Immature Domain adaptive strategies, the action is directed outward: once dispelled, it is no longer "my problem." Neither, however, is it available for working through to some better adaptive strategy. In the story, Hektor Acts Out his anxiety and suffers his death as a consequence.

In current clinical practice, especially where sociopathic patients are concerned, the term Acting Out often takes on many of the same negative connotations that sin does in Western theological models of human behavior. Thoughtless action can be destructive, turn other people away from us, and even result in social expulsion or imprisonment. Viewed clinically, however, it is important to put these aspects aside and to view it more as a phenomenon that can be recognized and treated in adults as a natural course in another phase of life. Like most human phenomena, Acting Out has to do with the personal history that has led to it.

As the product of a series of experiences that interact with an individual's genetic underpinnings, Acting Out—along with all of the other adaptive mechanisms, including those of the Immature Domain—requires the observer's understanding. The cardinal precept mentioned earlier will help balance the observations and ease negative connotations: at any given moment, people adapt to their inner and outer circumstances by using the *best* means available to them. We will visit this principle many times throughout this text because it informs recognition of adaptive styles,

---

1. Apollo, in Homer's story, sides with the Trojans; Hektor refers to him as the war god. Athena, goddess of wisdom and war, and for good measure the daughter of Zeus, the chief god, sides with the Greeks. In this setting, Daddy's girl trumps the march of the Sun across the sky every day.

as well as the aspects of differential diagnosis that they will call to mind in later chapters. For now, as an example, it allows us to explore one of the ways in which a functioning adult may have come to use an Immature Domain adaptive strategy. For this, let us consider the case of a more modern warrior.

COMBAT FATIGUE: ACTING OUT AND UNRELENTING STRESS

Major Edward C. "Mick" Mannock of the Royal Flying Corps flew bi-wing fighter against the Germans during the World War I. Although his number of "kills"—enemy planes shot down—remains unclear, he nonetheless was among the top, if not the top, fighter ace of the British pilots; his official number rests between 59 and 73, and his contemporaries regarded the higher number as an underestimate. The son of a corporal in the British Army, Mannock was born in County Cork, Ireland, where his father was stationed, and this gave him the nickname "Mick." He suffered an amoebic infection as a child that took part of his vision in his left eye; in our day, he would never have made it into pilot training. At the outbreak of World War I he was a civilian working in Turkey. He was imprisoned there and nearly starved to death when that nation allied with the German monarchy. A prisoner exchange repatriated him to England in bad physical condition, and, after recuperation, he joined the British Army and eventually the Flying Corps. He survived pilot training—by no means a small feat in those days. Despite his impaired eyesight, he had a talent for flying, as we will see again in Chapter 17, and was sent into combat in France in March 1917.

Early on, his thoughtful approach to combat flying—an entirely new form of warfare at the time—brought him the disrespect of his action-oriented colleagues, who regarded him as afraid to fly and to take on the German pilots. But his esteem steadily rose as the count of enemy aircraft downed both individually and through his innovative fighter tactics shifted the air fight to Britain's favor. In February 1918, as a veteran combat pilot and a decorated ace, then Captain Mannock took command of the newly formed 74 Squadron. Known for his supervision and training of the green pilots under his command, he brought the squadron into combat in France that March. In June 1918, he was promoted to major and sent home on leave. He wept openly on his departure.

While on leave, he was noted to have a visible tremor that would come over him along with profound tearfulness and salivation, both thought due to his "fatigue," a phenomenon we now think of as a form of posttraumatic stress disorder (PTSD). He was sensitive to the horrors of the Great War and once described himself in his diary as "a murderer" after seeing the corpse of a German he had shot down. On July 3, he returned to France to command 85 Squadron; he was, at age 31, one of the oldest combat pilots in the Royal Flying Corps. Over the previous year, he had seen a number of his friends and companions killed, beginning with Albert Ball in May 1917, and continuing through the McCudden brothers in July 1918.

In his last month, Major Mannock began behaving erratically, taking chances he would not allow others to take and would not have taken himself a few months earlier. He began flying low and raking the enemy crash sites with machine gun bullets to kill the already downed fliers. This brought him within range of ground fire on July 26, 1918, after he and his wingman had followed a German aircraft to the ground. He pulled up into enemy gunfire and his wingman saw that the plane's rudder stopped moving (Mannock 1966, p. 200). His aircraft caught flame and crashed.

A lapse in judgment, especially a dangerous one in an effectively functioning adult, calls up a question of adaptive failure. The prior question asks, what psychological adaptive mechanism did Major Mannock utilize during the last few weeks of his life? To answer this, let us apply the algorithm for recognizing psychological adaptive mechanisms. First, what was the stress involved? In this case, reason suggests more than a single stress. There appear to be a series of them in an unrelenting progression day after day, week after week, month after month. One stress was the continuing carnage of the World War I, to which Major Mannock was an eyewitness. In the diary he kept during his early months on the Western Front, he describes the horrors of the mass casualties and the trench warfare. We can add to this the continuing procession of the dead pilots that he knew as friends and students during his 15 months of aerial combat.

The recognition algorithm next asks whether the stress was sufficient to raise Squadron Commander Mannock's anxiety. It clearly was: like many pilots of the era he developed a continuing fear of being burned to death in his aircraft and carried a pistol with him as a means of killing himself rather than suffer the burns he had seen in other pilots. In his last months he spoke to his colleagues about his sense that he would not live through the end of the war. His anxiety, like the stresses that caused it, was ongoing: he regularly suffered nightmares along with tremors and physical nausea before a mission. In this context, we ask whether or not he perceived his anxiety as a problem. The answer here too is affirmative, especially in its physical manifestations. We reasonably conclude, therefore, that we have passed beyond the realm of the Primitive Domain adaptive mechanisms because those strategies do not admit the existence of the problem to begin with.

Did Major Mannock hold himself responsible for machine-gunning defenseless aircrews whose planes had crashed to the ground? There is little or no indication that he thought in this way in the last months of his second combat tour. His comrades recall their leader in his last months saying that it was not enough to destroy enemy airplanes: they had to kill the enemy pilots. But to do this, he chose a way that took his own person and aircraft needlessly into the path of danger, rather than away from it as would have been consistent with his rules for combat pilots. In behavior that was uncharacteristic of a leader who thought carefully and developed and taught rules for effective combat, in this instance he exemplifies an unexpected use of an Immature Domain psychological adaptive mechanism. In doing this, like Hektor of the shining helm, he utilizes the adaptive mechanism of Acting Out—moving directly into action in order to dispel all or part of the anxiety that reaches intolerable levels.

In Homer's example, Hektor responds with direct action rather than thought because, as Homer implies, his own narcissism cannot stand the assault of the anxiety itself. This is not the case with Major Mannock, who, by all accounts, was a man who, unconcerned with personal narcissism, happily gave away credit for downed enemy aircraft to other members of his squadron. Rather, he appears to have been turning a heavy load of intolerable anxiety into action. As we will see in further examples of his observable behavior in Chapters 17 and 18, Mick Mannock at his best consistently employed Mature Domain psychological adaptive mechanisms.

In the Great War, the clinical entity we currently diagnose as posttraumatic stress disorder was known as shell shock, and no one thought it applied to pilots. Characterized in a syndromal model by hyperawareness and an increased arousal to action in the setting of a perceived threat, PTSD itself can facilitate Acting Out. In this context, Edward Mannock's history further informs the present task of recognizing psychological adaptive mechanisms when considering one of the causes for the behavioral shift to Immature Domain mechanisms from those of the highest Domain. Not only an overwhelming acute stress, but also the increasing weight of an additive stress delivered continuously over a period of time can result in Acting Out as an attempt simply to get rid of the anxiety. This regressive process, as discussed below, can include all the Immature Domain mechanisms. It can reach all the way down to include the Primitive Domain adaptive strategies as well. There were no flight surgeons in Major Mannock's day. Had there been, he might have been taken off flight duty well before he descended into the ground fire that killed him.

THE INJUSTICE OF THE JUSTICE SYSTEM: ACTING OUT AND ACUTE STRESS

As in previous chapters, and those subsequent, we once again ask when Acting Out—moving from anxiety to action with no intervening thought—plays a normal role in psychological adaptation. Is Acting Out ever a normal adaptive style, and, if so, when and to what purpose? The reader knows that we already have a partial answer in the vignette that began this chapter: the 15-year-old on the skateboard. There, the stress involved was a positive one, full of excitement and adventure, if not particularly well thought out. Consider the following example of a very different valence.

A few months after passing a driver's education course and acquiring a license to drive a car independently, a young person's parents summon a family conference among the siblings. The subject of the conversation is a serious one. The parents quietly, but with a sense of concern for their children's feelings, inform them that one of the parents has received a diagnosis of a particular form of cancer and will begin treatment for that condition. They have discussed the problem with a cancer specialist: the prognosis is good, but the treatment will take several months and will involve changes in physical appearance. Normal appearance will return when the treatment finishes.

The young person listened quietly, and with an intent look, nodded periodically through the conversation and taking it all in. Not asking any questions on the topic, at the end of the discussion the youngster sums up his relevant feelings and thoughts very sincerely: "I have every faith in medical science to take care of this." The conversation concludes, and each of the family members goes about his or her business. But the parents feel uneasy. The conversation went too well, too rationally. In the old joke, there is a sense of waiting for the other shoe to drop, in this case the emotional shoe.

At work the next day, one of the parents receives a phone call from the obviously aggravated driver of the family car. The youngster begins railing about the local police who have just given out a ticket for speeding in a zone near school. "There's no justice in the world at all," the young person says with considerable force and energy. "They said I was speeding! I wasn't speeding! Or if I was it was maybe one or two miles per hour over the limit. I know how fast I was going, and I wasn't going fast enough for a ticket!"

The parent listens politely, asks whether there is any kind of an accident, and receives reassurance that none occurred. The parent asks about the youngster's whereabouts, and the latter replies, "At home," the destination at the time of the speeding ticket. The parent says to remain there and that the two of them will talk further later in the day. On the parent's arrival home, the young person sits quietly reading a school textbook. The youngster looks up, greets the parent and says in a calm tone of voice, "Isn't it too bad that some people would have to get cancer while nothing happens to this really awful person at school that I can't stand?"

To follow the recognition algorithm, we first identify the stress that perturbs the conscious sense of this adolescent's equilibrium. In this case, it is obviously the occurrence of a deadly disease in a parent.

The second step requires the observer to identify whether or not this adolescent recognizes the source of the anxiety. Listening politely and then making a comment about complete faith in medical science as being capable of taking care of the situation indicates this. The observer can also hear a sense of powerlessness in the son's words: trusting in medical science rather than being able to take care of the ill parent. This, like Hektor's powerlessness before Achilles' wrathful return to battle, challenges a sense of personal autonomy in the adolescent, one that still requires formation into an adult form. Powerlessness presses home anxiety as few other subjective perceptions can.

The youngster's first reaction—trusting in medical science—provides a partial answer to the third question, a key one in establishing the presence of any of the Immature Domain adaptive mechanisms. Does the anxiety—in this case, a sense of disaster at the prospect of losing a parent to a terrifying illness—belong to the adolescent? For a time, it remains at arm's length in the capable hands of medical science. But the next day action appears to be the only course when driving over the speed limit and meriting the attention of the police. Viewed in the clinical model psychological adaptive responses, the anxiety dissipates through defying the speed limit and then phoning to describe how unjust the police have been. By the time the parent returns home, the Acting Out adaptive mechanism has done its work and anxiety seems to have been capped, at least to some degree. The adolescent now meditates quietly on how unjust the world is, shifting from the police to the matter closer at home. Although the anxiety has not been resolved—and will not be until either the resolution of the illness or the acquisition of a Mature Domain mechanism—it has been put away for the time being. Acting Out is one of the standard adaptive mechanisms available to adolescents as they move from childhood into adulthood.

Fortunately, in this case, Acting Out did not result in any harm due to an accident or injury. This is certainly not always the case when adolescents take on risky behavior to dissipate their anxiety in response to some perceived stress. Nonetheless, adolescence itself is a necessary time of growth that must include the Immature Domain adaptive mechanisms for healthy, fully functioning, adult adaptation to occur subsequently.[2] If Acting Out becomes a usual adaptive mechanism in adult life, however, problems may follow, as in the next vignette involving a familiar figure.

THE SLEEPY INTERN AS PUGILIST

As so often happens to our long-suffering medicine intern in the course of this discussion, we once again find our protagonist in the wee hours of the morning with no sleep, a full load of seriously ill patients on the ward and a full load of critically ill patients in intensive care. A series of never-ending phone messages and pager alarms distract him from the continuity needed to attend for a sufficient length of time on one or another of the patients who depend on him. He has to hop from crisis to crisis through a very difficult night. This intern much prefers to move carefully and methodically, collecting evidence, sorting all of it at turns, and finally arriving at the specific decisions and treatment options in each carefully evaluated case. The situation of acute crises, all seeming to fall together about his shoulders, simultaneously wears away at his normal calm, efficiency, and control. He becomes increasingly aware of having to make decisions "by the seat of his pants," like a man vainly trying to stop several leaks in the roof of a house during a severe rainstorm. He manages to keep the house dry, but only just. One more leak and the floor will fill with water.

As happens to intern colleagues in most of the other chapters in this book, an urgent phone message arrives from the chief resident in the ER informing him that a new and very seriously ill patient will be arriving shortly for admission to the ICU. "Just who does he think I am?" the intern yells in consternation, to the startled dismay of the charge nurse on the ward. "Some kind of superhero?" The intern stands and rushes down the hall toward the stairwell. He runs down six flights of stairs,

---

2. In *Adaptation to Life*, Vaillant presents longitudinal, prospectively gathered evidence that when home circumstances did not allow a normal adolescent to use Immature Domain adolescent adaptive mechanisms during their teens and early twenties, the same mechanisms then occurred during their adult years. Immature Domain mechanisms at that stage then correlated with poor adult functioning in relationships, work, and play. By contrast, normal adolescents whose context supported the use of the tumultuous Immature Domain mechanisms at the age-appropriate time grew through them into the normal adult mechanisms and fared far better in measures of adult functioning. This observed contrast creates the strong impression that adolescent mechanisms cannot be skipped or bypassed: they must be worked through. Common circumstances that do not allow movement into the adolescent Immature Domain mechanism during teens and twenties include living with an alcoholic, drug-addicted, or otherwise unavailable parent. Conversely, available parents who tolerate their adolescent's tumultuous behavior through the teen years deserve congratulations and may find a sense of relief in the prospective data. See Vaillant (1998, Figures 3 and 4, pp. 333–334).

taking them two at a time. Reaching the lobby, he dashes past the vending machines, smashing a fist into one as though to move it out of the way. He bursts through the waiting room door of the emergency ward, wakes an elderly man who was sleeping in one of the chairs, and shoves a forearm into the door to the ER itself. At a very brisk pace, he rushes up to the chief resident, who leans against a counter, turned away from the intern, and taps him on the shoulder. As the chief turns, the intern delivers a hard right cross to the lower jaw. The chief resident drops to the floor in a daze while the security guards grab the shouting intern and restrain him with handcuffs. The intern is relieved of duty from that point forward and advised to seek mental health assistance and perhaps career counseling. The chief resident recovers and decides not to press charges.

Following practice with the recognition algorithm in respect to Immature Domain psychological adaptive mechanisms, the observer can identify the threat to our intern's mental and emotional homeostasis: it is the persistent, intense, and frequent demands of the environment. These lay waste to the intern's own inner sense of control. Here again, an intolerable anxiety makes itself known as it pierces, inside out, through the covering armor of deliberate, evenly paced behavior. As the armor breaks down, there is nothing to relieve the sense of disaster.

To locate the intern's reactions in the Primitive Domain of adaptive styles, the observer asks whether he perceives a problem. Unlike the strategy among the Primitive Domain mechanisms, this intern locates the problem in his own environment. That is, he acknowledges its existence. Following the stepwise inquiry, therefore, the observer asks whether the intern recognizes that the anxiety has to do with him. His response to the chief resident's phone message about the incipient admission answers this with a resounding *No*. In the intern's view, the problem is clearly not his own approach to the problems of a busy, acute medical service but the expectations placed on him by others, specifically by the chief resident.

To the intern, the problem is not inside himself—in his perception, he behaves in a reasoned and appropriate way in an unreasonable world. The problem is external, and he must strike it. From his point of view, this is the only way to dissipate the anxiety that, as intolerable as the thought is, he cannot keep up, that he cannot do a perfect job for each patient. But that his violent response results in injury and costs him his position—and possibly his profession—does not require thought in the moment between experiencing the horrible anxiety and moving directly into action. In the adaptation model, the intern's behavior suggests that the threat to homeostasis is a very deep one indeed and one that he can feel only with direct, impulsive action that dissipates anxiety. As with Hektor of the shining helm and the other examples in this chapter, the stress itself provides a very cogent threat to personal integrity. Although a number of other causes can result in Acting Out and the other Immature Domain adaptive mechanisms, the sense of powerlessness offers a useful formulation in considering this mechanism of psychological adaptation that we have defined as moving directly from anxiety into action.

As diagrammed in Figure 7.1, the common strategy of all of the Immature mechanisms locates the stress outside the self, as when the intern strikes the chief resident. That is, it locates the problem that raises the anxiety—and the responsibility for its resolution—outside the conscious person. Although on the surface this seems an easy strategy with which to blame external circumstances for internal inabilities, it may be better clinically to consider that the Immature Domain adaptive strategy has put the stress in a place where it cannot be addressed, namely as "not my problem." Schematically in Figure 7.1, an arrow points from the stress to "Not Me," that is, away from the conscious sense of oneself. As the reader may conclude from this diagram and the examples in this chapter, this adaptive stance is essentially static. It does not allow movement toward a resolution of the stress itself. In Acting Out, the adaptive mechanism points only to a temporary dissipation of the anxiety rather than to a solution. Adaptation at this level, therefore, addresses only the anxiety, not its cause. And Acting Out is only the first of the Immature Domain adaptive styles that utilizes the trick of acknowledging the stress to the individual person but locating it where it can't be dealt with.

REFERENCES

Cunningham, J. V. (1997). *The Poems of J. V. Cunningham*. Athens, Ohio, Swallow Press/Ohio University Press.

Homer. (1951). *The Iliad of Homer* (R. Lattimore, Trans.). Chicago, University of Chicago.

Mannock, M. E. (1966). *The Personal Diary of Major Edward Mannock*. London, Neville Spearman.

Vaillant, G. E. (1998). *Adaptation to Life*. Cambridge, Harvard University Press.

Primitive
Immature

CHAPTER 8
Passive Aggression

If anxiety can be transformed into action with a stroke like lightning, humans also have the ability to transmute it into the opposite: passive inaction. For an everyday example, one need only drive on a busy U.S. street or highway behind a slow-moving vehicle. Whether or not the driver of that vehicle actually intends to express his anger passively, suggesting both his or her social importance and little heed to others on the road, it is easy enough for the following drivers to regard it as Passive Aggression as they become more and more irritated at the slow moving driver impeding the road ahead. There appears to be some cultural overlay in this example with the idea in America of getting ahead—like F. Scott Fitzgerald's Jay Gatsby who "believed in the green light" (Fitzgerald 1925, p. 179), as compared to driving in Ireland, where the narrow lanes put a higher priority on cooperation rather than competition. But is passive behavior a psychological adaptive mechanism? If so, empirically speaking, we expect it to fit the working model of psychological adaptive styles.

As a beginning example, let us look again at the subject of *The Iliad of Homer*, namely the anger of Achilles. In Chapter 1 we learned the story of Agamemnon's public snub of his best warrior in denying him the spoils of war that Achilles believes he has justly earned. We learned, too, that this upset Achilles and, as Homer informs us, the Greek army (the Achaians) will suffer bloody conflicts and many men will die because of Achilles' anger. But how does this actually occur? We return to Homer's text and begin with Achilles'—referred to as Peleus' son in this passage—statement of his anger toward Agamemnon—here named Atreides, or son of Atreus—and then move to Achilles' curse on the Greek cause in their siege of Troy.

> But Peleus' son once again in words of derision
> spoke to Atreides, and did not yet let go of his anger:
> "You wine sack, with a dog's eyes and a deer's heart....
> And this shall be a great oath before you:
> some day longing for Achilleus will come to the sons of the Achaians,
> all of them. Then stricken at heart though you be, you will be able

> to do nothing, when in their numbers before man-slaughtering Hektor
> they drop and die. And then you will eat out the heart within you
> in sorrow, that you did no honour to the best of the Achaians."
>
> (Homer, *The Iliad*, Book 1, lines 223–225, 239–244)

Using the algorithm for recognizing psychological adaptive mechanisms, we focus on Achilles and first ask, what is the nature of the stress that has upset his conscious sense of well-being and resulted in his strong-voiced anger? This of course is his public humiliation—and the insult to his self-esteem—that he has suffered at the hands of his leader. Next we ask, does this perturbation raise his anxiety—that is, does it create in him a sense of impending disaster? Again the answer is *Yes*, although this will best be seen in his reaction to the anxiety as we explore it further.

In describing his response to the Primitive Domain of adaptive mechanisms, we want to know whether Achilles ignores the anxiety and stress that caused it. Judging from his angry invective at Agamemnon, nothing could be further from his mind. He certainly does not deny having been humiliated before the other warriors, project it onto the gods as their doing, or avoid the issue altogether. In the fashion of the ancient Greeks, he tells his feelings directly to Agamemnon and the company of the other warriors in assembly at the time. He is not functioning in a Primitive Domain adaptive manner.

Further ask, does he locate the responsibility for adapting to the anxiety, recalling this as a sense of doom or disaster caused by the social insult, within himself or send it outward as the responsibility of others? Recalling the subject of Chapter 7, for example, he does not instantly draw his sword and have done with Agamemnon by killing him, though this is well within his physical power to do so. Homer comments on this when he says that Achilles "did not yet let go of his anger" but somehow keeps it in. Although he does not release anxiety through Acting Out, neither does he move forward to resolve it.

Instead, he utters a curse in which he says that all of the Greek warriors, including Agamemnon, will one day regret this injustice done to him, this affront to his pre-eminence as the best Greek warrior. Those who did not rise up against Agamemnon's injustice will die in large numbers: theirs, not his, is the sense of impending disaster. He has projected the anxiety onto his comrades rather than work toward a resolution within himself. He tells them that they will die because he will leave the battlefield and he will not return to it until Agamemnon's injustice has been reversed. As the story unfolds, the anger of all the others, and even the cunning persuasions of Ulysses, leave him completely unmoved. He knows that the Trojan warriors will have the advantage once he has left the field, and he says so. He underscores his view with the passively angry statement that they will all eat their hearts out from sorrow at the tragedy that will befall them. And this, according to the story, plays itself out as Achilles goes to his tent, sulks there, and refuses to return to the battlefield until the end of Homer's narrative poem.

Like the driver impeding traffic, according to our adaptive mechanism model, Achilles has made his anger everyone else's problem by behaving in such a way that everyone else feels it, suffers because of it, and returns the anger to Achilles himself.[1] In this process, he locates the responsibility for his own anxiety outside of himself and in the lap of the others of his warrior group. In doing so, he fulfills the algorithmic criteria of the Immature Domain adaptive mechanisms: he locates the problem outside of his sphere of responsibility to do anything about it. Achilles' anger is someone else's problem from his point of view.

This particular adaptive strategy uses passive expression of anger or aggression in such a way that others not only perceive it but direct it back at the person him/herself. That is the definition of Passive Aggression. From the person's own point of view, everyone else's anger is just too bad and it is their problem, "not mine." His or her own anxiety has lessened internally, and the problem belongs to everyone else.

In the story, the passively angry Achilles sulks in his tent until the death of his friend Patroklos, much later in the narrative poem, results in his return to the battlefield when the fury of revenge for his friend's killing outweighs his personal irritation. Until then, as we have seen in Chapter 7, the Trojan warriors have the advantage on the battlefield and, on his return, fall victim to their own Immature Domain adaptive mechanism, rather than exercise their option for a more effective adaptive behavior, as we shall see in Chapter 17.

PASSIVE AGGRESSION IN DYSFUNCTIONAL FAMILY LIFE

For now, let us leave the mythic realms of the Greek siege of ancient Troy to consider Passive Aggression in a more domestic, and more modern, context. Consider the following "micro" story, "November," by Ursula Hegi:

> When my daughter finds me standing in the swimming pool, water up to my ribs in November, the beige of my wool dress darkened with moisture, she'll cancel her wedding. Even when she was a girl, she could be stubborn, but I always knew how to stop her. Sometimes just words—*you're making my heart ache*—and holding onto my chest. Once, when she wanted to buy that foolish motorbike, I pushed the bread knife into her hand—*you might as well slash my throat*. Now she insists on marrying. She's barely 31, and I told her there is no rush, even broke my crystal glasses and stepped on them with my bare feet. But she only walked away and locked herself in her room at the end of the hall.
>
> Arms raised straight out from my side, I stand in the icy water, my palms inches above the cloudy surface. My legs and feet feel numb, swollen, as though they belong to someone else, but my belly is warm. I wake to the sound of my daughter's car, the slapping of her tires against the pavement, the reassuring latch of her car

1. In another model, some might say that Achilles exemplifies—even symbolizes—the emphasis on the individual that characterizes the mythology of ancient Greece. In that context, he appears as a metaphor for individual conscience and even civil disobedience against the unjust actions of his social group. Although this is interesting to explore, Homer's description of his emotional state entices exploration of Achilles in our adaptive model. Great fun either way.

door. She'll come running toward the pool and cry out my name, kneel down and offer both hands to me.... But it is quiet. Only the sky comes closer, the hazy dome tilting across the edges of the pool.

(Hegi 1996, pp. 90–91)

Calling to mind the recognition algorithm, we first identify the stress that impinges on the consciousness of woman who narrates while standing fully dressed in a swimming pool on a cold November day. We learn in the first paragraph that her daughter is about to leave in order to marry and that this may have something to do with the mother standing in the pool. From the mother's point of view, her daughter behaves unrealistically: she is only 31, and it is still early for marriage. The reader infers that the situation looks different from the daughter's point of view for at least one reason: the end of her childbearing years may not be far over the horizon. But this telling detail does not seem to have come to rest in the mother's consciousness, suggesting that the mother sees things only from her own point of view.

Next, what does the mother do about the anxiety from the thought of having to live alone, without the support of her daughter? As in Achilles' case, anxiety resulting from the perturbation of the mother's conscious equilibrium, too, seems to have been turned outward. But unlike Achilles' immediate furious reaction, in this instance it has taken on a pattern, having occurred at least three times before—when she feigned a heart attack, requested that her daughter stab her, and walked on broken glass—and now she is freezing in a swimming pool in November. Each of these responses happened not coincidentally, but in response to the narrator's need to "stop" her daughter in one or another action. One can nearly feel the relief of the mother's own anxiety each time she has blocked her daughter's movement away from her—at least until the present moment.

Referring to the recognition algorithm, the narrator clearly acknowledges her daughter's impending departure and makes no attempt to ignore it as might be expected were she using one of the Primitive Domain adaptive mechanisms. Consistent with an Immature Domain adaptive style, the mother sends her anxiety about the situation outward, waiting for her daughter's anxiety to drive her to come rescue her mother from the pool. She locates the solution to both the stress and its intolerable anxiety outside herself, the prime characteristic of the Immature Domain adaptive strategies.

When asked to identify what emotion she may be aiming toward her daughter, we find our first clue in the feelings that the story generates in us as we read it. Something makes us very angry at the mother as she waits for her daughter to kneel—suggesting subservience—and pull her out of the pool. Finding it hard to summon a sense of compassion for this mother—another characteristic of the Immature Domain adaptive mechanisms—most readers very likely identify with the daughter who has not arrived and, as the second paragraph suggests, is not likely to. Putting ourselves in the daughter's position puts us in the realm of the mother's passive anger, and that will only escalate, as it has done in the course of the four instances the author gives us. This mother tries to control her offspring with behavior that relies on generating anger on the daughter's part. The narrator behaves by putting herself passively at risk—real or imagined—and always blaming the daughter for having done so. Sending one's anger out in this way such that it comes back from others tells us that the adaptive mechanism at work here too is Passive Aggression.[2]

A characteristic of this adaptive mechanism, one shared with all of the others in the Immature Domain of psychological adaptation styles, rests in its effect in driving people away, as the missing daughter in this case illustrates. When the person sends anxiety and anger outward for others to experience, others perceive this as an unnecessary irritant. When the Immature Domain adaptive mechanisms locate the problem where it can't be solved, outside the conscious sense of oneself, as illustrated in Figure 7.1, others are expected to solve it. Of course, they cannot do so any more than they can live someone's life for them and often resent the implication that they are responsible for someone else's problem. As a result, the members of the social network around a person who regularly uses an Immature Domain mechanism tire of the continuing irritation and either give up on the person or extrude the person into a social institution—such as a psychiatric clinic—for professional help. The person using the Immature Domain mechanism rarely seeks help on his or her own because the Immature Domain adaptation mechanism holds the anxiety at bay. The person, him- or herself, perceives no pressing difficulty so long as anxiety lives elsewhere. The professional psychotherapist in this setting, therefore, must constantly return the anxiety to the person's own conscious perception in the interest of beginning to move to a higher, more effective psychological adaptive mechanism through which the person gains an ability to resolve problems rather than simply cast them outward.

With the knowledge that Immature Domain psychological adaptive mechanisms irritate, rather than act as social lubricants, what possible use can they serve as they characteristically push others away? Stated differently, is Passive Aggression ever normal? Consider the following imaginary snapshot from another adolescent.

OH, *THOSE* CHORES: PASSIVE AGGRESSION AS NORMAL ADAPTATION

Beginning at age seven, and weekly thereafter on successive Thursday nights for the next six years, the oldest child of the family has taken out the garbage. Dutifully, he has wheeled the large plastic cart full the family's refuse down the driveway of their suburban home and left it at the curb for the garbage truck to empty and leave the container behind the next day. When he began this duty, the physical task itself challenged his ability to navigate with the large cart. Truth told, he needed some help for the first few months and got that from his father, who was touched with

---

2. Pondering this in another context and another time resulted in the author's following epigram:

> Here lies *Passive*, the least of earth's harried,
> By his good friends aggressively buried.

the boy's sense of responsibility and his work at the task of growing up. There were times when his father, lying awake in those few minutes before drifting off to sleep at night, recalled visions of the boy managing his trek to the curb in the trailing light of sunset, and he himself filled with parental pride.

So it came as a surprise on the day after the boy's 13th birthday when the father looked out the front window of their home in the early evening and did not see the garbage container resting on the curb as it normally should on a Thursday. Relying on his son's sense of pride of responsibility, however, he said nothing and went about his own projects in their house. An hour later, however, glancing again toward the curb and finding the same lack of placement, he goes to find his son, who is in his room text messaging his friends. The father mentions casually that is Thursday night and time for the garbage to be taken out. Looking at his father with a sense of vague mystification, the son says, "No problem, Dad, I'll get to it in a little while." Knowing his son's careful attention to detail, the response satisfies the father, who returns to what he was doing.

Another hour goes by, it is early dark now, and the father still does not see the garbage can or its shadow in the light of the street lamp, where it should be. He goes again to his son's room, to find that he is still talking with his friends, and this time, with a firm but gentle voice, gives an order: "Take out the garbage in a little while." His son responds in much the same way, as though hearing the news about Thursday and the garbage cart for the first time. And his father, mostly confident in his son's ability to shoulder his commitments, goes about his business.

Still another hour deepens the evening, and still the garbage container has not reached the curb. The father now walks briskly to his son's room and tells him, "Go take the garbage out. It's late."

"Sure," his son says. "I'll get right to it in just a minute."

"That's what you said before."

"I never said that before. I only just said it now. Besides," he adds, "why can't somebody else do it?"

"Because it's your job around here. That's why," the father adds in a stern tone of voice. Believing he has made his point, the father goes about his business once again, this time getting ready for bed.

After nearly another hour, however, the garbage still not taken out, the father stomps to his son's room, throws the door open and tells his son, "Take the garbage out, NOW," with an explosion on the word *now*.

The son looks at his old man as though he had just flown in from Jupiter and didn't really understand the rules of Earth and says, "I'm going. I said I would and I am. I'm going. What is the matter with you?"

The father looks at him and yells, "Now MARCH!"

The son gets up, looks at him with a derisive sneer and says, "All right, all right. I'm going. You don't have to yell. That doesn't help at all."

With the garbage cart in its resting place, and the son sleeping quietly in his bed, the father now tosses and turns, wondering what came over him, what the matter is with his son, and why he can't seem to fall asleep.

Although it is easy to see the father's increasing upset through the course of the evening in this vignette, his irritation is only a response to that of his son's. The recognition algorithm, therefore, asks what stress besets the son's conscious sense of equilibrium. In this case, it is the continuing work of the transition from the dependent childhood to independent adult functioning, which is to say, the process of adolescence. A shift in importance has occurred from being the dutiful son to the requirements of active communication with one's peer group. The peer group conversation is an exciting one that will help the son move forward, while the weekly duty of taking out the garbage is a well mastered item of the past. From the adolescent's point of view, everyone else, especially adults, should understand this change. And, when pressed, no one ever does, which most adolescents find irritating. Anxiety of beginning to find one's own way serves as the generator of the son's adaptive mechanism that the passage illustrates.

Recalling the algorithm, does the son in this vignette ignore the stresses of adolescent growth? Rather than denying or avoiding their existence—and remaining forever in childhood—the son in this case appears to luxuriate in the oncoming change, so much so that when others ask him to cease participating in this context, as for example in his father's unreasonable request to take the garbage out on time, and he refuses to do so in the interest of his own priorities, others become remarkably angry. The son himself is, of course, not angry at all at his father's implied insistence that he continued his childhood duties and never grow up. But by a strange coincidence, he makes his father angry when he refuses to go along with his old man's formulation.

This exemplifies normal Passive Aggression and its service in the transition from adolescence to adulthood. In one view, in order to walk on their own, youngsters in the adolescent transition years must gradually push away the supports that have sustained them during their childhood. As the vignette suggests, this requires adjustment for both the adolescent, who begins using Immature Domain psychological mechanisms in the service of adapting to independent life, and the parents, who find the placid waters of school-age children changing into the turbulence of fast flowing psychological development. Fortunately for all concerned, in the vast majority of cases, the Immature Domain adaptive mechanisms, with their projection of anxiety outside the conscious sense of the adolescent's self, remain time-limited. The functioning adult gives up the Immature Domain mechanisms in favor of those that locate day-to-day problems within his or her sphere of control and toward resolution as discussed in subsequent chapters. As this occurs, adolescence becomes a colorful, and perhaps creative, memory.

In some cases, however, especially those in which the normal "turmoil" of adolescent development may be thwarted or unavailable, Immature Domain mechanisms of adaptation become much more difficult to work through or to give up. In this regard, they may remain as the primary adaptive mechanisms in adult life for some period of time. When this occurs, the person may not reach appropriate adult levels on the measures of normal healthy psychological functioning. One such common measure, if not always applied systematically, includes work performance, as in the following description of our ongoing character.

INTERN COUCHANT

Once again midnight is three hours past, and the sunrise is several hours away. The sleepy intern finds himself on duty during a busy night in the hospital. Three of the eight patients on the general medical ward have been getting worse and may be edging toward the ICU, while four others admitted in crisis have stabilized earlier in the day. All are under the intern's care, and he feels that he has kept up with them, although they clearly will prevent him from getting any sleep and he does not find any of their ailments particularly interesting. At this juncture, he receives a call from the chief resident in the ER saying that they have another very acutely ill patient who needs to be admitted to the ICU and will be moved up shortly. The intern says that he appreciates the phone call and asks whether they can stabilize the patient in the ER for an hour because matters upstairs are inordinately busy. The chief resident agrees.

The intern goes down the hall to the on-call room lies down to take a nap for an hour. He is awakened 90 minutes later. The chief resident is on the phone asking if he is ready to accept the critically ill person. The intern begs off, saying that the ICU is even busier than it was before and a few patients on the medicine ward are going sour. Could the chief resident possibly wait another hour and a half? The chief resident reluctantly agrees.

The process repeats itself another time, two hours later, with the intern once again begging off. Finally, just before daybreak, the chief resident comes upstairs and finds the intern fast asleep in the on-call room. He learns from the nursing staff that the intern was nowhere to be found all night. The chief resident shakes the intern vigorously, wakes him, and tells him to get to work. Rather than express his anger any further, the chief advises the training director of the intern's behavior. The latter person notes that the intern has behaved in this way before and that it is now time for him to leave the program. The intern receives his termination notice later that day.

Applying the recognition algorithm, the stress once again lies in the added work burden in the middle of the night. Its effect is to raise anxiety in the intern, who must meet the challenge. In this case, however, our intern relates to the work itself in a passively angry manner, finding it neither interesting nor worthy of robbing him of his needed sleep. His adaptive response, nonetheless, does not include denying the existence of the challenge or distorting it as not being real. His response is not that of a Primitive Domain adaptive mechanism.

By contrast, however, the intern views the new admission, like the rest of his patients, as uninteresting and beneath him. It is a situation that is simply not worth losing sleep over. Having to be in this position at all raises his dissatisfaction—the perturbation of his conscious sense of himself. As this rises, so does his anxiety and anger. But his behavior does not address his own dissatisfaction in his career choice, a much larger issue requiring an active examination and thought. Rather, his behavior aims at assuring his sleep and having as few as possible responsibilities in his job. From his perspective, there are more than enough people around to take care of his patients: let the patients be their problem for a while. In this respect, passively assigning his responsibilities to others without their knowledge or acceptance describes an Immature Domain mechanism in his adaptation to what he perceives as a situation that fills him with intolerable anger but that, in the adaptive model, the intern can express only passively.

Feeling devalued and put upon in his own situation, he behaves in a passive way, delaying the admission of the new patient through the course of the night and ignoring his communications with the nursing staff in respect to those already in hospital. The intern employs Passive Aggression as his primary adaptive mechanism—sending his anger outward through his behavior in such a way that it comes back at him. The chief resident, who begins by taking the intern at his word with respect to the busyness of the service, later becomes furious and feels taken advantage of when he finds out the intern's true behavior. Like the daughter in the story of the woman in the swimming pool, he has had enough. Rather than act on the anger he feels, the chief resident appropriately reports the intern's behavior to the training director. Like the chief resident, the intern's social context, in this case the training program, too, has had enough. It extrudes the intern from its midst, not with a sense of anger but in a cold judgment of the intern's inadequacy in shouldering the responsibility for the health and well-being of very ill people.

PASSIVE AGGRESSION AND THE BRAIN: A CLINICAL DIFFERENTIAL

The examples of Passive Aggression so far have implied that this Immature Domain adaptive strategy emanates from psychological sources that best fit with models of the mind—based in experience and development—rather than those of the brain and its chemistry. For adults like Achilles, the mother in the pool, and the passively furious intern, that model best fits, although future enlightenment from neurobehavioral research may well expand our knowledge in this regard. Clinically, however, as with all of the Immature and Primitive Domain adaptive mechanisms, Passive Aggressive behavior may also call forth a model of brain dysfunction. This occurs in the differential diagnosis of proximate causes and their treatment, especially when the behavior has not been a previously characteristic style of the person using it. Consider this example from the high-risk setting of solid organ transplant surgery.

Five days after a 48-year-old male received a liver transplant, the surgical team called in a psychiatrist consultant to see him. His native organ had failed because of autoimmune hepatitis, a rare condition in which his body produced immune antibodies against his own liver as though it were an infection from outside. After receiving the consultation request through the electronic record system, the psychiatrist contacted the resident on duty for the transplant service in order to focus the surgical team's question optimally. During the conversation the psychiatrist sensed that the resident was himself very angry at the patient, referring to him as a "slugabed that everyone here knows is obstinate, uncooperative, and just plain lazy." Asked who "everyone" was, the resident listed the surgical team, the nursing staff on the postoperative transplant unit, and "everyone else" who has come in contact with the patient. He made special mention of the respiratory therapist, who voiced her concern over the patient's lack of cooperation in keeping his lungs healthy with deep breathing exercises designed to prevent postoperative pneumonia. The team had heard similar concerns from the physical therapist, who stated that the patient would not cooperate with exercises aimed both at preventing possible blood clotting conditions and regaining the physical stamina needed to walk and to carry out the normal activities of daily living. When the psychiatrist asked whether the surgical team had let the patient know that a psychiatrist would be stopping by, the resident replied affirmatively adding, "See what you can do for him, but honestly I don't think you're going to get very far. This is the way he treats everybody."

The psychiatrist first reviewed the patient's medical record, including the very assiduously detailed pretransplant evaluation in which a series of clinical observers described the man as pleasant, engaging, and cooperative. He never had any difficulty in adhering to the medical regimens that his internists prescribed in their efforts to prolong the life of his native liver. There were no reports of frank confusion or other mental symptoms from his liver failure, although his wife of 25 years noticed that at times he had difficulty remembering recent conversations and occasionally mislaid objects about the house. He had worked successfully as a manager in a construction firm and was welcome to return to that job when his health permitted. He and his wife had raised two grown children, who were both doing well and living in distant cities. Other than autoimmune hepatitis, he had no other illnesses requiring treatment. A careful assessment of drug and alcohol use history was negative and corroborated by the patient's wife.

At interview, the psychiatrist introduced himself to this middle-aged-appearing male with some graying hair but with normal ruddy skin tone and no yellowing of his eyes that might suggest either excessive blood loss or liver failure, respectively. The patient was awake and alert, and could focus his attention on the conversation. He gave clear and appropriate answers as to why he was in the hospital and what his doctors were doing for him; he stated that he was feeling well following the operation. Asked why he was having a hard time with the breathing exercises and with the physical therapy needed to regain his stamina, however, he looked at the psychiatrist with a puzzled expression and said, "I try to do everything that people tell me to do. I haven't noticed any trouble with exercises." As he said these words, however, they sounded flat and emotionless, with little energy behind them. The psychiatrist too noticed his own transference reaction itself as including a sense of puzzlement, reflecting the patient's own apparently befuddled state of mind. Contrary to expectation, the patient gave no indication of either passive or active anger that the psychiatrist could notice.

At this point the doctor conducted a careful assessment of the man's thinking capacities and found that he often had to redirect the patient to the tasks at hand when his motivation for participating in the interview appeared to wane from time to time. In addition to difficulty sustaining his motivation, the examination also brought out impairments in judgment and in planning, all evidence that pointed to a slowing or impairment of the thinking processes mediated by the frontal lobe of the brain. In addition to these, he had difficulties with memory tasks and adding numbers of increasing complexity, functions that involved the temporal and parietal lobes of the brain, respectively. On physical examination, the patient had a mild tremor of the tongue on protrusion. His knee reflexes appeared abnormally brisk and crossed to the opposite side with both legs jumping when psychiatrist tapped his reflex hammer on only one side.

The psychiatrist diagnosed the man as suffering from a very subtle form of delirium—a syndrome characterized by an impairment of the thinking—or cognitive—processes of the brain, as well as other parts of the nervous system. Delirium may result from myriad underlying medical conditions and requires a careful consideration of the causes that can be treated. In this case, the psychiatrist recognized that it most likely resulted as a side reaction to the anti-immune medicines needed to preserve this patient's new liver from a rejection reaction by his own body. The anti-immune medicine used in this case crosses into the brain and engages with its own set of chemical receptors there. Because the medicine was lifesaving to the patient and his new liver, the psychiatrist advised targeting the delirium symptoms themselves and continuing the necessary anti-immune coverage. He recommended adding a very small dose of a dopamine-blocking agent aimed at restoring the patient's higher order thinking capacities that were now in disarray. The liver transplant team did so and found that the next day their slugabed patient appeared chipper, attentive to all of his instructions, and was now working well with his postoperative recovery program. The psychiatrist advised stopping the dopamine blocker after three days and the patient did not suffer a return of his thinking difficulties.

As discussed throughout this volume and highlighted again in Chapter 22, observed change from the higher adaptive Domain mechanisms, especially from observed Mature Domain mechanisms, to the lower, less flexibly adaptive Domains brings the necessity of considering differential diagnoses. The detective work of the differential diagnosis systematically labors to establish underlying causes for the behavioral changes, when possible, and to direct treatment. As seen in Major Mannock's case in Chapter 7, prolonged, inescapable stress can drive psychological adaptation down to lower Domains, and we shall see in Chapter 22 that overwhelming acute stress can do so as well. Neither obtains in this case, however. If anything, the liver transplant recipient appears remarkably stress free, in large part because his anti-immune medicine has impaired his motivation and judgment, leaving him to appear indifferent to his own care and unable to understand the concerns of others. Because of this, the liver transplant team members find themselves angry at this uncooperative patient, leading to a behavioral interpretation of his being Passive Aggressive. In this instance, however, his altered brain chemistry serves as the culprit. As the dopamine-blocking agent puts this back in order, the patient returns to his previous adaptive level, as well as to normal cognitive functioning.

Specific treatment in this case required neurochemical intervention aimed at the delirium. Specific treatment of the Immature Domain adaptive mechanisms, when these occur as characteristic behavior patterns in adult life, often requires behavioral treatment alone or sometimes combined with medicinal treatment, rather than neurochemical treatment alone. Combination treatments may be needed in cases in which adaptive Domain regression occurs in response to the degree or chronicity of stress, as when treating some forms of posttraumatic stress disorder (PTSD). Behavioral treatment may constitute the treatment of choice in cases that do not involve profound or prolonged stress and in which the diagnosis of brain disorder remains negative. In this setting, treatment should target the lack of development *beyond* the Immature Domain adaptive mechanisms in the first place, the province of Character or Personality Disorders in the model of the statistical manuals. Individually in such cases, the hard work of continuing psychological development and the human energies that push it forward may flower best in the setting of psychotherapy, as in the next example.

PASSIVE AGGRESSION: TREATING THE IMMATURE ADAPTIVE MECHANISMS

A well-educated, intelligent man in his late 20s arrives for a first visit at the office of an experienced and well-respected psychoanalyst known in her professional community for successfully treating character and personality disordered patients. At the appointed hour, she invites the young man to sit opposite her desk while she goes over his responses on an information form. She learns that the new patient is a graduate student in the government school of the internationally prestigious university located in their northeastern college town. When she compliments him on his accomplishment in gaining admission, he replies, "I look very good on paper." The psychoanalyst notices a sense of lassitude, of sluggishness that suggests her own need for increased energy in maintaining her attention in listen to this patient. A passive quality about him puts her off, suggesting that this may have the same effect on others. He dresses conservatively and carries a subtle look of contempt in his facial expression that the analyst notices as well. His face is otherwise blank, and he appears to go out of his way to avoid eye contact.

Asked why he has come to the office today, the new patient states in even tones that he himself has no particular interest in talking with the analyst. He has come to the appointment because his wife has said that he must get help or she will leave him; they have been married for three years. He has not had any contact with mental health professionals before and has no belief that they do any good. Nonetheless, he takes a written list out of his pocket and hands it to the analyst with the explanation that his wife has jotted down the things he does that irritate her. They spend most of the hour talking about the items on the list and about his wife. At the end, the analyst advises him that in her opinion, he should return for a weekly session each of the next six weeks so that he can learn for himself whether the sessions are useful and judge whether he makes any progress. With mild disdain, he asks, "Why should I?" and looks out the window.

"You can stop the sessions today," she responds, "and your wife will leave you. Or, you can try them out and see if they help. The choice is yours. What would you like to do?" As she says this, he makes eye contact with a flash of anger and looks away again. He waits in silence and then says, "I'll see what I can do."

"I am putting you down in the appointment book for this same hour next week," she adds. "I require 24 hours notice if you find you can't make the appointment. Otherwise, I'll charge you the full price whether you arrive or not." His eyes flash again in a very angry look, but only momentarily. He nods to her, grumbles something inaudible and leaves the session. She perceives two reactions in herself as he leaves: first, a sense of relief at his departure, and second, the feeling that she would like to roll him up into a ball and throw him 50 yards down the sidewalk with a splatter against the side of an office building. She makes note of both of these as transference reactions involving the anger that originates in the patient himself. They inform her work for the next six sessions: she must find ways of articulating this patient's anger to him in a way that will allow him to begin to regard that emotion as his own. Her task is to introduce the doubt that everyone else in his world is at fault for of all the angry discomfort he feels.

When, in the course of adolescence, Immature Domain adaptive mechanisms do not wane but remain in use as adulthood unfolds, observers may regard them as part of the character of an individual. In this respect, they are often referred to as Character styles and, in models that note only phenomenology, result in symptomatic attributes that allow diagnosis of the Character or Personality Disorders. For example, Passive Aggression, in our current model, resembles the Passive Dependent Personality Disorder in the context of diagnostic and statistical manual editions (World Health Organization 2012; American Psychiatric Association 2000). Although particularly challenging in the context of psychotherapy, adult life instances of Immature Domain adaptive mechanism use call forth an approach of steady, continuous work in recognizing the anxiety source as having at least some part that is within the patient's control. Psychotherapy of this nature employs an alliance with a professionally trained outside observer who can comment on the consequences of behavior with the aim of expanding the sphere of the patient's own control over his or her behavior. Although this approach is often difficult, requires a great deal of patience, and may sometimes be amenable to group therapy efforts, it lies within the nature of human psychological adaptation to move forward to more flexible, more creative adaptive mechanisms.

This psychotherapy case illustrates the nature of that kind of psychotherapy. Of first note, and true of the Immature Domain adaptive mechanisms as a class, the patient arrives at the therapist's office not because he necessarily perceives anything to be wrong but because his social network, in this case his wife, has extruded him there. Part of the work will include his beginning to apprehend his own reasons for paying attention to his behavior along with the pain of his own anger that others reflect back to him. Recalling the recognition algorithm, he perceives that there is a problem somewhere in his life, and he does not ignore it, as would be characteristic of the Primitive Domain adaptive mechanisms. But, in his view, his wife perceives it rather than he; therefore it must be her problem. He has no particular investment in considering otherwise, having located it outside himself, in the style of the Immature Domain mechanisms.

The other person in his network, the professionally trained therapist, however, immediately senses both the off-putting way he has in dealing with others, and the anger that occasionally flashes from beneath it. Both occur as transference reactions—her capacity, developed over many hours of professional training and practice, to tune in to his emotional state. First, she notes his keeping his difficulties at arm's length for others to deal with rather than engaging with his problems himself. And second, she senses the profound anger that he lives with and finds painful. Because he locates his anger outside of himself, it remains unavailable to him as an energy source for change. The therapist notes directly in her reaction to this patient, first, how hard it is to want to pay attention to his passivity, and second, his anger in the office that he likely evokes everywhere else. If all the others in his social network react to him personally—rather than professionally—in the same manner, he leads a very lonely and unsatisfying life indeed. But she notes her reactions to him—rather than acting on them in the style of Chapter 7—and looks for a way to use them constructively in the therapy. Her goal is to help him see his anger and its ramifications as his own.

The patient still finds the idea of change painful and gives only a passively negative answer about returning for a second session. The therapist responds by outlining his choices: he can go no further in therapy and his wife will leave him, or he can return and see whether the process is useful. He manages a brief facial expression of anger and returns to a Passive Aggressive stance of I'll-Think-About-It. In a businesslike, matter-of-fact style, she puts his name in the appointment calendar and tells him that he can break it only with 24-hour notice. In so doing, she has not reacted to him with overt anger, which is to say she has not cooperated in his Passive Aggressive adaptive strategy in which he perceives his anger as belonging to others. At the same time, she has made it clear that the patient, not the therapist, will be making the active decisions in his life. If he chooses to do so, he will be working toward an active, rather than a passive, psychological adaptive strategy in respect to his own, barely tolerable, anger.

In his late 20s, rather than his mid- to late teens, the patient, viewed in the adaptive model of this volume, continues his work on moving out of the Immature Domain Passive Aggression mechanism and into the adaptive styles that characterize adulthood. In clinical experience, this kind of psychotherapy may often be slow going from his point of view, with hard-won steps toward more flexible psychological adaptive mechanisms. His therapist will recognize this and tailor her expectations to the patient's ability to achieve them: the first, in this case, being whether to show up at the next session. The therapy itself will remain a continuing process of staying out of emotionally charged confrontations and constantly articulating the choices before the patient, and then asking which among them he chooses. This kind of work is often difficult, whether in individual sessions or in groups, and not all therapists will find that it matches their interests or talents. Its promise lies in the continuing psychological energy—to use that term in lieu of a better one—that is inadequately explained in the present day: the energy that humans have not only to adapt to their inner and outer circumstances psychologically, but to pursue *better* adaptive strategies through the course of life. Even in the setting of Immature Domain adaptive mechanisms in adult life, the human organism/self can move forward. The promise of therapy lies in its ability to speed the process such that our patient in his late 20s can gain an adaptive maturity that might be unavailable to him until his late 40s or beyond. In the present model, systematic clinical recognition and serial assessment of psychological adaptive mechanisms may assist empirical demonstration of expedited change through psychotherapy relative to the Immature Domain mechanisms.

REFERENCES

American Psychiatric Association. (2000). *Diagnostic and Statistical Manual of Mental Disorders* (4th ed., Text Rev.). Washington, DC, American Psychiatric Press.

Fitzgerald, F. S. (1925). *The Great Gatsby*. New York, Scribner.

Hegi, U. (1996). "November." In *Micro Fiction: An Anthology of Fifty Really Short Stories* (J. Stern, Ed.). New York, Norton.

Homer. (1951). *The Iliad of Homer* (R. Lattimore, Trans.). Chicago, University of Chicago.

World Health Organization. (2012). *ICD-CM* (9th ed.). Philadelphia, Saunders.

CHAPTER 9
Hypochondriasis

The ability of human beings to convert stressful situations into physical symptoms has enjoyed a long and distinguished history in the annals of modern medicine. Among the European neurologists of the 19th century, when medical science began to develop an increasingly precise view of the neuroanatomic connections between the brain and other parts of the body, the work of Jean-Martin Charcot focused on muscular paralysis. He wanted to know why in some people muscular paralysis followed the anatomical patterns of nerve damage, while in others, paralysis appeared to occur in the absence of any damage and in patterns that did not reflect the neuroanatomic structure of the body. This led him to the remarkable discovery that while under hypnosis, the latter group exhibited normal muscular functioning that returned to a state of paralysis when they woke. Sigmund Freud, a young and ambitious neurologist of the era, studied this condition—then called "hysterical paralysis"—with Charcot, and from this work developed his clinical observations on the unconscious. Jung, who worked with very psychotic patients as a resident under Eugen Bleuler in Switzerland, followed this with his empirical observations on how the brain keeps track of its perceptions. And Anna Freud, as we have seen, added the idea of psychological homeostasis, expanding on her father's idea of the ego defending itself. It is only recently, however, that unexplained physical symptoms as evidence of a specific psychological adaptive mechanism has come into the clinician's consciousness.

Unexplained, or "hysterical," paralysis is relatively infrequent in our era but still occurs, as seen in the next case example. However, less dramatic varieties of aches, pains, complaints, and chronic unrelieved symptoms occur every day, especially in the practices of primary care doctors. Some physicians regard such patients as frustrating: they never seem to get better, and the physician's own sense of feeling responsible for a "cure" thereby takes a beating.

Others, who can begin to view hypochondriacal symptoms as playing a role in adapting to human life as the patient experiences it, find themselves feeling much less responsible for providing an immediate resolution to them. This perspective frees them to ally with patients in the professional relationship for the purpose of keeping track of the symptoms and perhaps introducing the possibility that they may in some way be related to the stresses the patient may be experiencing. As Charcot—and others since—have shown, the symptoms often resolve on their own because there truly is no neurological or other physical damage involved. In many cases, however, this may require a long view, because many of the symptoms may persist for significant periods of time, as well as change in their character, location, or frequency. The physician's primary objectives in that case include (1) ruling out any of the known pathological conditions that require medical or surgical treatments, (2) avoiding practices such as long-term opiate or sedative use that may do harm, and (3) continuing the professional relationship with the patient even though clinic visits may be relatively infrequent.

THE JILTING MAN: PHYSICAL SYMPTOMS AS ADAPTATION TO SOCIAL STRESS

To illustrate the above statements in application of the model of psychological adaptive mechanisms, let us consider the case of a man in his 30s who is brought to a hospital by ambulance after having collapsed in the factory where he assembles parts for electronic recording units. Sitting on a stool at the assembly line, his coworkers noticed him slip off and fall the approximately 2½ feet to the concrete floor. Landing on his tailbone, the patient told those around him that he had no feeling in either of his legs. When they tried to assist him to stand, he found that he had no control of his legs and could not move them to stand up. The neurological examination at the hospital found that his sensory responses were intact and that his leg muscles had normal tone even though he could not use them. There was no flaccidity on either side that would characterize a stroke or some other untoward neurological event. In the hospital he underwent a computed tomography scan of the brain. That too showed no changes in the brain structure that might indicate a pathological cause for his symptoms. The next day, a psychiatrist was called to see him for the purpose of assessing whether he was fabricating his symptoms, a common referral question in such cases.

At interview, the patient appeared calm, attentive to the conversation, and somewhat unconcerned about not being able to move his legs. He nonetheless made a point of saying that his paralysis was "not all in my head" and that he truly was unable to use the muscles in his legs. The psychiatrist said that he was glad to hear that the neurologist had ruled out all of the terrible causes for symptoms of this nature and that people generally get better even though sometimes that might take a while. When the psychiatrist offered that it would be helpful for him to know exactly what had occurred, the patient agreed to go over the incident. In the process, the patient described himself as growing up as a middle child in a large family. He had learned to fend for himself while his parents devoted time to the crises of his older and younger siblings. As a result, he considered himself an independent person who functioned well on his own and rarely had to ask others for help. He could not recall any particular stress in his life other than the pleasant fact that he was to be married in three days. He felt badly now, however, because both families would have to call off the wedding until he felt better. "When I leave that church, I want to walk down the aisle under my own power," he said. The patient was discharged from the hospital the next day with the assistance of a wheelchair, and his wedding was postponed. About five months later, his intended bride announced that she had found someone else. He noticed the beginning of a return of the use of his legs and found a full recovery about one month after that.

To apply the recognition algorithm for psychological adaptive mechanisms, we first ask what the stress might be that leads to the anxiety that requires an adaptive mechanism. On the surface, it may appear that the unexplained paralysis itself is a stress, but the patient's own reaction to it with a relative indifference suggests that some other stress is that work. Only after the interviewer has set aside the concerns about paralysis as being "all in the patient's head," or "psychosomatic," to use that unfortunate term, the conversation leads to a more likely source of anxiety, namely the patient's impending marriage.

The algorithm next asks whether he recognizes the anxiety or approaches it in the way of a Primitive Domain mechanism by denying its reality, avoiding it, or projecting it onto some unseen power. Clearly none of these are at play. He does not sit in the hospital and claim that he has no paralysis and can walk, he does not avoid discussion of it with the neurologist or the psychiatrist, nor does he say that his legs have been poisoned, for example, by some extraterrestrial force in the universe. His adaptation style rises beyond the Primitive range. He is able to discuss the facts that his legs do not "work" and that he is engaged to be married.

The algorithm next asks whether he can recognize that the current anxiety has something to do with him. More specifically, does he recognize that his anxiety has to do with his wedding in a few days? He clearly does not: he does not speak of the upcoming wedding with particular concern or emotional distress. Rather, he talks about it matter-of-factly, saying that it will have to be postponed until he is feeling better. From the interviewer's point of view, the anxiety seems oddly absent and the patient seems much less upset about the fact that his legs appear to be paralyzed than most other people, as for example after an auto accident with documented spine injury.

What accounts for this? Where has the anxiety gone? The answer to this provides the key to understanding Hypochondriasis as an adaptive mechanism against psychological distress: the patient has projected the anxiety—not outward or toward some other person—but into his body. Consistent with the adaptive strategy of Immature Domain mechanisms as diagrammed in Figure 7.1, the anxiety is not consciously available to him—that is, to his ego, which we have defined as his conscious sense of himself.

Earlier psychoanalytic models might define his avoiding his wedding due to the paralysis in his legs as his *secondary gain* from the physical symptoms—that is, avoiding a difficult situation. *Primary gain* in those models has to do with getting rid of his anxiety. Although the current model shares something with the latter idea, it focuses more on the patient's maintaining equilibrium in his conscious state. In this view, the cause of the anxiety, namely the marriage for which he may not be ready, has not gone away, nor has the anxiety reached a resolution in the patient's consciousness.

He would need to do much work for that to occur. His symptoms, meanwhile, abate after the stress itself departs.

SUPERWOMAN: BEYOND HYPOCHONDRIASIS

Although its clinical formulation is relatively recent, the process of transforming stress into physical symptoms has most likely characterized human experience since conscious awareness began.[1] As one instance, far more recent than ancient times but well before Charcot, let us consider the words of the redoubtable nun who reformed her religious order on her principles of prayer that modern observers have referred to as mystic or meditative. In doing so, Teresa of Ávila angered the Spanish Inquisition and reputedly made God laugh,[2] the only person in the cultural metaphors of Western civilization reported to have done so. She did not begin as a saint, however, according to her autobiography. She was born to a wealthy family and had an attractive sister who married well. She herself, judging by the one contemporary portrait we have of her, was probably not considered one of the great beauties of the time. Rather than marrying, in those days when marriage had much to do with social contracts that could assure family standing, she went to the convent.

We learn that after arriving there, she was beset by a very serious, though not fatal, illness. She describes it in part early on in an early chapter of her writing:

> My tongue was bitten to pieces, and my throat was so choked from having eaten no food and from my great weakness, that I could not even swallow water. My bones seem to be wrenched out of their sockets, and there was a great confusion in my head. As a result of all those days of torture I was twisted into a knot, and unless someone moved them for me, could no more move, foot, hand, or head than if I had been dead. All that I could move, I think, was one finger of my right hand.

---

1. In quoting from St. Teresa of Ávila's account of her illness in this section, I ask the reader to depend more on the view of applying the clinical model of psychological adaptive mechanisms to the experiences she describes rather than to regard the discussion as attempting to establish "proof" that that remarkable personage of 16th-century Spain actually suffered from a psychosomatic illness. Although some of the details she describes can fit with the modern attributes of a somatic disorder—for example, her mother's illness as a symptom model, her symptom descriptions as not always fitting what we now know of anatomy and illness, and her release from her physical condition as her own sense of self-sufficiency develops—the historical data she presents simply are not sufficient to provide for modern-day diagnosis. Rather, the consideration of St. Theresa from a "what if" point of view allows us to play with the adaptive style recognition model, as it were, and to learn from an application of the recognition algorithm to her case. The discussion intends to complement, therefore, her marvelous personality and the description she left for us to consider in our time of analogous, but often very different, views on the context and causes of human experience. She will instruct us again in Chapter 19.

2. According to lore, St. Teresa complained to God about the difficulty she found in doing her religious work. God replied that he always sent difficult trials to his most capable friends. St. Teresa shot back, "That is why you have so few of them!" The heavens thundered with God's laughter.

> …My extreme weakness is beyond description; I was nothing but bones. As I have said, I remained in this state for more than eight months, and my paralysis, although it grew less, continued for almost 3 years. When I began to crawl on hands and knees, I praised God.
>
> (Ávila 1995, p. 45)

This appears as a remarkable illness indeed, to have been so starved and so paralyzed for so long a time, and still to live through it. Other commentators have ascribed her symptoms to different physical causes, including malaria and other infectious processes. Because there is no way of establishing the actual truth of any diagnosis, for this chapter's discussion we will develop a working hypothesis that her illness may have represented an adaptive mechanism for her. In this regard, she offers us some other tantalizing descriptions that might be consistent with this view. For one, consistent with a modern diagnosis of some psychosomatic disorders, she had in her life someone else from whom to model her own symptoms. Here is her description:

> My mother too was a woman of many virtues, who endured a life of great sickness, and was extremely modest. Although she possessed remarkable beauty, she never showed the least signs of setting any store by it. Although she died at 33, she already dressed like a woman advanced in years.
>
> (Ávila 1995, p. 23)

Further, as she leaves her illness behind, she provided us with an interesting formulation of both its cure and its cause:

> As my own health was so bad, I was always hampered and useless until I decided to take no notice of my body or of my state of health; and now I bother very little about either.
>
> It pleased God to let me see this trick of the Devil's. Then, whenever he suggested that I was making myself ill, I would answer 'It doesn't matter if I die!' and 'Rest! I don't need rest but the Cross,' and so on. I clearly saw that although I am very sickly, in most cases my illnesses were temptations of Satan, or arose from my own weakness. Since I have given up caring so much for my ease and comfort, my health has been very much better. It is very important at the beginning, when we embark on prayer, not to be frightened by our own thoughts.
>
> (Ávila 1995, p. 90)

In a spirit of useful imagination, therefore, our algorithm approaches St. Teresa's symptoms by first asking what stress might have triggered her anxiety such that she needed an adaptive response. We might imagine a vivacious and strong-willed young woman who enjoys the company of others being relegated to the consolation prize of a lifetime in the convent, perhaps because of the arranged marriages of the time. A stress of this magnitude may well be expected to bring a sizable force of anxiety, perhaps reflected in the magnitude of the symptoms that follow from it.

Does she avoid consideration of her fate? Her narrative provides evidence that she does not. She does not, for example, say that she never went to the convent, avoid writing about her experiences there, or insist that convents are the homes of beings from Venus. Her adaptive mechanism does not live in the Primitive Domain.

The next step on the algorithm asks, during the period of her illness, does she describe being sent to a nunnery as something that she would have to come to terms with? She makes no mention of that in her writing, and for our imaginative purposes we can say *No*. Instead, she suffers a terrific illness that renders her completely incapacitated for a very long time. She adds the remarkable detail that she was paralyzed throughout her body with the exception of one finger on her right hand. Again, with our imagination going forward, the reality of this bears no resemblance to what we now know of the innervation of the hand. This allows us to suggest the possibility that the stress and anxiety she suffered from her social fate might have found expression in her body and its symptoms. According to our model, we can imagine her as adapting through the psychological mechanism of Hypochondriasis in the Immature Domain of adaptive mechanisms. It locates the psychological stress as projected into her body by way of her physical illness, a place where the stress cannot be gotten at, let alone resolved, until it goes away on its own.

When that occurs, in our hypothetical rendition, she describes her own behavior in taking control of her illness: the less she thinks about it, the less illness she suffers, and when she does have a symptom, she can ascribe it to the Devil and thank God for the insight because it puts her in closer touch with her Creator. The center of dealing with her stress and its anxiety has shifted away from the illness she can do nothing about and into her own consciousness, where she can use her beliefs. Her new adaptive behavior resembles the adaptive mechanism of Reaction Formation, discussed in Chapter 16 of this volume without reference to St. Teresa. But she continues to describe the process of her growth in her autobiography and will appear again in a very different setting that requires much less imagination on our part when we meet her again in Chapter 19. As readers of the communications she left us from a much earlier age, however, we may see her sense of relief in the waning of her physical symptoms and in the description of her growth in developing new, and better, adaptive styles. Hypochondriasis can indeed be a very painful psychological adaptation, as portrayed in a passage written about 300 years after St. Teresa.

CRIME AND ITS PUNISHMENT: REGRESSION INTO HYPOCHONDRIASIS

Rodion Raskolnikov, an impoverished young Russian intellectual, has planned and carried out the murder of an old woman to whom he owes money and who holds his only valuable possessions in pawn. He kills her by driving an ax through her skull. While rifling through her apartment looking for his possessions, her younger sister enters and finds him. He kills her too with the ax. He then escapes back to his own tiny room, drops down on his sofa, and remains there through the night in a dazed state with brief periods of sleep. As he begins to waken and recall his actions and their consequences, he notices his body:

> In the first few moments he thought he must be going mad. A dreadful chill enveloped him, but this was partly the result of a feverishness that for many weeks had always accompanied his sleep. Now, however, he was seized with such a violent fit of shivering that his teeth chattered uncontrollably, and every limb shook. . . .
>
> He sat down exhausted on the sofa. And at once an unbearably violent shivering shook him again. Mechanically he took up from where it lay on the chair beside him the old winter overcoat he had worn as a student, which was warm even if ragged, covered himself with it and surrendered himself once more to mingled sleep and delirium.
>
> Not more than five minutes later he sprang up again and rushed back to his clothes. . . .
>
> The conviction that everything, even memory, even the simple power of reflection, was deserting him, had begun to torment him unbearably. . . .
>
> Now a strange idea entered his head: perhaps all his clothes were soaked and stained with blood and he could not see it because his mental powers were failing and crumbling away. . . .
>
> But instead, his head declined once more towards the pillow; once more a sudden chill congealed his blood; once more he drew his greatcoat over him. . . .
>
> He sprang up and sat on the edge of the sofa. His heart thumped so heavily that it was painful.
>
> (Dostoevsky 1995, pp. 84–87)

Dostoevsky wrote his famous novel in order to explore what he regarded as the innate psychological processes that would punish human beings when they transgressed basic social mores, in this case the proscription of murder. In doing so, he puts the first round of punishments in Raskolnikov's body. The punishment that he will suffer through the rest of the book begins with physical pain.

The first step in applying the recognition model for psychological adaptive mechanisms asks us to identify the stress that raises anxiety in conscious experience. What is it that perturbs the ego? Like a scientist lighting the blue flame of a Bunsen burner, Dostoevsky describes Raskolnikov's stress as his brutal ax murder of two defenseless older women. More specifically, however, the murder violates every attribute and value of Raskolnikov's own personality. He is an idealistic, young graduate student who is trying to better himself in living in the world. Under normal conditions, in better circumstances, the thought of murder would not enter his mind. But in this portrayal, he is wracked with poverty, unable to retrieve his few paltry possessions that he has pawned, and still in need of more money to provide for basic needs like food. Dostoevsky uses the social circumstances—the "boy next door" hungry, cold, and with no options for living—to get at what happens to the spirit as it tries to right itself after committing an act of horrendous violence. The stress that interests Dostoevsky involves the good guy having to think of himself as an ax murderer, followed by the sense of both disaster and oncoming doom—that is, the anxiety—that the stress provides.

The next task for the observer is to ascertain whether Raskolnikov ignores the stress and anxiety or somehow acknowledges it. Again Dostoevsky leaves no doubt. As soon as he kills the two women, Raskolnikov searches for his possessions and then quickly leaves, covering his tracks as much as and as quickly as he can. He does not wait for the police to come along and then claim nothing has happened when the two sisters are really dead. He is beyond the Primitive Domain of psychological adaptive mechanisms.

In considering the scene quoted above that occurs immediately after Raskolnikov's escape, the algorithm next asks, does he consciously perceive an anxiety from having taken two other lives, having done that in a brutal and uncharacteristic fashion? On returning to his room, his body throws him into fatigue and something like sleep. But it is not untroubled or restful, and it lasts only a little while. His body wakes him first with a fever, then with a series of pains, and then with confusion. He begins to doubt his own perceptions and even his own memory. The physical sensations crowd his consciousness and he reacts to them. There is no mention of a sense of anxiety or even directly of the killings. As Dostoyevsky portrays him at this instant in time, the anxiety and to some extent the deed itself are not present in Raskolnikov's consciousness. The physical sensations of his body crowd out any consciousness of psychological anxiety. As with the above examples, Raskolnikov has projected the anxiety of his unacceptable actions into his body. However flexibly, however maturely, his adaptive mechanisms may have helped him to adapt to his life before this point, and he now employs an Immature Domain psychological adaptive mechanism. His immediate conscious problem is not himself or his act, but his body that is full of sickness. Even the beating of his heart, normally a consistent symbol in describing relationships with others, is now painful at every beat. Raskolnikov's immediate adaptation exemplifies Hypochondriasis in response to a severe, acute psychological stress. Dostoevsky's character will go on in the novel to reach higher level adaptive styles as he works to reconcile his person and his violent act. But, for our purposes, his adaptive starting point—the best he can do at the time—projects his anxiety into the pain of his body.

IT ISN'T CANCER: HYPOCHONDRIASIS AS NORMAL ADAPTATION

Do only ax murderers project their anxieties into their physical well-being to this extent? Asked another way, is Hypochondriasis ever a normal way of adapting to the stress experienced in living? To answer this, we follow a 14-year-old ninth grader to his pediatrician's office during after-school hours on an afternoon in the early spring. When it's his turn, he goes in to see the doctor—a middle-aged man wearing a long white coat, tan slacks, a blue button-down shirt, penny loafers, and the characteristic bow tie common among male pediatricians. This fatherly figure asks the young man what has brought him to the office.

"This right here," the young man says, pointing to a red, sore-looking lesion on the side of his nose, one that just appears to be forming pus. "I think it's cancer! My grandma died of cancer. Can this kind of cancer be cured?"

Without batting an eye or even giving way to the most subtle form of a smile, the pediatrician takes his patient seriously and says, "Well, let's have a look." He sits the young man down under a spotlight and examines the lesion. Then he says to the boy, "In my professional opinion, having seen a number of these kinds of lesions over my years, this is not cancer. I'm very sorry to hear about your grandmother and her experience with cancer. But if it's any reassurance to you, you don't have cancer."

The boy pauses for a moment or two as if in thought and asks, "Are you sure it's not cancer? Because I don't want my friends to see me with cancer."

"Your friends?" the pediatrician asks. "At school?"

"Yes. My friends at school, I mean," the young man says, pausing again, and then adding, "my friends and some other people too."

"Other people?" The doctor asks again, "Like at church or somewhere social?"

Another brief pause and the boy says, "Like someplace social. Like there's this dance on Saturday—they call it a mixer—and I want to go to it but my friends are going and if I have to go to it, I don't want to go there with cancer."

"A mixer," the pediatrician says. "I've been to a few mixers in my time. If I remember right, there are usually girls at a mixer. I see what you mean about cancer. A fellow wants to look his best at a mixer. Fortunately, what you have isn't cancer. It's called a pustule. That's its scientific name, and we can fix it in the next few days between now and the mixer. I'm going to write out a schedule for you to soak it at home with warm soapy water two or three times each evening. When it gets ready, it's going to open up all by itself and then you soak once or twice more after that and then it'll heal up by itself. I don't want you squeezing or pressing on it because that can make it worse. And I'm going to give you a little packet with some cream medicine in it. If it's still red when the mixer comes around, just put a dab of the cream on your littlest finger tip and gently rub it onto the pustule. That way it will blend in and no one will know that you've actually had a pustule."

The young man nods seriously, suitably impressed with the world of science. He follows the directions the doctor gives him to the letter and manages to get to and from the mixer, conscious of the girls looking at him there all the while, but all the while cancer free.

As we regard this adolescent boy from the point of view of the recognition algorithm, the social stress involved—namely going to a dance where members of the opposite gender will be present—results in as being acutely aware of his physical appearance. This common stress in early adolescence, especially among those who may be slower to develop than their confreres, provokes this young man's anxiety. Going to the mixer brings with it a sense of impending disaster. His pediatrician, a fatherly sort familiar with the various disasters of this age, recognizes this.

Does the young man in this vignette revert to Primitive Domain mechanisms of adaptive behavior? He clearly does not avoid the issue, deny that the mixer is going to go on anyway, or ascribe his distress to his younger siblings who have no idea what he's talking about. Although the possibility of having an actual cancer may have the desired effect of keeping him home from the mixer, along with bringing the admiration of his friends who would perceive him as near death—a state of mind reminiscent of Tom Sawyer's imaginings about how important he would be to those around him if he actually passed away—reality suggests otherwise.

Rather, the pediatrician's adolescent patient presents himself to confirm the diagnosis or, if that can't be done, to seek treatment for a physical ailment. He does not perceive consciously his own sense of anxiety but focuses that on the skin lesion that indicates to him the likelihood of cancer. He presents, therefore, an age-appropriate Hypochondriasis as his adaptive mechanism to this particular stress of social growth. The doctor recognizes this and meets him on his own terms. He diagnoses a "pustule" rather than calling it a pimple, a far more mundane diagnosis that carries a certain demeaning sense with it. The young man is grateful for the scientific diagnosis and proceeds both to a successful treatment as well as to his first experience of mixers. He survives both with flying colors. And as he continues through his adolescent journey, he will outgrow the Hypochondriasis in favor of more mature adaptive mechanisms. Clinically, adolescents negotiating the rapid changes in their bodies that occur over a few brief years commonly worry about having cancer. Lumps, bumps, spots, and pains of all kinds serve the purpose and require evaluation when the youngsters complain of them. They very rarely have to do with cancer and much more frequently indicate something of the stressful, if creative, turmoil of growing up.

IT ISN'T CANCER EITHER: STRESS-DRIVEN HYPOCHONDRIASIS

As we have seen, whether in normal adolescence or in response to intense social conditions, Hypochondriasis can flower forth into the symptoms that project the anxiety of a stress into one's body. This can also become a characteristic pattern in meeting anxieties of adult life, as we learn in another visit with our sleepy intern.

We again find our intern in the small hours of the morning tending to the eight patients on the medical floor and the four others in the ICU. He has been working hard but finds the night's duty particular difficult. First, the nurses called him to see one of the floor patients—a middle-aged, thin-looking woman with a thyroid condition. Her pulse rate has skyrocketed. While timing her pulse that was indeed rapid, he began noticing his own heartbeat: it seemed to be just as rapid and felt like a pounding in his chest. He politely excused himself, went out into the hallway, and took his pulse. The rate was normal but he still felt as though his heart was pounding. He asked the nurse to take his pulse and she too found it was normal. He returned to the patient and told her he would give her some medicines to bring her pulse rate down and that she would be feeling better. He left again feeling his heart pounding and worried about having some sort of heart attack himself. At the same time, he noticed the vague sense of a headache starting near the back of his head.

Then our intern got a page message to see another of his inpatients: an elderly man complaining of severe pain from the arthritis in his fingers. While examining the man's fingers with his right hand, the intern noticed that two of his own fingers on his left hand, following the ulnar nerve distribution, were beginning to tremble on their own. Soon they too clenched in a spasm of pain that seem to move up his left arm. He excused himself and went down to the nurses' station. Rather than show them to the nurse, he rubbed the two fingers for a minute or two until the pain eased. Then he asked for a nonsteroidal anti-inflammatory tablet. He ordered medicine for the patient's arthritic pain and then went along to answer another call to examine a patient in the ICU.

There he encountered a man in his 40s with a 20-year history of heavy drinking. The man was doubled over in the bed with severe pancreatic pain, claiming that it was as though someone had hit him in the stomach with an ax. As the man writhed from the pain with his knees pulled close to his chin, the intern began, nervously, thinking what to do next. At the same time, he noticed his own abdominal muscles tightening, followed by a sharp pain that stretched across his abdomen at the level of his belly button, along with a feeling of nausea as though he would soon vomit. Excusing himself again, he wrote orders for pain medicines for his patient and then stood in the hallway until his symptoms began to subside—all except for the headache, which seemed to have gotten worse.

Alarmed now, he walked along the hall with one hand on the wall in case he were to fall or have a seizure, eased himself onto the elevator, and went down to the ER. He quietly found the chief resident, told him about the headache—especially because it was occurring in the early hours of the morning as headaches often do when they're associated with brain tumors—mentioned the tremor of the two fingers in his left hand, and requested that the chief order a brain scan for him. The chief resident listened politely but said he would not do so because the resident had already had a brain scan when he was last covering the hospital three days ago. He also had one two weeks before and, in fact, another four weeks before that. As far as the chief knew, he held the record for the most brain scans for any intern ever in the program. The chief resident politely suggested that he pull himself together because they were about to send him another patient for the ICU, a woman in her 20s who had had a seizure and probably did have a brain tumor. He reassured the intern that he was a good doctor and would do fine with the new admission. The intern's face turned ashen, and he fainted. When he awoke a few minutes later, the chief resident admitted him to the hospital. The intern was discharged two days later after a negative medical evaluation. He accepted a mandatory leave of absence from his clinical residency.

Training in the medical professions does not create immunity against hypochondriacal symptoms. In fact, a regular occurrence among medical students when they begin learning about disease states includes their finding many of the symptoms reported in textbooks in their own experience. With time, more knowledge, and the perspective of clinical experience, this classic phenomenon falls by the wayside in the vast majority of cases.

Not so for this chapter's intern. Applying the recognition algorithm, we recognize the surface stress is over work and lack of sleep. But here also we find a glimpse of a deeper, more profound source of stress. The object of the internship—the first year of training in any clinical specialty—includes the basic requirement of learning to take on the responsibility for someone else's life and physical well-being. This transforming year of accelerated professional growth takes an individual from the academic learning of the medical student and delivers an autonomous physician capable of making medical decisions and managing the care of others. Most grow through this transition year, although some, like the intern in this chapter, find the stress overwhelming.

The recognition algorithm asks whether the intern recognizes the source of anxiety or ignores it. He clearly struggles with it, rather than denying its existence, avoiding its reality, or claiming that his distress is the fault of some imaginary being. He does not employ the Primitive Domain adaptive mechanisms.

Does he perceive, according to the next step in the recognition algorithm, that the anxiety to which he tries to adapt is located in his conscious self, or is it somewhere else? As portrayed, he does not reach a conscious apprehension of anxiety as he attempts to shoulder the responsibility for someone else's well-being. Rather, he identifies with each of their symptoms in succession and finds himself increasingly convinced that he is physically fragile and approaching the point of death. Symbolically, the sense of doom he experiences is that of a physical doom as indicated by his symptoms. He does not recognize it as a conscious sense of anxiety. His adaptation projects his anxiety into his body in the form of his symptoms. Following the definition of the Immature Domain psychological adaptive mechanisms, his Hypochondriasis makes up his best adaptation in this stress-filled environment. Unlike some of the other cases mentioned above, however, his adaptation appears far more indurated, as it can become in some people for whom it takes on the properties of a standard, repeated behavior.

Through processes that have yet to be fully understood, Hypochondriasis, like all the other immature Domain adaptive mechanisms, may become so much a part of the personality as to resemble what are described as "character styles" in other models and their nosology.[3] In the present model of psychological adaptive strategies, the observer can note that Hypochondriasis—that ability to project anxiety into the perception of one's body—occurs with greater or lesser degrees of relative permanence, from normal adolescent development, on the one hand, to chronically impaired function, on the other. The latter occurs frequently among primary care practices, for example, but does not always receive attention as an adaptive process. Why Hypochondriasis occurs at all in only some people and not in many others, and why it sometimes persists in debilitating forms in this person but not in that one, constitute useful topics for clinical investigation.

REFERENCES

American Psychiatric Association. (2000). *Diagnostic and Statistical Manual of Mental Disorders* (4th ed., Text Rev.). Washington, DC, American Psychiatric Press.

Ávila, T. (1957). *The Life of Saint Teresa of Ávila by Herself*. London, Penguin.

Dostoevsky, F. (1995). *Crime and Punishment*. New York, Oxford University Press.

Reich, W. (1980). *Character Analysis*. New York, Farrar, Straus and Giroux.

World Health Organization. (1990). *International Classification of Diseases, 9th Edition, Clinical Modification*. Washington, DC, US Government Printing Office.

3. American Psychiatric Association (2000); World Health Organization (1990). See also Wilhelm Reich's (1980) formulation.

Primitive

Immature

CHAPTER 10

Schizoid Fantasy

Human beings have not only the ability to live in the world but also the ability to reflect upon it. The capacity to dream during waking hours allows us to imagine about ourselves and the world, and indeed the universe and beyond. It offers us many more useful functions in life than merely adapting to our surroundings or to our own inner forces and emotional states. With this ability we can cast our fantasies beyond the limits of time and space and causality. For example, we can imagine traveling beyond the speed of light to the farthest edge of the material universe and back again even though in our physical existence this is a clear impossibility. But what fun it is to imagine that we could.

In the myths that humankind has constructed over the history of its existence as a conscious being—myths that are themselves imagined constructions of human experience—the ability to imagine, to make believe, puts us in touch with that which in everyday life we describe as the Eternal. This is the part of life that humans experience as beyond time, or outside of time, in which human phenomena such as love, compassion, self-sacrifice, and the life of the spirit all abide. We will have much more to say about this area of human functioning in Chapter 20. But for now, we may reasonably ask, how does this very vibrant human function come to be classed in our model as an Immature Domain psychological adaptive mechanism that has something to do with that pathological-sounding word *schizoid*?

Although *fantasy* conjures up products of the imagination, *schizoid* has to do with withdrawing from other persons and contact with them, especially emotional contact. The term *schizoid fantasy*, as Vaillant uses it and as we shall use it here, describes withdrawal into one's imaginary life, into one's fantasies, as a way of adapting to the stresses and strains of the world. "Reality always disappoints me. My fantasies never do," so to speak.

Rather than building imaginative works that engage other people with our ideas and our feelings, here such productions remain inside, known only to the person who experiences them. Both the emotional and cognitive contents that the mind produces or with which it reacts remain unavailable to others, leaving the impression of withdrawal into a subjective state of being. Rather than engaging in the hustle and bustle of everyday life, including everyday pain and finding ways to adapt that connect us with others, a schizoid fantasy world serves to isolate. In terms of adaptation, however, a schizoid fantasy world offers far more of the apparent security that comes from living in a controllable internal environment, although an extremely limited one. If, as the Buddhists say, all life is sorrow, schizoid fantasy as a psychological adaptive mechanism says that life within one's own fantasies can shut out much of the sorrow, if at a heavy cost. In effect, from the point of view of a person who uses this mechanism, "Life in here is better than life out there," in which *better* means less stressful and therefore less filled with anxiety.

MISS HAVISHAM REGRETS: STUCK IN ADAPTIVE SCHIZOID FANTASY

Charles Dickens, that designer and describer of what others have called "flat,"[1] or unidimensional, characters each presented for the purpose of delineating a specific human attribute, provides us a useful example in the figure of Miss Havisham in his novel *Great Expectations*. Jilted on her wedding day by an inconstant lover, she remains in her decaying house from young womanhood through middle age, wearing her wedding dress and locked in the fantasy of her wedding day, knowing that her marriage will never take place. Pip, the hero of the novel, describes his first encounter with Miss Havisham when she introduces him to Estella, her ward and a girl Pip's age, both children.

> Miss Havisham beckoned her to come close, and took up a jewel from the table, and tried its effect upon her fair young bosom and against her pretty brown hair. "Your own, one day, my dear, and you will use it well. Let me see you play cards with this boy."
>
> "With this boy! Why, he is a common laboring-boy!"
>
> I thought I overheard Miss Havisham answer—only it seemed so unlikely—"Well? You can break his heart."
>
> "What do you play, boy?" Asked Estella of myself, with the greatest disdain.
>
> "Nothing but Beggar My Neighbor, Miss."
>
> "Beggar him," said Miss Havisham to Estella. So we sat down to cards.
>
> It was then I began to understand that everything in the room had stopped, like the watch and the clock, a long time ago. I noticed that Miss Havisham put down the jewel exactly on the spot from which she had taken it up. As Estella dealt the cards, I glanced at the dressing table again, and saw that the shoe upon it, once white, now yellow, had never been worn. I glanced down at the foot from which the shoe was absent, and saw that the silk stocking on it, once white, now yellow, had been trodden ragged. Without this arrest of everything, this standing still of all the pale decayed objects, not even the withered bridal dress on the collapsed form could have looked so like grave-clothes, or the long veil so like a shroud.
>
> So she sat, corpse-like, as we played at cards; the frillings and trimmings on her bridal dress, looking like earthy paper. I knew nothing then of the discoveries that

1. See E. M. Forster (1927, Chapter 10).

are occasionally made of bodies buried in ancient times, which fall to powder in the moment of being distinctly seen; but, I have often thought since, that she had looked as if the admission of the natural light of day would have struck her to dust.

(Dickens 1998, pp. 54–55)

Applying the diagnostic algorithm to this portrayal, we first ask whether Miss Havisham perceives any difficulty in her life. In Dickens' description, she has no doubt that her bridegroom left her at the altar. In this sense, her adaptation is not that of a psychosis or of the Primitive Domain adaptive mechanisms. Nor does she, as Dickens presents her, think that the marriage actually will take place any moment now, a delusion that would make us think of what we currently regard as a major psychiatric disorder. The character speaks logically to the other characters in the book and without any sense of psychotic false beliefs such as we have seen in others of Dickens' characters, Mr. Dick in *David Copperfield*,[2] for example. Miss Havisham's portrayal reaches beyond the Primitive Domain styles of adaptation.

We next ask, does she see her own role in adapting to the world around her in such an extremely isolated manner? Or does she hold herself blameless for the responsibility of her isolation and her solitary relationship with the world? Does she see a part for herself in respect to the pain she experiences, including her relationship and what might have been her own role in her lover's jilting of her? Dickens makes it very clear that she does not. All the blame lies in the falsehood of her bridegroom's actions, and she perceives herself as having no control over them.

By retreating into the frozen safety of her never-ending, never consummated, wedding day, Miss Havisham adapts to, but never resolves, her broken heart. She has located any resolution outside of her own power to grasp it. It is a telling detail, however, when she seeks a vicarious revenge in arranging matters for Estella to break Pip's heart. Miss Havisham prefers the isolated fantasy of her decaying life, and a revenge on males of the species, over the pain of having to bring her circumstance within the purview of her own responsibility. She prefers to regard herself as the blameless and heroic victim of this nuptial tragedy rather than accept the painful possibility of change from within. Well in advance of any of the present formulation, Dickens portrays Schizoid Fantasy as a psychological adaptive mechanism. Miss Havisham prefers the confines of her own repetitive fantasies to engagement in a life outside her mind and the give-and-take of experience that would broaden her imaginings and allow contact with others.

In recognizing a stress and its anxiety, yet accepting no responsibility for one's participation in it—we identify the strategy common to all of the Immature Domain

---

2. Mr. Dick is a completely concrete thinking and yet both lovable and admirable character who suffers the continuous delusion that King Charles I, beheaded in London 200 years earlier in 1649, controls his thoughts; specifically that King Charles' head does. The term "King Charles' head" from the novel became a catch phrase in the late 19th century, referring to intrusive, obsessive thoughts. In Bleuler's typology (1911), Mr. Dick would have been classed as a "simple" schizophrenic: quietly, and chronically, crazy, harmless, and capable of low-stress work. In the resolution of David Copperfield, Mr. Dick takes on more heroic proportions.

psychological mechanisms through which they provide their adaptive value. All of them locate the stress outside the affected person—the so-called externalizing mechanisms—where the stress can't be gotten at. From the person's own point of view, the stress is somebody else's problem. For the people in that person's social network, this irritates, as it does to some of the other characters in *Great Expectations*, or at least puzzles, as we heard Pip describe above.

DIFFERENTIATING FROM THE PRIMITIVE

One might reasonably ask, how does this mechanism of Schizoid Fantasy differ from the Primitive Domain mechanism of Avoidance/Distortion? After all, Miss Havisham simply avoids the complications of life by remaining in her fantasies. The answer lies in the differentiating characteristics of the Primitive versus the Immature adaptive mechanisms. The two Domains are separated by the relatively simple phenomenon of whether or not the person recognizes that the stress exists in the first place. In Primitive Avoidance, the stress simply isn't there when other things distract the person's attention. From the person's point of view, "If I don't look at it, it isn't there." So we saw in Chapter 5 that King Lear prefers the distraction of the thunderstorm over his otherwise unrelieved anguish where his daughters are concerned. Instead of having to recognize the matter itself, Primitive Avoidance characteristically focuses on other things not laden with anxiety triggers.

By contrast, Dickens' character Miss Havisham does not avoid the fact that the groom fled on their wedding day. She appears, instead, not only to recognize it—or to resolve it—but to perpetuate it as a horrible fate. Another model—one of post-traumatic stress disorder—might suggest that her perpetuating the trauma of her wedding day has made it a permanent part of her character and her focus in life. For change to occur, persons who characteristically use the Immature Domain mechanisms must to begin to doubt whether the problem really does belong to others. Taking responsibility, and thereby control, makes up a central attribute of the Neurotic Domain psychological adaptive mechanisms as we will discuss further on. For now, let us return to the Immature Domain.

THE SECRET LIFE OF THE SLEEPY INTERN: STRESS DRIVEN TO SCHIZOID FANTASY

Our sleep deprived intern, in the middle of the night in the hospital, has dozed off for a nap and then awakens suddenly when the phone rings. Struggling back into consciousness, the ER resident at the other end of the line announces that another case will be coming to the service forthwith and going directly to the ICU, where the intern must conduct an evaluation and write treatment orders. Our intern hangs up the phone with the realization that this announcement has nothing to do with him. Yes, the patient will be coming up to the ICU, but someone else must take care of the patient, probably the ER resident whom the intern does not like very much anyway.

The new patient is someone else's problem, while the intern is content to drift back into the fantasies of being a successful musician, something he considered before ever deciding to try a career in medicine. He plays the violin. He is a concert violinist. With technique and feeling, he negotiates both classical symmetry and romantic upheaval in piece after piece. With an agile left hand on the strings and a deft liveliness on the bow that no other virtuoso has ever approached, he fills the audience with the electricity of his playing. After each piece, the applause increases, each more deafening and longer lived than the last. He is clearly the most beloved violinist who has ever touched the instrument. He responds with encore after encore. The night goes by, the ICU nurses are unable to contact him, and the ER resident must cover the admission to the ICU on the patient's behalf. The next morning, the intern is found, still in his reverie, which is broken by an interview with the chief resident, who reports the incident to the medical attending staff. They relieve the intern of duty on the spot, suggesting that he take medical leave to assess and correct his behavior before any reinstatement.

In this vignette, our intern has met an increasing stress in an Immature fashion by preferring to drift off into fantasies rather than to take charge of the new admission. Referring to the recognition algorithm, the added stress of the new admission, and the anxiety it provokes, results in our intern retreating from the edge of his fantasy life to a place deep within its bounds. He recognizes the stress and therefore does not qualify as using a Primitive Domain adaptive mechanism. But he sees the new admission as someone else's problem and does not discuss it with anyone else. His own fantasies keep him from feeling any responsibility for his actions in the situation. Responsibility for the acute situation—in this case, for the care of a very seriously ill patient—shifts to someone else, as is often the case even in lesser situations in life. This very specific social situation, however, allows no tolerance where other people's lives may be endangered, and the social network, namely the training structure, moves the intern out of the situation because it no longer trusts his judgment or actions. This too is indicative of an Immature Domain psychological adaptive mechanism: rather than connecting us with others in our social networks, the Immature Domain mechanisms push others away. They result in actions that limit the extent to which others, who must interact with the person using an Immature Domain psychological adaptive mechanism, will tolerate their behavior.

WHEN I GROW UP: NORMAL FANTASY

In common consideration of all the Immature Domain mechanisms, we can now ask, when might an isolating behavior that pushes others away serve a useful purpose? As with all of the Immature psychological adaptive mechanisms, a strong fantasy life too can be a normal part of adolescent development in that heroic passage that young people must traverse from the starting point of dependent childhood to the endpoint of independent adulthood. In this process, they naturally push parents away in the effort to gain their own psychological autonomy. But it is one thing to push away the parents upon whom they depend and another thing to have some replacement handy on which to rely. Very personal fantasies of this nature often serve the purpose on the causeway to adulthood.

Common examples of adolescent fantasies include the following: What will life will be like when I am grown up and can make my own decisions? What kind of work will best satisfy me and allow the world to appreciate my true talents? What wonderful person will I marry and build a home with? A fantasy life at this age looks forward, rather than backward, and usually contains within it the excitement of someone starting out on a journey. It is a general phenomenon that has been commented on throughout recorded human history.

As one example, early in Homer's *Odyssey*, the goddess Athena—who for our purposes is herself a fantasy in the mind of Odysseus' son Telemachos—appears to Telemachos and tells him that he must go find his father, the hero of Homer's wandering epic. Disguised, as fantasy beings often are, as one of his father's friends from another kingdom, she tells him,

> But for yourself, I will counsel you shrewdly, and hope you will listen.
> Fit out a ship with twenty oars, the best you can come by,
> and go out to ask about your father who is so long absent.

And a few lines later she adds,

> You should not go on
> clinging to your childhood. You are no longer of an age to do that.
> (Homer, *The Odyssey*, Book I, lines 281–282, 296–297)

Symbolically, Telemachos' father represents the adult course of life and someone who has pursued his own role both personally and socially. The war goddess Athena appears to him as a symbol of his own strivings: she tells him that it's time to leave his childhood and enter the adult warrior world. Again symbolically, the father leads the way in life with regard to the outer world, and the son must begin a path toward his own destiny with his father's path as an inkling or blueprint on what to expect. More generally, the mythological stories of the "father quest" involve coming to an understanding of what one's career is or where one's sustaining interests lie as young people move into adulthood. Imagining what that might be or what it might entail allows a young person's imagination and perceptions to stretch, to include, to discard, and to work through this time of life.

A strong advantage of adolescent fantasies obtains precisely because they require no responsibility: they are only fantasies and can be gotten rid of when a better one comes along. At the same time, such productions are intensely private. Although the word *schizoid* is probably a misnomer in this context, most adolescents certainly don't want their parents to know anything about the kinds of things they imagine. And parents, for their part, feel somewhat irritable about being shut out of the thoughts of this young person who was previously their buddy and took them into confidence. The adolescent's fantasy life thereby serves a dual purpose: it helps the parent realize that this young person is becoming independent, and part of that is a letting go on the parent's side of the equation. As adolescent maturity continues, and the irresponsibility of imaginings turns naturally into the responsibility of young adult actions, parents find their own responsibility lessening and, concurrently, their own freedom increasing. Such is the shared dance in the parent-offspring relationships of human development.

THE SECRET—AND TRAGIC—FANTASY LIFE OF WALTER MITTY

The energy of adolescent development pushes on with the assistance of the alluring fantasies of great heroes taking on great adventures in the great world. At that young age the course of life appears experimental, and therefore full of adventure. But what if experiencing the great world is actually banal, humdrum, gray, and ultimately uninteresting? James Thurber asked that question in his famous short story. We join his characters as they fly through the middle of a terrible thunderstorm:

> "We're going through!" The Commander's voice was like thin ice breaking. He wore his full-dress uniform, with the heavily braided white cap pulled down rakishly over one cold gray eye. "We can't make it, sir. It's spoiling for a hurricane, if you ask me." "I'm not asking you, Lieutenant Berg," said the Commander. "Throw on the power lights! Rev her up to 8,500! We're going through!" The pounding of the cylinders increased: ta-pocketa-pocketa-pocketa-*pocketa-pocketa*. The Commander stared at the ice forming on the pilot window. He walked over and twisted a row of complicated dials. "Switch on No. 8 auxiliary!" he shouted. "Switch on No. 8 auxiliary!" repeated Lieutenant Berg. "Full strength in No. 3 turret!" shouted the Commander. "Full strength in No. 3 turret!" The crew, bending to their various tasks in the huge, hurtling eight-engined Navy hydroplane, looked at each other and grinned. "The Old Man'll get us through," they said to one another. "The Old Man ain't afraid of Hell!"
>
> "Not so fast! You're driving too fast!" said Mrs. Mitty. "What are you driving so fast for?"
>
> "Hmm?" said Walter Mitty. He looked at his wife, in the seat beside him, with shocked astonishment. She seemed grossly unfamiliar, like a strange woman who had yelled at him in a crowd. "You were up to fifty-five, "she said. "You know I don't like to go more than forty. You were up to fifty-five." Walter Mitty drove on toward Waterbury in silence, the roaring of the SN202 through the worst storm in twenty years of Navy flying fading in the remote intimate airways of his mind.
>
> (Thurber 1942, p. 47)

Nonsensical commands and all, the Commander's rakish demeanor, his sheer courage in the face of adversity, and the crew's belief in his experience as a seaplane pilot in the face of the storm, all seem to Mr. Mitty preferable to keeping his speed down in obedience to Mrs. Mitty's orders while driving her to the beauty parlor in a Connecticut suburb. The thunderstorm in all its glory takes him away from boredom and puts him in the realm of exciting action, with the particular advantage of not actually being in a dangerous thunderstorm or flying a plane through one. He can leave the storm and the plane at will, as he does when his wife interrupts his reverie. As readers, we find the situation comical and the Walter Mitty fantasy amusing, especially hearing the ta-pocketa-pocketa-pocketa-*pocketa-pocketa* in the background for added effect. And this is Thurber's intent at this point in the story.

But our own deft shift of reference allows us to apply the model of psychological adaptation mechanisms to the portrayal of Walter Mitty. Following the recognition algorithm, our first task is to ask, what anxiety-provoking stress calls forth an adaptive mechanism? To answer this, we pay attention to the other fantasies that engage Thurber's character through the course of the story. Mitty appears as a specialist consulting surgeon to the rich and important, as the righteous defendant in a murder trial with a beautiful young woman falling into his arms, and as a British infantry captain in World War I about to begin a risky mission with a stiff upper lip, a spot of brandy, and more pocketa-pocketa-pocketa in the background. Against these, we find the real Walter Mitty in Waterbury driving his car into the wrong lane of a parking lot and giving the keys to an attendant who doesn't trust him to park the car himself, trying to recall the shopping list of drugstore items that his wife had given him, and, after a struggle, remembering that he had to find a shoe store to purchase overshoes. In the portrayal, Mitty's stress does not arrive in any specific crisis—as compared to Dickens' Miss Havisham—but by way of the continuing, uninteresting, and unengaging experience of his day-to-day life in which he seems only partially competent to manage his affairs. The anxiety behind the comedy, subtly integrated into the story, includes the sense of a life being, if not wasted, lived somewhere well short of its fullest potential, something most people wonder about themselves at one time or another.

The next step asks whether Walter Mitty perceives this stress, that is, the humdrum repetitiveness of his life. We learn that he hates the weekly drive to town with his wife, that he sees the people around him as cocky and demeaning, and at one point that he considers putting his right arm in a sling in order to get more sympathy from others. By contrast, were he to use the Primitive Domain adaptive styles, his life would be just fine, with the U.S. Navy seaplanes controlling his thoughts, or he would avoid the whole question of stress altogether. As it is, he feels a sense of discomfort at every turn through real-world experience, even in Waterbury, Connecticut. His portrayal does not include the Primitive Domain approach to psychological adaptation.

The next step in the recognition algorithm calls for an assessment as to whether James Thurber's character perceives the banality of his life as something over which he has some measure of control or whether the tenor of his existence is simply out of his hands. The Walter Mitty of the short story bumbles through his trip to Waterbury with no conception that things might be any different in any place other than his own fantasies. His portrayal does not include the turmoil of addressing an experience of life that he does not like and finding ways to change it. Were that the case, Thurber would have written a different story about a very different character. But his Walter Mitty adapts to the life around him by retreating into schizoid fantasies that bring him a far greater sense of purpose and heroism than he will ever experience without them, and for us as readers, a far greater sense of comedy as we read and reread his fantasies, finding new layers of hilarity each time through, until the final one:

> Walter Mitty lighted a cigarette. It began to rain, rain with sleet in it. He stood up against the wall of the drugstore, smoking.... He put his shoulders back and his heels together. "To hell with a handkerchief," said Walter Mitty scornfully. He took one last drag on his cigarette and snapped it away. Then, with that faint, fleeting smile playing about his lips, he faced the firing squad; direct and motionless, proud and disdainful, Walter Mitty the Undefeated, inscrutable to the last.
>
> (Thurber 1942, p. 51)

The comedy catches us at first glance, and it is a funny picture indeed. The wall of the drugstore in Waterbury transforms in an instant to the wall of a prison in a Romantic novel in which the imaginary Mitty will face down even his own death as a hero, unbowed and with a sneer of self-confidence. But there is more to it. In the content of each of the other fantasies both Mitty and the reader always see a way out: the Commander manages the seaplane, the doctor saves a life, the murder defendant assaults injustice, and the infantry captain may well come back from his dangerous mission. But in this fantasy, Mitty the Hero dies at the hands of a firing squad and against a prison wall—both of his own making. On one level, the final scene continues the hilarity of the story. But at another, it recalls the ancient Greek definition of tragedy as the expression of the hero's fatal flaw.

Thurber's Walter Mitty has no way out, either symbolically as the prisoner before the firing squad or in reality as a character who locks himself into his own imaginings. The story's underlying sense of a life being wasted—its connection to a sense of compassion with a universal source of human anxiety—here provides a useful comment on the nature of Schizoid Fantasy as a psychological adaptive mechanism. While living in one's mind has its uses in adolescence, like the other Immature Domain adaptive mechanisms, it takes on the attributes of a prison if it remains as a primary adaptation mechanism in adult life.

One problem in Schizoid Fantasy as an adaptive mechanism lies in the person's own recognition, or lack of it, that the fantasy life actually limits them. From the inside out, with no alternative viewpoint or experience, isolating fantasies may not seem like a prison, but its opposite. This may last indefinitely for some, but for others the natural push of individual psychological growth may bring new viewpoints and the possibility of change, as in the following, more mundane, clinical example.

THE LIBRARY WALLS: GROWING OUT OF SCHIZOID FANTASY

A woman in her mid-30s has met with three other women from her book club for a late breakfast on most Saturday mornings for nearly two years. The book club meets only one evening a month, but the woman and her friends have found that they enjoy the intelligent morning discussions among the four of them, sometimes triggered by their readings and sometimes not. The woman herself finds imaginative fiction particularly interesting, especially when it involves female characters. She works as a research librarian in a large municipal library. With her graduate degree in information science, she is especially adept at ferreting out hard-to-find books and articles. Scholars from the local universities and colleges value her expertise in finding arcane references from national library holdings, and local businesses often ask for her assistance in finding government sources on ownership and tax codes. Referrals for the library research services do not generally occur in person but come through the library's e-mail system. As a result, the research librarian spends most of her time during the day working at a computer and sometimes in the library's vast book repository. She prefers working in library research to working with other people and has turned down several offers of promotion. Where others describe the library as a large dusty collection of books that is slowly being overtaken by the electronic media, she regards it as an exciting place inhabited by authors and characters that for her live nowhere else. While at work, she often thinks of her favorite literary personalities as accompanying her at her job. Her friends and acquaintances include plain Jane Eyre, the goodhearted governess who triumphs romantically in the end, and Queen Guinevere whose name from an earlier time—Ginover—seems somehow more appropriate to describe the misunderstood woman whom most regard as a symbol rather than as a human being.

At age 31, she met a man 10 years older than she who brought a referral for a library research project to her office in person. He described himself as an administrative assistant in a large, prestigious legal firm that he joined after receiving a business degree in college. With low pay and no hope of promotion, he nonetheless took pride in the prestige that the firm held in the community. He and the librarian went out socially but infrequently over the next year and surprised each other when he proposed, and she accepted, his offer of marriage. Only his widowed mother attended the civil ceremony before a judge. Her parents, several states away, wished her well and sent money as a wedding gift. After living on their own in her apartment for six months, they moved into his mother's home, citing more room and less expense as their reasons. After that, she began taking on more work and spending longer hours at the library—in her view the more exciting of the two principal locations in which she lived her life. Her husband, although not an intellectually challenging man, was nonetheless kind to her and did not object to her long hours elsewhere. When they made love, every six to eight weeks on average by her calculations, she found him not unacceptable but in her mind preferred the company of Rochester or Lancelot. Her mother-in-law, likewise, was not at all overbearing and seemed neither particularly upset nor particularly pleased at her presence in the household. Of late, however, she had begun to ask her son whether they would be producing any grandchildren. When he mentioned this to her, she politely declined without letting him know that she felt completely repulsed at the idea. At the same time, however, she found herself wondering what Rochester's or Lancelot's offspring might look like. New for her, something in her mind suggested this as a sign that she needed more people in her life. She sought out, and found, the local book club for women through a local professional association.

She found herself especially pleased by reading books and having the opportunity to discuss them with others, although she made no mention of *Jane Eyre* or *Morte D'Arthur*. Her favorite book over the previous two years was Walker Percy's *The Moviegoer*. She liked the idea of larger-than-life people on screen but found something vaguely troubling about the book at the same time. As the Saturday morning brunches continued, however, she found herself increasingly drawn to the conversations with others, something she had not found of particular interest before that. Although the other members of the small group might miss a Saturday morning from time to time for one excuse or another, she never did. Over the past year, she had begun very slowly to share a few of the details of her life with her Saturday morning friends. As this went on, one of them commented one day that, like some other women, she had "married well beneath herself." The other two, in her perception, while not chiming in, had nonetheless not disagreed. Without voicing her feelings, this left her mortified and with a sense of embarrassment. To her surprise, her inward embarrassment did not go away over the next several Saturdays and in fact seemed to increase with each meeting. Finally, without meaning to, one Saturday morning she asked her friends what they had in mind by "marrying beneath herself" and broke down in tears, causing her to feel even more embarrassed. As they listened to her describe her situation, all three reacted in concert with the sisterly suggestion that this might be something that required the help of a professional, someone with training beyond their scope. Sensing a precariousness that none of them had noticed before, they added that they valued her and wanted to keep the Saturday morning brunch discussions going. A month later, the librarian sought out the help of a professional therapist, choosing one of the same gender.

Considered from the point of view of the recognition algorithm, the woman in the story has lived for a very long time with her fantasies as the best part of her everyday experience. Raised in the emotionally cold home of her parents—they send her money rather than attend her wedding—her fantasy life becomes more dependable than the people around her. Yet, to her credit, she does not function at the Primitive Domain level: there is no indication of ignoring or distorting her worldly circumstances or projecting them onto bizarre productions of a psychotic nature such as plots by angry gods or extraterrestrial beings. Rather, she finds a way to continue her preferred life of fantasy and still make a living. She finds a line of work that allows her the company of favorite literary characters during a day's time rather than the company of real people, whom she finds much less colorful and less interesting by comparison. She even manages to contract a marriage in the latter half of her childbearing years with perhaps a sense of its being something that she ought to do. But to an outside observer, her choice of a partner and their living circumstances continue the inescapable prison-like grayness relieved only by idealized romantic fantasies. From her point of view, however, life flows in much the same manner as before and her fantasies continue to save the day. Consistent with the Immature Domain mechanisms, all is well so long as any threats to personal equilibrium remain outside her conscious experience, while her fantasies keep anxiety, that personal sense of impending disaster, at bay.

The possibility of real offspring jars this equilibrium and does so very deeply, as one might expect from a part of human existence that has been continuously conserved in the biological evolution and psychological adaptation of human life over many millennia. Although her fantasies make a valiant attempt at managing the sense of an impending disaster in having children with this partner, they are simply not up to the task. Her Schizoid Fantasy psychological adaptive mechanism begins to fail her and leaves her with the sense of needing to talk to other people as a way of managing it. She goes on to find three "outside observers" with whom she becomes friends over a period of two years. Trust among them develops to the point at which they can share opinions and her friends' comment about marrying beneath herself strikes an emotionally resonant chord. Recalling the recognition algorithm, it is at this point that her adaptation to the stress of bringing new life into her world, both literally and symbolically, moves from Schizoid Fantasy "out there" to an emotionally charged problem in her own consciousness, one that she can share with her real friends rather than literary characters. Perceiving both her pain and their limits, her friends suggest that she look into professional assistance. After some consideration, she does so, rather than retreat into fantasies that no longer seem as useful as before.

This clinical example, focused on the point of adaptive change, illustrates the usefulness of the algorithm not only in recognizing adaptive mechanisms in the present moment but, as well, in systematically charting their growth along the recognition algorithm as a person moves from a lower to a higher Domain of adaptive functioning. In this case the shift is from Immature Domain Schizoid Fantasy to the higher Neurotic Domain mechanism of Repression, the subject of Chapter 12, in which emotional content arrives in waking consciousness while its cognate thought content remains to be explored. In this example, the librarian's tears flow forth now, although her understanding of their origin will require work with a well-trained therapist, a professional outside observer.

CONTINUING ON: SCHIZOID FANTASY AND ADJUSTMENT TO SEVERE ILLNESS

In instances of the previous kind, we look naturally to the progression and growth of human experience as it moves along the courses of individual lives. Progression brings with it the greatest sense of hope when considering our capabilities of adapting to the world around us. There may be times, however, recalling the clinical principle that people engage in the highest level of psychological adaptive mechanism at their disposal in the face of stress, that even the Immature Mechanisms provide significant adaptive value, and hope, as in the following clinical example.

The medical staff of a tertiary care hospital accepts the transfer of a man in his early 60s who requires stabilization of his vascular system after having suffered a stroke. Occurring on the right side of his brain in the area that manages control of the voluntary muscles in the arms and legs, the stroke has resulted in profound weakness on the left side of his body, leaving him with only a very small degree of motion in part of his left hand. In the process of evaluating him, the resident on the medical team notes that he makes occasional statements about "dying anyway" that seem to have the ring of passive suicidal intent to them. She asks for a psychiatric consultation to assess this.

At interview with the psychiatric consultant, the patient describes himself as a "loner" who prefers to live by himself in a remote area. He has a brother living 30 miles distant whom he visits infrequently because he can't stand the brother's heavy smoking. The patient himself is overweight and does not exercise much. He spends his time in an unstructured manner, largely "policing the area" around his rural home, by which he means raking leaves, tending the lawn, and other light outdoor activities. In the evenings he watches television. He relates having a few friends in the area that he sees perhaps one or twice a month when they meet for hamburgers near a local grocery store where he buys food.

When the doctor mentions that sometimes people feel down or blue after having a stroke of this nature and wonders whether that might be his case, the patient answers *No* and that he feels just fine. He says further that he has no suicidal thoughts and doesn't know why anyone would think so. The psychiatrist follows this by asking what his plans might be when he leaves the hospital. The patient answers that when he returns home he will buy some deep fat frying equipment and build a business selling fried turkey legs to his neighbors. He expects to make enough money from this to move down to Mexico, where he will "live a life of ease." Despite the unrealistic sound of this plan, the psychiatrist notes that bedside tests of his ability to think properly are normal for his age and education level and do not appear to have been affected by his stroke. The consultant thanks the man for their interview and asks his permission to keep in touch while he is in the hospital. He agrees to this and the interview ends pleasantly.

The man in this case, recalling again the recognition algorithm, has lived a very isolated existence with interpersonal problems and other such stresses kept far distant, even insofar as his living arrangements are concerned. He functions at the Immature Domain level with problematic matters located "out there" until, quite literally, they occur "in here" when the vascular system in his brain fails him, resulting in his stroke. As with any injury or condition involving the brain, the psychiatrist wisely checks out whether there has been a failure in cognitive ability that might have an impact on the patient's adaptive status. In this case, there is none and the focus shifts to the patient's outlook in the face of very severe illness. Despite innuendos to the contrary, he himself notes no particular evidence of a depressed mood, for example the classic triad of hopelessness, helplessness, or worthlessness. As the interview proceeds, however, it becomes clear that this patient locates even this proximate physical injury as "out there" when he describes his fantasy of starting a new business, making money from it quickly, and relocating to a warmer climate where he will live like an aristocrat.

The psychological stress, in this case, emanates from the fear that naturally occurs following a very serious injury and loss of function. Anxiety, that impending sense of doom, is never far away from consciousness in such situations. In this case, both the sense of fear and its anxiety serve as the basis for the compassion between the patient and the interviewing psychiatrist. That compassion allows an alliance in which both will recognize the Schizoid Fantasy that keeps the anxiety at bay, and both will treat that adaptive response in a mutually respectful manner. Fantasies of this nature sometimes call forth a desire in observers to tear them asunder in the name of truth and reality. Considered in the framework of our adaptive model, even fantasies of this nature serve as "true" psychological adaptive mechanisms and thereby make up their own "reality."

As in the case of the librarian whose Schizoid Fantasy adaptation begins to fail her in the service of a more mature adaptation, in this case too the responsibility for change does not rest with the outside observers. Rather, recalling the analyst-patient interaction in the case of the graduate student in Chapter 8,[3] it rests only within those who engage their own psychological adaptive mechanisms in what they perceive as the useful effort to manage stress and anxiety. Although clearly not the most flexible group of adaptive mechanisms, as this volume continues to illustrate, even the Immature Domain mechanisms, those that are most irritating to others in the patient's life, serve an adaptive purpose. The wise clinician will engage the recognition algorithm in a systematic assessment of the psychological adaptive mechanisms used by the patient who sits before him or her. The assessment then informs the processes toward support or toward change, as the patient indicates. In the case of the man with the stroke, in the setting of serious illness and few social resources, support is the wiser choice.

REFERENCES

Bleuler, E. (1911). *Dementia Praecox or the Group of Schizophrenias*. New York, International Universities Press.

Dickens, C. (1998). *Great Expectations*. Oxford, Oxford University Press.

Dickens, C. (1994) *David Copperfield*. London: Penguin Books.

Forster, E. M. (1927). *Aspects of the Novel*. New York, Harcourt.

Homer. (1967). *The Odyssey of Homer* (R. Lattimore, Trans.). New York, Harper and Row.

Thurber, J. (1942). The Secret Life of Walter Mitty. In *My World and Welcome to It*. New York, Harcourt, Brace.

3. See the section "Passive Aggression: Treating the Immature Adaptive Mechanisms" in Chapter 8.

Primitive

Immature

CHAPTER 11

Neurotic Projection

If anxiety can be politely tucked away in fantasies, or immediately acted upon without thinking, or sent inside to torture the body, it can as easily be directed outward—aimed at others whom we regard as the cause of all our troubles. Miss Eudora Welty, 20th-century American novelist and short story writer, lived nearly all of her life in her family's home in Jackson, Mississippi. Visitors who dropped by to see her of an afternoon could expect a kindly reception with tea and cookies. It seems both an irony as a person and a tribute as a writer that this gentle woman would introduce us to the horrors of Neurotic Projection as she takes us into the mind of a murderer, one who commits a killing based purely on race. Miss Welty wrote her story shortly after the murder of Medgar Evers, a civil rights worker and among the first to integrate the University of Mississippi, who was assassinated in 1963.[1] The killer speaks in this excerpt:

> Never seen him before, never seen him since, never seen anything of his black face but his picture, never seen his face alive, any time at all, or anywheres, didn't want to, need to, never hope to see that face and never will. As long as there was no question in my mind.
>
> He had to be the one. He stood right still and waited against the light, his back was fixed, fixed on me like a preacher's eyeballs when he's yelling "Are you saved?" He's the one.
>
> I'd already brought up my rifle, I'd already taken my sights. And I'd already got him, because it was too late then for him or me to turn by one hair.
>
> Something darker than him, like the wings of a bird, spread on his back and pulled him down. He climbed up once, like a man under bad claws, and like blood

---

1. Eudora Welty herself writes in the preface to her *Collected Stories* (1980, p. xi), "That hot August night when Medgar Evers, the local civil rights leader, was shot down from behind in Jackson, I thought, with overwhelming directness: whoever the murderer is, I know him: not his identity, but his coming about, in this time and place. That is, I ought to have learned by now, from here, what such a man, intent on such a deed, had going on in his mind. I wrote a story—my fiction—in the first person: about that character's point of view, I felt, through my shocking revolt, I could make no mistake."

could weigh a ton he walked with it on his back to better light. Didn't get no further than his door. And fell to stay....

I stepped to the edge of his light there, where he's laying flat. I says, "Roland? There was one way left, for me to be ahead of you and stay ahead of you, by Dad, and I just taken it. Now I'm alive and you ain't. We ain't never now, never going to be equals and you know why? One of us is dead. What about that, Roland?" I said. "Well you seen to it, didn't you?"

(Welty 1980, p. 604)

In applying the recognition algorithm to this passage, our first task, as always, is to look for the anxiety-raising stress that occasions the psychological adaptive mechanism. The unnamed killer, a white man, tells us specifically. He articulates the idea of a black man getting "ahead" of him and, for him, the intolerable condition of him and any black man being "equals." By verbalizing this comparison of himself to others in terms of worth as human beings, we immediately know that his sense of his own worth is at stake. At the same time, he thinks neither of himself nor of the black man he kills as unique, human individuals. Were he to do so, there would be no need for comparison in respect to being "equals," or "ahead," or behind; each would simply be a separate individual. But in considering both himself and Roland, each, as racial stereotypes. the figure of the black man represents all black people. The "you" in "for me to be ahead of you" can be read as plural—encompassing a whole race—as well as singular.

The fact that he must compare himself to others, and prove in every instance that he is better than they, tells the reader of his anxiety that this is not true. Using Carl Jung's model of the Self as one formulation, the conscious need of this man to prove that he is better than the man he kills reflects the unconscious content of what Jung calls the Shadow;[2] this is the equivalent of Freud's concept of the personal unconscious. In Jung's model, the Shadow is the repository of all the aspects of oneself that the conscious mind cannot tolerate. As an exercise for the reader, paying attention to all those things you don't like in other people—that is, in respect to one's judgment of someone else's worth—often provides a good catalog of what lurks in one's own Shadow. The Shadow—that is, the unconscious content—is unavailable to the conscious self unless it is specifically looked for. The resulting anxiety from the intolerable unconscious contents, however, is very much a conscious perception and one that appears triggered by people we don't like simply as people.

As a trivial example, Mr. Jones can't stand to be around other people who have red hair because at an unconscious level he thinks his own red hair makes him look particularly ugly. Consciously, however, he becomes very anxious and uncomfortable around people with red hair because he finds them particularly ugly and unappealing. In models of the mind that posit the unconscious as part of human makeup, including Jung's and Freud's, humans project their own unwanted attributes onto others in this way. So it is that Eudora Welty's murderer experiences his own anxiety—previously defined as a subjective sense of doom or disaster—as coming from a race

2. See Jung (1959, pp. 20–21).

of people he regards as inferior. According to Jung's model, the murderer's Shadow contains the unexpressed perceptions of and beliefs in his own inferiority.

Putting this back in the model of psychological adaptive mechanisms, the stress to which the murderer responds with conscious anxiety begins in the unconscious belief that he himself has little or no worth as a human being and that he cannot get "ahead of" or even be "equals" with anyone else. Eudora Welty adds a cultural inflection to this when she describes him sighting down the barrel of his rifle and finding his victim's back "fixed on me like a preacher's eyeballs when he's yelling 'Are you saved?'" She describes the preacher found at a fundamentalist Protestant revival meeting. According to the tenets of fundamentalist belief, man is born in human depravity because of Adam's Original Sin; this is viewed so literally, rather than symbolically, that it is often nearly palpable. So it is that Miss Welty's murderer starts out in a world that tells him he is evil. Add to this his poor grammar, suggesting poor education and perhaps low intelligence, and we can deduce that he lives in poverty, is poorly educated, suffers the unconscious belief of his own sinfulness as a symbolic blackness of his soul, and faces every day a world that points out how everyone else is better than he. He cannot get ahead of them and cannot even be their equal. No wonder a sense of doom walks never far away from him in his consciousness.

Having identified the stress, an unacknowledged one emanating from the unconscious in this case, and the not-so-subtle conscious anxiety that results from it, the recognition algorithm next asks whether he ignores the anxiety through use of a Primitive Domain adaptive mechanism. Where an adult in a psychosis due to a neurochemically imbalanced brain might pull the rip cord of denial and ignore the anxiety, or avoid it altogether, or blame it on signals from outer space, Eudora Welty's murderer does not suffer from such a neurochemical imbalance that might apply a psychotic distance between him and the anxiety. Rather, he suffers a long lasting, painful perturbation that does not go away.

Because he employs none of the Primitive Domain adaptive styles, the algorithm next asks whether he owns responsibility for his anxiety: whether he locates the stress that causes it as being inside or outside himself, with the latter characteristic of the Immature Domain adaptive mechanisms. Eudora Welty leaves us in no doubt when her character says that there was only one way for him to stay "ahead" of his victim and that was to kill him. The murderer remains alive, and his victim is dead. Because of this, they will never be "equals." And as a last confirmation, the murderer sees the fault in the killing as belonging to the man he gunned down for trying to be better than him: "Well you seen to it, didn't you?"

Eudora Welty gives us an unforgettable window on Neurotic Projection in her handling of this character. Projecting the unconscious "badness" onto other people and then perceiving them as making us anxious—conveying to us a sense of disaster or doom—is the nature of Neurotic Projection. In a more striking way than the other Immature Domain psychological adaptive mechanisms, Neurotic Projection locates the stress well outside the self where the affected person cannot resolve it with conscious effort because it is simply not recognized in consciousness. The projected "bad people" that this adaptive style judges as such are always "out there." Reasoned judgments make up an important component both of critical thought and of the processes needed for moving thought into action. Judgments based on unconscious projections, by contrast, never have to do with critical thinking because they come from the Unconscious, by definition never the home of critical thought. It is in this respect that one might hear St. Matthew's written version of Jesus' careful injunction to ignore the mote of anxiously projected dust in one's neighbor's eye and to pay attention to the unconscious beam of wood in one's own, as we might paraphrase it today.[3]

The psychological adaptive mechanism model of Neurotic Projection allows insight in respect to the nature of judgments and how to begin to recognize when they are reasonable and when they are not. This adaptive mechanism and its relation to unconscious projections mistakenly construed as conscious judgment provides a psychological basis for human prejudice. The root of the word *prejudice* entails a prejudgment, one formulated prior to conscious thought. Miss Welty's murderer projects his own unconscious horrors onto a whole race of people. In the history of human life, the same phenomenon has targeted ethnic groups, nationalities, religions, the poor, the rich, the middle class, the sick, and myriad other groups of people or individual persons who may become the object of someone else's unconscious projections. In part, this is what Carl Jung meant when he said that the unconscious can get us into all kinds of trouble if it is not understood and worked with properly.

Some politicians of our day consciously exploit the same phenomenon when they seek to engage and manipulate a block of voters who share the same anxiety derived from unconscious projections. Common examples often center around hateful feelings for some foreign group. The prejudgment process invites those in the local group who agree with the unconscious projections to join the political demagogue who seeks to take advantage of them. But this, like Neurotic Projection itself, is not a new phenomenon in the world of public affairs, as the next example demonstrates.

WHITHER CLEON?

Scholars argue as to whether the description of the Athenian politician Cleon, whom Thucydides hands down to us in his account of *The History of the Peloponnesian War* (431 B.C.), is an accurate portrait of the man. In the present discussion, we shall not be able to offer any clarifying data and, in the cause of full employment for historians, must remain content to let the scholars argue until new information emerges. But we can make use of the description of Cleon as it stands.

The date is about 429 B.C., shortly after the death of Pericles, Athens' wisest and best leader, in a plague that swept over the city. During the years of Pericles' rule,

3. "Stop judging that you may not be judged. For as you judge so you will be judged, and the measure with which you measure will be measured out to you. Why do you notice the splinter in your brother's eye, but do not perceive the wooden beam in your own eye?" (Matthew 7.1–7.3, NAB). And, alternately, "Do not judge, so you may not be judged. You shall be judged by that judgment by which you judge, and your measure will be made by the measure by which you measure. Why do you look at the straw which is in the eye of your brother, and not see the log which is in your eye?" (Matthew 7.1–7.3, NT).

Athens steadfastly adopted a defensive policy in preserving its empire against the Peloponnesian league led by Sparta. Having for many years opposed Pericles in a minority that argued for aggressive attack against Athens' enemies, Cleon and his faction now come to the fore. Pericles, from an old Athenian noble family, is a friend of the writers, philosophers, and scientists of his era; but Cleon, the son of a successful tanner, has very different views of educated people. Thucydides records one of Cleon's speeches before the Athenian assembly: a plea for force as opposed to Pericles' use of diplomacy.

> You forget entirely that your empire is a despotism and your subjects disaffected conspirators, whose obedience is ensured not by your suicidal concessions, but by the superiority which your own strength, not their loyalty, gives. The most alarming feature in the case is the constant change of measures with which we appear to be threatened, and our seeming ignorance of the fact that bad laws which are never changed are better for a city than good ones that have no authority; that steadiness without education is more helpful than cleverness without character; and that ordinary men usually manage public affairs better than their more gifted fellows. The latter are always wanting to appear wiser than the laws, and to overrule every proposition brought forward, thinking that they could find no more important field for their intelligence, and by such behavior too often ruined their country; while those who mistrust their own cleverness are content to be less learned than the laws, and able to pick holes in the speech of a good speaker; impartial judges rather than competing disputants, they are generally more successful. That is the type to which we should conform, and not be led on by cleverness and intellectual rivalry to advise her people against our real views.
>
> (Thucydides 1960, pp. 159–160)

Applying the recognition algorithm in our model of psychological adaptive mechanisms, what stress is involved as Cleon goes about his speech to convince the members of the Athenian assembly that they must act with force rather than wisdom? To answer this requires first an examination of the dichotomy he sets up in his speech between intelligent people and those who do not consider themselves as intelligent. In this translation, he demeans the first group by calling them "clever" rather than wise, and elevates the second by calling them "ordinary," the equivalent of a present-day, idealized "Common Man." He goes on to say that educated people who write good laws don't use their authority because they think too much: therefore intelligent people make bad governors. However, at the same time, ordinary people who do not consider themselves clever regard themselves as no smarter than the laws, and are content with bad laws and a stable government. He is careful not to insult the ordinary people by calling them uneducated and takes care not to call them unintelligent, calling them not "clever," the demeaning epithet he applies to his opponents.

Cleon aims his words at those of his fellow Athenian citizens who think that educated people look down on them, that intelligent people can't be satisfied with the simple law and order of ordinary people, and that educated intelligent people are too weak to use force to maintain the Athenian Empire. He voices a prejudice, in short, against intelligence and education that he hopes will raise the anxiety of his hearers sufficiently for them to vote in a way that will quell their sense of doom or disaster, that is, vote his way. The stress, in this case, lies in the intolerable unconscious projections of his Athenian fellows who vote—and there must have been a lot of them for Cleon to use this approach—and who see doom as coming from the educated, intelligent Athenians who look down on them. It may well be that Cleon himself, the less educated son of an upwardly mobile businessman, voices his own prejudice in this regard. If so, he was clever enough to see this in others and to manipulate it for his own purposes.

Referring again to the recognition algorithm, do either Cleon or his target audience pay attention to the anxiety generated by his argument that intelligent, educated people look down on them and make poor leaders? The answer is clearly *yes*. They not only pay attention to it, but they go on to make it a unifying political cause for their faction. If they had been responding to the anxiety with Primitive Domain adaptive styles, Cleon would be talking to a remarkably disinterested group who deny its existence or avoid it altogether. The group's adaptive style in response to their prejudices toward intelligent, educated people is beyond the Primitive in our model.

The algorithm next asks whether the roots of the prejudice toward educated intelligence can be recognized as originating within its holders or are ascribed only to external factors. Cleon's words leave no room for complexity in understanding the prejudice he articulates against intelligence and education in his Athenian colleagues. The speech, coming from his conscious self, reflects only the perception that the intelligent and educated are the bad guys who sneer at us and think they're better than everyone else. He gives no voice and no quarter to the unconscious fears of those around him, and perhaps of his own, that the members of his faction may not have the proper tools of government that can result in careful diplomacy and save both the Athenian Empire and the lives of its citizens. There is only the prejudgment based on reaction rather than careful critical thought. Locating unconscious fear externally, where it must remain unaddressed and unresolved, as in this case, identifies it as Neurotic Projection in the Domain of the Immature psychological adaptive mechanisms.

As the historical situation unfolded, Cleon and his faction were voted into power and tried to control the Athenian Empire with the use of military force at the cost of many lives on both sides. Not until Cleon himself and his Spartan counterpart died in battle a few years later, in 422 B.C., did a negotiated peace follow. Owing to the ubiquity of unconscious fears and the need to control the anxiety they create at a conscious level by projecting them onto others, Cleon and his faction do not constitute the last example of Neurotic Projection in the political arena. One need only think of the 20th-century examples of Nazi Germany and its persecution of Jewish people and other groups, and of totalitarian Soviet Russia and its pogroms against enemies of the state, that is, anyone who did not adhere to Communist Party thinking—resulting in the organized murder of many millions. At this writing, in the early 21st century, religious-based terror groups reminiscent of Eudora Welty's murderer employ the same mechanism.

In the context of the horrible examples discussed thus far, it seems entirely unlikely that Neurotic Projection could ever serve as a normal, useful psychological adaptive mechanism in human life, one that conserves or promotes health rather than destroys it. But this, as with all the Immature Domain adaptive styles, remains true in that tumultuous period of human development that we think of when we use the word adolescence. We consider this again in the next example.

EWW! GROSS! NEUROTIC PROJECTION AS A NORMAL ADAPTATION

Until recently, a 14-year-old girl has regarded herself as fortunate to have been born into such a fine family and to have lived under the same roof with her parents. But now she is not so sure. Where they used encourage her creativity and initiative, now they seem to have become remarkably testy, especially in her choice of clothes. "And, oh my God, as if they had any taste in clothes themselves!" For years, while puttering around the house in warm weather, her father wore polo shirts, Bermuda shorts, black socks, and tan sandals. "Black socks? Nobody wears black socks. How geeky can you get?" And her mother seems recently to have developed a nervous laugh that she voices at the end of any sentence that she thinks is particularly clever. None of them were clever, her daughter was certain, but that doesn't stop her mother, who thinks that every other sentence demands a giggle, a chuckle, or worse—a snort.

A few weeks before her birthday in late June, therefore, when her parents began talking about a birthday party to which she could invite all of her friends, she became ominously silent. "A birthday party! On a weekend! Black socks, snort laughs! Why don't they just buy a vanilla cake with pink frosted roses on it and the word 'Gross' written in cursive pink icing across the top?"

Clearly something has occurred here that involves the young lady's perception of her parents as having changed from people of whom she was once proud into people she now finds embarrassing at best. We can apply the recognition algorithm in order to gain a better understanding of this change in her parent's status from admiration to something less. First, we note that the stress, as in the other adolescent responses we have discussed in considering the Immature Domain adaptive mechanisms, lies in the normal physical and psychological development that ushers humans from childhood dependency to independent adult living through the creative transition period of adolescence. The transition requires addressing the anxiety it provokes that, were it continuously and always a conscious experience, would quickly become debilitating. As a result, although the stress of growing up lies out of touch in the adolescent unconscious, anxiety in day-to-day life requires an adaptation in waking consciousness.

For the great majority of adults, the Primitive Domain adaptive mechanisms that were once normal in early childhood have long since served their purpose and fallen away. The young woman in the above vignette does not deny the process of growing up, nor does she avoid it or ascribe it to some supernatural power. She does not use any of the Primitive Domain adaptive mechanisms.

To the contrary, she is acutely aware of the fact of growing up and as part of this becomes especially aware of social appearance in her peer group. Like most young people of her age, she wants to be cool in the perceptions of her age-mates and become part of their group. To her horror, she discovers that her parents have suddenly become the exact opposite of cool: black socks, snorting laughs, and all. To an outside observer, there has been little, if any, change in the parents themselves. The change, rather, occurs in the adolescent girl's perception of her parents, and has all the hallmarks of a projection. It is a judgment that seems to come out of nowhere; it does not match any objective change in her parents or their habits, and it appears to be driven by anxiety rather than any carefully thought out process of arriving at a conclusion. As a projection, it seems to say that if my parents are uncool at a conscious level, I in my unconscious self am terrified of not being cool and, worse yet, of appearing as such to my friends. That would be a fate worse than death.

In our recognition algorithm, therefore, similar to the other examples so far discussed in this chapter, an intolerable unconscious content transmutes itself into conscious anxiety that then has to be sent outward. It must be unconsciously projected on to the most appropriate target, in this case the young woman's parents. This adaptive maneuver serves at least four purposes. First, it renders the anxiety immediately tolerable rather than creating a constant threat to her equilibrium. Second, it allows the young lady to manage her unconscious stress-generated anxiety in workable doses as she moves, over a number of years, to an apprehension of her parents as surprisingly competent adults. Third, it allows the unconscious stress itself to work its way slowly into manageable consciousness as our heroine learns to question and think through her judgments with respect to what is cool and what isn't, when peers are important and when they are less so, and how geeky qualities may or may not characterize her parents. Fourth and last, like all of the Immature Domain psychological adaptive mechanisms in normal adolescent use, it serves the very necessary purpose of pushing her parents away in the service of her own independence and eventual functioning as an adult woman. She uses Neurotic Projection in a healthy way, therefore, leaning upon this Immature Domain adaptive style only for a time. Like the Primitive Domain styles of early childhood, Neurotic Projection too naturally drops away as part of a healthy jettisoning of adaptive styles that are no longer needed and have been replaced with more mature versions. As in the two cases mentioned before, however, continuing use of Neurotic Projection as a principal way of adapting to the stresses in adult life signals a psychological pathology, in those cases and the one that follows.

THE CHIEFS OUT THERE: NEUROTIC PROJECTION KEEPING THE INTERN DOWN

Once again it is 3 A.M., and the sleepless intern prowls the hallways of the hospital. His mobile phone has rung incessantly with questions and text messages from the nursing staff about the five patients in the ICU and the remaining eight out on the medical floor. One of the patients on the floor, an elderly man with heart failure, is doing poorly and may need to be moved to intensive care. Wherever he looks, the intern is filled with dread. It is as if people suffered illness just to torture him and take him beyond the limits of any reasonable physical stamina and far beyond the boundaries of ordinary compassion. A text message arrives instructing him to phone the ER resident, who this night happens to be one of the chief residents from a sister hospital in the same training program. The intern phones and learns that another critically ill person is on the way up to the ICU. Another torture meant for him.

He speaks few words, and utters those in an unemotional tone, and then hangs up the phone. "Don't give them any ammunition. They haven't got a leg to stand on, and they know it. All those chiefs, they talk to each other all the time. Who do they think they are? Lording it over us every chance they get. I'd like to see them get up here and do my work. They couldn't do it, and I know it, and then I'd lord it over them and see if they liked it. I'd watch their every move and tell them about every mistake, and I know they'd make a bunch more than I ever do. And do they compliment me? No. But all those other jackasses in my class suck up to them. You can see it every day. And who gets a pat on the back and the good ratings? Sure as hell not anybody who tells the truth. And they just can't stand that. I tell them when some other jackass makes a mistake when we talk over the cases in rounds every morning. I make sure they know I know. And then they just say some pansy thing back like, couldn't I be a little more diplomatic, spend a little more time on the feelings of others? What do they think this is, some kind of lonely hearts club? The feelings of others. We are to fix these people, and they are to get well. Any jackass who can't do that ought to be selling insurance, and they ought to learn that, the sooner the better. Those chiefs who stand around buttering up everybody else and look at me like I'm from Mars. Just who do they think they are?"

The intern finishes his shift at eight o'clock that morning. The next day, after a night's rest, he is summoned to his own chief resident's office and informed that his contract won't be extended into a second year. He just hasn't demonstrated the capacity to work well with others. The chief resident advises him to contact the psychiatry department and get help with his difficulties in his work relationships. The intern replies, "Drop dead," struts out of the office, and leaves the hospital for the day. When he returns to work the day after, his training director informs him that he no longer has a position at that institution. He leaves and never pursues or accepts any psychotherapeutic help after this or any of several subsequent occasions when it is suggested.

We recognize the intern's stress in this instance as an unconscious one: namely the sense that he is not good enough to accept the responsibility for other people's lives, a sense lurking in what Carl Jung would call his Shadow self. Because it is too terrifying to bring into conscious examination, he too, like the other cases in this chapter, experiences only its by-product—namely a potentially debilitating source of unrelieved anxiety. He too has to come to terms with it in some adaptive way.

Once again, we do not see him employing Primitive Domain mechanisms in this case. He does not distort his situation as unreal, or enter into a psychosis in which he blames his predicament on the messages left on the license plates of buses as they go by the hospital, nor does he deny that he ever acquired a medical degree and joined a training program in order to learn how to take care of patients.

Rather, as in the other cases of this chapter, he evidences an awareness of being in an intolerable predicament but blames that on other people, in this case a conspiracy of chief residents to undermine his excellence as a physician and to keep him from promotion. Reminiscent of Cleon's "ordinary man," he believes that the chief residents conspire to demean him and, like Eudora Welty's murderer, they will never let him be their equal because they know he will be better than they. By noting reflections of the content of his projected biases toward the chief residents, to the outside observer he creates a mirror image of the contents of his unconscious Shadow: he, not the chief residents, is incompetent at his job. They, not he, consistently tell the truth. He, not they, will never allow him to be a chief resident. He, not they, must consider that he is not good enough.

With catastrophic potential of intolerable unconscious content to upset already compromised psychological equilibrium even further, bringing matters of this nature into conscious thought is a tall order in any circumstance. So it is that when the chief resident counsels the intern to get help for his psychological difficulties in relating to others, he refuses. His Immature Domain psychological adaptive mechanism, Neurotic Projection, will not allow it. In this respect, he presents a clinical dilemma characteristic of this style of psychological adaptation: those who project their anxieties on to others whom they judge as inferior will very rarely, and sometimes never, regard themselves as needing help from inferior beings.[4] It is not until they begin to doubt the judgment that others are inferior and begin to entertain the idea that perhaps they themselves have some responsibility to question their views of other people that they will seek help.

This describes the natural process among adolescents as they move from their innate certainty of their parents as living on Mars to the slow appreciation a few years later of their parents as actually reasonably constructed Earthlings. If it is not an easy process, or a quick one, for adolescents, it is far less so for adults locked into Neurotic Projection as their primary psychological adaptive mechanism in daily life. And for many in that predicament, it may never change. However, for others, as in the next case, it may begin to do so with the passage of time and the continuing, if slowed, energy that humans possess toward psychological development.

I'VE LEFT WORD: A CLINICAL CASE

Twenty-two years after the end of the Vietnam War, a white man of average size and medium build arrives for an appointment in the alcohol and drug clinic of a federally supported hospital. He sits in the waiting area, his back to the wall of the room, and eyes those about him with a suspicion honed from long and frequent use. And like a well-worn tool, its substance has thinned. He cannot put his finger on the reason for it, but lately he has begun to wonder about his life and why it is that some of the people he knows seem to have an easier time trusting others than he does. He often finds himself fearful of others, for example the heavyset Asian man about

---

4. In another model of mental functioning, they may be given the title of personality disorder, paranoid type. See DSM-IV-TR (American Psychiatric Association 2000), as of this writing the current standard, with a fifth edition on the way.

10 years younger than he who looks like a sumo wrestler, who padded into the waiting room and sat down opposite him and is working hard to catch his breath. The Vietnam vet makes little noise and is nearly motionless as he tracks others coming and going through the waiting room. Finally, from a door farther down the hall, a doctor walks to the waiting room and calls his name. The doctor introduces himself, offers his right hand, and the man shakes it firmly as though a test of strength, and yet only briefly.

The desk in the doctor's office is perpendicular to the door and rests against the wall in an opposite corner. The man seats himself in a chair next to the door. When the doctor invites him to tell why he has come to the clinic, the man first says, "I want you to know that I told my sister I'm coming here today. I figured on being an hour to get here, an hour to be seen, and an hour to get back home. If my sister doesn't see me in three hours from when I started out, she knows to call the police and tell them to come get me out of here." The doctor senses a fearfulness in himself that he recognizes as coming from the patient who is sitting calmly with no evidence of danger. When the doctor asks why it is that the man thinks anyone would want to keep him in the hospital against his will, he replies, "Because that's what you people do." The doctor points out that this occurs only when someone wants to kill him- or herself or kill somebody else and asks whether the man has any intent in either case. When the man answers *no*, the doctor says, "Then there's nothing to worry about on that score. Perhaps you could let me know why you've come to the clinic today." The man begins describing a problem with street drugs that he hasn't used in over three years but now has become worried that he might start using again. The doctor suspects, however, that there may be something more going on that this man is finding difficult to talk about, perhaps something about his military service that seems buried deep in his past and well covered by a trail of illicit drug use.

They meet weekly over the next several months, and the man's discomfort in discussing his past gradually eases as his trust in talking with the doctor grows. They discuss the first few years of his return from Southeast Asia and the difficulties he had working in the civilian world after his tour in a combat zone as an Air Force mechanic. "It's like nobody I worked with stateside understood anything. They'd laugh. They'd joke on breaks. They'd just chortle like a bunch of damn fools not knowing that I could snuff them out in an instant and that anybody else could. What's wrong with these people? I kept asking myself. Where do they live their lives? Who do they think they are? It was like they lived on some other planet than I did."

"You kept watch on them," the doctor commented.

"Sure," the man replied, "somebody had to watch those dumb bastards. They sure as hell weren't watching themselves."

"Watching like that takes a lot of work," the doctor commented again.

"All the time," the man replied, "The only relief I got was from the drugs. And then they started to wear off by themselves few years ago."

"Maybe you didn't have to watch quite so much or so often," again from the doctor.

And the two continued in this sort of conversation for several more months. Then, on a Wednesday afternoon, the man came to his appointment seeming edgy and distracted. He had had a hard time sleeping for the past week, catching only a few hours nightly. He had begun to be bothered by memories of his combat buddies in the Air Force. The recollections would arrive when he tried to drift off to sleep at night and then made it impossible for him to quiet himself from wakefulness. The doctor, noticing this time a sense of profound sadness in his own reaction to this patient, quietly asked whether he had thoughts of killing himself. The man's eyes widened, filled with tears, and he choked out a *yes*. The two of them agreed to admit the man to the hospital, where he stayed for a couple weeks. The doctor saw him twice a week during this period, and they focused on memories of his buddies. In the process, he learned that the man had considered himself the inadvertent cause of the death of one of his comrades. When they exchanged lighthearted insults on the flight line one day, his buddy was sucked into a jet engine. The subsequent inquiry had cleared him of any fault in the matter, but that meant nothing to him, then or now.

In considering this case in the context of the recognition algorithm, our first task remains to locate the stress that flowers forth in anxiety in the conscious mind. In this case, the stress ascends to the surface in waking consciousness only after many months of careful, trust-building work in the doctor's office, a setting that one psychotherapist has called "a safe place."[5] Both doctor and patient learn that the perturbation lies in the long-ago death of the man's comrade in military service, a death that the patient believes he himself caused. Recalling Leo Tolstoy's statement that wartime comradeship creates closer bonds than even those of the family provides the perspective to understand that this death was the emotional equivalent of fratricide—the killing of a beloved brother. For many years its content had lain repressed (see Chapter 12) as a specific memory lurking in the unconscious Shadow, like an explosive waiting in a tightly closed bottle. But the contents of Jung's Shadow/Freud's Unconscious will always have their effect in waking consciousness in generating the sense of impending disaster that the person knows as anxiety. And that, applying our model to this case, the stress of causing a brother's death, even inadvertently, and its resultant anxiety requires an adaptation in the service of maintaining a psychological equilibrium.

Next the recognition algorithm asks whether the Primitive Domain psychological adaptive mechanisms are at work in this man's case. Although he presents to the doctor initially as someone who is worried about being kept against his will, this does not possess the character of a formed delusion that would qualify as Psychotic Projection. While the belief may be irrational, its source is not bizarre, that is, outside of everyday human experience: it does not come from hallucinated voices, from TV programming intended only for the patient, or from special directions emanating from the kitchen toaster, for example. It comes, rather, from the patient's apprehension in going to a clinic where he will talk to a psychiatrist knowing that that psychiatrists have the ability to commit people to a hospital against their will. As we shall see shortly, there is something of a projection in this apprehension—that the psychiatrist will think he is crazy—but it does not have the character of a Primitive Projection. Considering the other adaptive mechanisms of the Primitive Domain, we find no evidence that this man distorts his own perceptions of his anxiety or ignores them altogether. His adaptation is at a higher level on the algorithm.

5. See Havens (1989).

We next ask whether he locates the difficulties in his life inside, or outside, his conscious sense of himself. Only at the very end of his clinical progress does the perception of his anxiety—a conscious sense of doom reflected in his suicidal thoughts—appear as having something to do with him. Until that time, and for a great many months, his adaptation located the sense of disaster outside himself. Disaster is always on its way, and he is always watching for it. He sits with his back to the wall in a dangerous world. He is mystified, and somewhat resentful, that the people he works with in civilian life have no perception of life's fragility or its danger. They simply do not understand that life's disasters can always be trusted to occur and that the only hope lies in constant vigilance. And he comes to the doctor wary of a commitment order, of someone drawing down behavioral restraints that may limit his ability to respond to a disaster. Badness—that sense of doom that he feels—comes from "out there," just over the horizon, always waiting to occur. His adaptation is clearly in the Immature Domain, the psychological adaptive mechanisms that locate anxiety outside one's conscious self where it can neither be addressed nor resolved.

Within that Domain, what evidence do we have that the man in this vignette adapts by using Neurotic Projection? For one, as in the previous examples, he makes rapid prejudgments of others: they perceive inaccurately, while his own perceptions reflect the true reality of living. For another, the common theme of badness or doom carries through all his concerns about others misperceiving the dangerousness of human life. Only stupid people, those who are too ignorant to see the badness, surround him, and therefore they can't be trusted. For many years, his drug abuse distracted him from the disaster out there. Having given up drugs, however, he finds the sense of the badness "out there" returning and causing him to worry about resuming his dependence on chemical agents to relieve it. Like the other cases in this chapter, the problems are not his. They belong to the other people who live out there. This defines Neurotic Projection as his psychological adaptive mechanism.

As with any projection of this nature in adapting to intolerable stresses, the greatest importance lies in understanding what it is that the person sends outward, that is, the content of the projected judgments and beliefs. In this case, again looking at the snap judgments and his suspicion of oncoming disaster as mirror images of an unconscious Shadow content, the badness out there reflects an intolerable badness deep inside the man's self. The attributes that he ascribes to others are those that he applies to himself at the same unconscious level: that he is stupid, incompetent, and unable to prevent oncoming disasters, even to the extreme of causing them. As his case unfolds in the professional relationship with his doctor, this perception moves closer and closer in from its outside locale until it threatens to hurt him: to the point of being overwhelmed by his own badness and considering his own self-destruction as its natural course. After all, this same badness resulted in the death of his friend.

So it is that in the extreme forms of Neurotic Projection that are sometimes connected to the harm or death of others, when they move to more flexible, more internally located psychological adaptive mechanisms they may risk the very dangers that the person projects out on to others. Eudora Welty's murderer, were he to address his anxieties over his inferiority as something within him, would have to risk murdering himself, literally, in the process. The risk, however, brings with it the potential to resolve the stress that has lain untouched before.

The case of the doctor's patient above adds the understanding that one adaptive style—in this case Neurotic Projection—is falling away. It no longer works as a resolution, any more than the drugs did in this case. Something in that patient pushes him to move toward more creative, more flexible, more useful adaptive mechanisms that will offer much more control over, and satisfaction from, living his life. But the new adaptive mechanisms have not yet put themselves in place. And in the interim, there occurs a profound sense of vulnerability—very reminiscent of the "hopeless, helpless, worthless" triad of mood symptoms seen in different forms of depression. This carries its own dangers, including that of having very little reserve with which to meet threats of self-destruction. In this case, a hospital and an ongoing clinical relationship served to support the continuing change and growth that this man experienced.

This kind of depression, unlike other, more neurochemically based forms of that syndrome, also provides an indicator of a positive process and a good prognostic sign: change is underway. Even the most severe adult-life adaptation through a Neurotic Projection—often the most recalcitrant of the Immature Domain styles when it comes to seeking help—may include the potential for growth with the proper help. Psychotherapy with this mechanism and all of its Immature Domain cognates requires a careful, very patient clinician and continuous attention to reflecting the possibility—time after time, contact session after contact session—that what is "out there" may have something to do with what is going on inside. As adaptation mechanisms shift toward the positive, the psychological adaptation model can find use in both observing and measuring change. Humans remain capable of change, and for the better. But sometimes, as in the more severe cases of Neurotic Projection and the other mechanisms of the Immature Domain adaptive styles, change occurs with very great risk.

REFERENCES

American Psychiatric Association. (2000). *Diagnostic and Statistical Manual of Mental Disorders* (4th ed., Text. Rev.). Washington, DC, American Psychiatric Press.

Havens, L. (1989). *A Safe Place: Laying the Groundwork of Psychotherapy*. Cambridge, Harvard University Press.

Jung, C. G. (1959). *The Archetypes and the Collective Unconscious*. Bollingen Series, Vol. 20. Princeton, Princeton University Press.

Matthew. (1970). *The New American Bible*. Iowa Falls, World Bible.

Matthew. (1996). *The New Testament* (Richmond Lattimore, Trans.). New York, North Point Press.

Thucydides (1960). *The History of the Peloponnesian War*. Oxford, Oxford University Press.

Welty, E. (1980). Where Is the Voice Coming From? In *The Collected Stories of Eudora Welty* New York, Harcourt, Brace, Jovanovich.

Primitive
Immature
Neurotic

CHAPTER 12

Repression

The term *Repression*, like *Denial* and *Acting Out*, has found frequent usage in common speech; it usually means that something has been forgotten. "Oh. I completely repressed the fact that my taxes are due on April 15," or "I should have remembered that there was a social gathering this evening, but I must have repressed it." While this has some resemblance to the way we will use the word in the setting of clinical recognition of psychological adaptive styles, we can both define it and use it with a much greater degree of precision in the interest of recognizing Repression in our clinical work with patients and in other settings where recognition of adaptive styles proves useful. Let us first begin empirically with an example from a medical setting.

GHOSTS: REPRESSING PAINFUL THOUGHTS IN PTSD

An attractive, neatly dressed 45-year-old woman, accompanied by her husband of 20 years, arrives at the psychiatrist's office, having been referred there by her cancer specialist, who has advised her to undergo a bone marrow transplant procedure as the best treatment option for her particularly devastating form of Hodgkin's disease. The psychiatrist comments on her ruddy, healthy complexion, and the patient says that the chemotherapy she has received so far has put her illness into remission. Her oncologist, however, advises that this will not last, however, and the patient indicates that she and her husband have arrived as requested as part of the routine referral for the actual bone marrow transplant procedure that will be done in another state. Neither the patient nor her husband had consulted a psychiatrist before, and the doctor endeavors to set them at ease by explaining the routine and outlining the questions that he will cover.

During the course of the interview, the doctor asks whether she has ever encountered any physical traumas, such as bad accidents or injuries, that subsequently resulted in unwelcome thoughts that intruded in her usual daily activities, or resulted in experiencing flashbacks during which she appeared to relive the trauma, or gave her nightmares that woke her from sleep with a sense of terror. In response to this, she sits quietly as if thinking about an answer, and then, with gentle prompting from her husband, gives her reply. She relates that 25 years earlier, while traveling in Europe as a college student, she had been involved in an airplane crash. She had been sitting in the last row—"the cheap seats," as she said—of a small jetliner that had tried to land on an icy runway during the second of its four planned airport stops. The plane had skidded to the end of the pavement and through a barrier, breaking the aircraft apart forward of the wing section. Sitting within the relative protection of the aft section of the aircraft, she had escaped through the rear door and suffered no physical injuries. The next day she read in a newspaper account that the plane had caught fire and that many of the people in front of her were killed, maimed, or badly burned, something that she herself did not remember seeing. After telling the psychiatrist of her ordeal, the patient then goes on to say that she has no intrusive thoughts, flashbacks, or nightmares relating to the incident.

As she finishes this terse description, however, her eyes fill with tears and she begins dabbing them with a tissue, though she stops short of sobbing. In response to the psychiatrist's inquiry, she states that she feels sad. When he asks what might be causing this, she says, "Oh, I was just thinking about my Hodgkin's disease." When he inquires further as to whether her sadness might have something to do with her description of the airplane crash, she replies, "There may be ghosts there, Doctor, but if there are, I won't let them live. That happened such a long time ago. If there were ghosts, they would've flown away by now. Do you believe in ghosts, Doctor?" The doctor listens courteously and replies that people can mean many different things when they say the word *ghosts*. Taking a cue from her mention of Hodgkin's disease, he then directs the conversation back toward the evaluative process.

It is time again to apply the clinical algorithm with the goal of identifying the appropriate Domain that will account for the psychological adaptive mechanism the Hodgkin's patient displays in this vignette. Our first question is, what is the stress? Because we are now in a complex adaptive situation, the answer to the first question is likewise complex. On the surface there is a clear stress: the occurrence of Hodgkin's disease in an otherwise healthy, middle-aged woman. Who wouldn't regard the diagnosis of this subtle, and often dangerous, form of cancer as stressful? But to approach a clinical recognition of the appropriate Domain that this patient exemplifies, we will need more than an obvious cognitive statement meant to describe the stress.

Rather, in identifying the stress that accounts for the adaptive mechanism, the observer must pay attention to both the affect—that is, the emotional presentation the patient expresses—and the cognitive content—the idea the patient expresses, or again the thought he or she describes—that occur in association with each other from the observer's point of view. Stated more simply, we ask, what stress is associated with the combination of thought and feeling before us? In this case, for example, the patient's emotion expresses itself at the end of a very terse description of a tragedy long ago. The emotionally laden stress, in this situation, is likely not the Hodgkin's disease, contrary to the patient's statement, but the airplane crash. From the doctor's point of view, the woman's feelings made themselves known as she described the incident, suggesting a working hypothesis that her emotional expression has to do with the accident.

According to the clinical recognition model, therefore, we must pursue the stress as being the airplane crash and first ask, following the algorithm, whether the patient recognizes the incident as a stress or whether she treats it with concrete and utter avoidance, as in the Primitive Domain. When the doctor asks, she describes the incident, leaving no doubt that she recognizes and remembers it as a stressful occasion. No Primitive Domain adaptive strategy is at work here.

Referring to the algorithm, we next ask whether she perceives the stress as something that occurred to her and that engenders an anxiety that she must deal with. Or, by contrast, does she approach the stress of the incident as belonging to some other person or place, as we have seen in the Immature Domain of adaptive mechanisms. From the doctor's point of view, she clearly locates the stress in her own experience and acknowledges that it lives in her recollection, if only in a "ghostly" form, as she puts it. According the algorithm, therefore, she has progressed beyond both the Primitive and Immature Domains of psychological adaptive mechanisms. Our next task is to see whether she has ascended to that Domain of mechanisms, common in adult life, that Vaillant terms "Neurotic." To do this, we will have to add an extra layer of complexity to our diagram of the adaptive mechanism model. Figure 12.1 illustrates this.

NEUROTIC ADAPTIVE MECHANISMS DEFINED

As in the previous renditions, we begin with the stress occurring in a way that perturbs the conscious sense of oneself, that part of each human being that we have called the Ego. As before, this results in an increase in anxiety that, in part, signals to

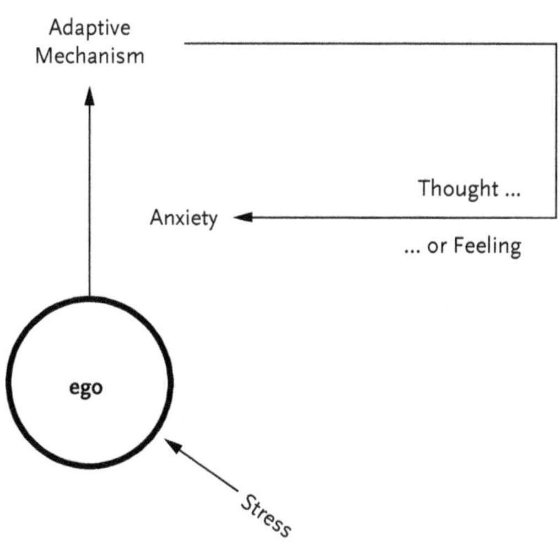

Figure 12.1
In the Neurotic Domain strategies depicted here, stress activates anxiety that calls forth the Neurotic Domain psychological adaptive mechanisms. These adaptive styles recognize the existence of the stress and locate the necessity of dealing with it within the Self. However, the painful thoughts and painful feelings that the stress occasions do not work together. The arrow separating thought and feeling represents this. Because they are unintegrated, they cause further anxiety and result in a circular process in which anxiety may continue but in which the stress itself is never resolved.

the person that there is a perturbation to be dealt with. The psychological adaptive mechanisms then engage to cap—that is, to moderate—the anxiety such that the associated physical and mental energies can be directed toward a solution to the problem the stress brings. By contrast, the Primitive Domain adaptive mechanisms do not acknowledge the stress, and the Immature Domain mechanisms, while acknowledging it, perceive it as having nothing to do with the Ego, such that its resolution belongs elsewhere. But to consider the Neurotic Domain adaptive mechanisms, we need something more.

We must now enlarge the model so as to consider that, from the point of view of the target Ego, the stress itself has two components. Put another way, the person responding to the stress notices two different experiences directly related to the stress involved. First, the person perceives it cognitively. That is to say, the stress presents an idea or thought content or cognition—using each of those terms interchangeably and equally—that specifically characterizes this stress, both as compared to all others as well as in relation to all others.

As an example, let us recall the Darwinian situation of a human walking in the woods and encountering a bear. Viewing the presence of the bear as stressful, as would be appropriate in a wild setting, the cognitive content of the stress would be something like, "Here comes a bear." The cognitive content of the stress—in this case the perception of the bear's presence—serves to identify the stress in conscious thought. Without that the human being would have no means of recognizing either a threat or any other kind of occurrence in his/her outer environment.

The same is true of stresses emanating from a person's internal environment, whether from unconscious sources or from conscious memories. For example, a college student awakens on a Tuesday morning feeling very bad and wonders whether she has the flu. As she continues to waken, she recalls that she learned the day before that she flunked a mathematics examination and feels even worse. The idea content of the stress might be something like, "I'll never learn this," or simply, "I flunked the test." She may then go on to think, "No wonder I feel lousy," as the cognition sinks in. There is no external "real" bear in this case, but the internal perception of inadequacy qualifies as a stress.

The phrase "sinks in" leads us to the second component than makes up the person's perception of the stress. That is the emotion, the affect, or the feeling—again each of these terms used in an interchangeable manner—to denote the second component of the perceived stress. In the case of the college student with the bad test score, the feeling may be one of personal inadequacy, frustration, or even anger, or some combination of these and others. The affect "sinks in" to the cognition, so to speak; the feeling "sinks in" to consciousness along with the thought.

In the case of the person out walking and meeting the bear in the woods, the affective content may be much simpler and more direct: stark terror. To the statement "Here comes a bear," affect adds an emotional valence: "Good God Almighty, here comes a bear!" In the cases of both the woods walker and the underperforming college student, the situations carry negative emotional valences—terror and inadequacy, respectively. As we have noted before in Chapter 7, however, emotional valences can be positive as well and still be part of the human perception of a stress.

Examples include "I'm getting married!" or "This is my newborn baby!" in which the affective content may be one of joy.

With the two components—the affect and the cognition—of the perceived stress in mind, our model of psychological adaptive mechanisms now asks whether they work together in an integrated manner in the Ego's perception, or whether they are separate, not integrated, and unaware of each other, so to speak. The disjunction of idea and affect—that is, the separation of thought and feeling—makes up the definition of the term Neurotic, both traditionally and as used in our present model. In Figure 12.1, the arrow from Adaptive Mechanism splits Thought and Feeling on its way back to Anxiety, rather than addressing the stress. This symbolizes the lack of integration between cognition and emotion. The model now arrives at a greater degree of clinical subtlety as it explores the relationship between idea and feeling. How does this relationship manifest itself in observable behaviors that we can characterize as psychological adaptive mechanisms? To answer this, we will return to the interview with the woman requesting a bone marrow transplant for her Hodgkin's disease.

In the process of taking a psychiatric history that, among many other factors, surveys for indication of stress disorders, the doctor finds that this patient becomes tearful after she relates a brief description of a traumatic accident in her past in which she saw other humans burned, killed, and maimed. The immediacy—the freshness—of the emotion in her expression tells the observer that her feelings—the affective content of the horrible stress—remain present and observable. This is a clinical indication that it has not been resolved—that the stress remains active in some way in her consciousness. The emotion from that terrible stress long ago may have lain out of consciousness for some time as she has gone about her life, but now it has surfaced in her present circumstance during the interview with respect to treatment for her own potentially mortal illness. The doctor sees the affect and gently follows it when he asks about its relation to the recollection of the aircraft accident.

There, however, in the woman's perception, the trail turns cold. In her perception the cognitive content of the event itself does not make itself available to her: she does not remember seeing what happened to the other passengers. She talks about the accident as "a long time ago" and insists that the "ghosts, if there are any," would have flown away. The doctor senses that the cognitive ghosts cannot be approached in the evaluative interview and does not press the issue. The patient's asking him whether he believes in ghosts suggests that at some level the ghosts have not departed and that the patient would benefit from an integration of the available emotions and the unavailable details of the thought recollections. This takes work, however, and in the doctor's judgment would best occur after the crisis of the Hodgkin's disease and the marrow transplant have passed. At the end of the interview, he sums up by saying to the woman and her husband that she may find some relief in reconsidering her ghosts at some future time if they trouble her.

Viewed in the psychological adaptive mechanism model, this woman's case presents the specific definition of Repression as we shall use it: in response to the stress, the emotion—the feeling content—is present in the person's conscious perception, but the cognition—the associated thought content of the stress—remains many miles outside the person's conscious perception. The idea content—the cognition—is repressed out of ordinary consciousness. It is in this sense that the two subjective components of the person's adaptive response to the anxiety of the stress—the idea and the feeling—do not function together in an integrated manner. In Repression, only the emotional content remains available in the subjective consciousness of the person using that adaptive mechanism.

To an observer, however, such as the doctor in this vignette, both feeling and idea may appear in obvious manners, as they often do. In this case, the tearful expressions of facial affect immediately observed and the horrible experiences that the patient read about but does not consciously recall both present themselves. In the setting of Repression, the doctor acknowledges the presence of the emotions the patient expresses. At the same time he recognizes both the thought content associated with her sadness and the fact that it is unavailable to her, and therefore knows that it is unavailable to him to voice in the conversation. Moving the thought content into closer intrapsychic proximity with the associated conscious emotions requires the focus and the hard work that an appropriate psychotherapy can provide.

The achievable goal of integrating the two provides the solution to the dilemma that their separation occasions. Until then, the stress itself is never really examined. In Figure 12.1, the arrow pointing back toward Anxiety symbolizes this diagrammatically. In this case, the patient acknowledges the lack of a resolution when she refers to her subjective perception of the chasm between feeling and thought in a metaphor: the disjoined feelings and thoughts are her ghosts. Symbolically speaking, her ghosts take on a repetitive quality because she has never put them to rest.

Clinically, this repetitive, never resolved pattern of continuing affective and cognitive disjunction constitutes another of the principal characteristics of the Neurotic Domain psychological adaptive mechanisms. Persons coming to treatment in this context frequently describe repeating behaviors that they do not enjoy or find troublesome, and yet that they feel powerless to change. Unlike the Primitive and Immature mechanisms, persons suffering from the repetitive effects of the Neurotic Domain mechanisms both recognize their pain and do not blame it on others. Because the pain itself occurs in consciousness, persons stuck in the Neurotic Domain cycles of promise and unrequited resolution will often seek help as patients. They do so in the hope of reaching that integration of feeling and thought that will allow for relief and for more effective functioning. In recent times, persons suffering in this way have often been described by the demeaning epithet "the worried well." The wise clinician will remember that psychic pain is debilitating and that humans function much more effectively without it.

REPRESSION, EMOTIONAL AVAILABILITY, AND GENDER STEREOTYPES

Because the availability of emotions to conscious perception defines Repression as an adaptive mechanism, and because women are frequently stereotyped as "emotional" and men as "unemotional," popular characterizations assume that Repression is an adaptive mechanism of choice, as it were, among women. Some take this to an even more extreme, if unproven, conclusion, namely that Repression is a more common defense among females largely because of their genetic and therefore physiologic differences from males. Conversely, males, by the same illogic, more often present intellectually based adaptations of the kind discussed in Chapter 13 on Isolation of Affect. While, to the author's knowledge, no large population surveys of psychological adaptive mechanism frequencies by type and gender currently grace the scientific literature to substantiate or refute stereotypes of this kind, in the present model each gender is equally capable of using Repression. The author makes no claim to being the first to note this. Others have done so, as in the following example from English literature.

Writing in the exact middle of the 19th century, Charles Dickens, who had an eye for characterizing the attributes of human nature, presents a scene near the end of *David Copperfield* that is apropos of our discussion. Over the course of the novel, the reader has gotten to know Dora, Copperfield's young wife who is alternatively known as his Rosebud. Called by this name that forecasts fragility and a short span in the blossom, we find Dora slowly dying from one of the unnamed wasting illnesses that seems to have claimed a disproportionately large number of Victorian heroines. But Dickens takes us inside the mind of this title character, who narrates the scene:

> It is night; and I am with her still. Agnes has arrived; has been among us, for a whole day and evening. She, my aunts, and I, have sat with Dora since the morning, altogether. We have not talked much, but Dora has been perfectly contented and cheerful. We are now alone.
>
> Do I know now, that my child-wife will soon leave me? They have told me so; they have told me nothing new to my thoughts; but I am far from sure that I have taken that truth so hard. I cannot master it. I have withdrawn myself, many times today, to weep.... I have tried to resign myself, and to console myself; and that, I hope, I may have done imperfectly; but what I cannot firmly settle in my mind is, that the end will absolutely come.
>
> (Dickens 1994, p. 626)

And a few paragraphs later, he describes his reaction at her death:

> It is over. Darkness comes before my eyes; and, for a time, all things are blotted out to my remembrance.
>
> (p. 628)

Applying the recognition algorithm, Dickens delineates Copperfield's stress in no uncertain terms. It is the death of Rosebud. Similarly, there is no doubt that Copperfield experiences this as anxiety: an oncoming doom that he can feel but not apprehend. Dickens does not write "Copperfield suffered anxiety." Instead he gives a deft portrayal of a man struggling with a reality that is before him and at the same time sensing that he is not up to the struggle. In this case, Copperfield recognizes that he is vulnerable to the anxiety and it troubles him. He does not blame his own response on anyone else. He is very sure that it is he, not the others in his environment, who finds Dora's incipient death difficult to comprehend. As with our Hodgkin's disease patient, Copperfield has passed beyond the Primitive and Immature ranges.

The next task in recognition is to ask what characterizes the cognitive and emotional components of the stress Copperfield encounters. For the reader, both are relatively simple. As outside observers, we apprehend the cognitive content: Dora will be dead soon. At the same time, we easily note that this is a very sad occasion for all involved, and especially for David Copperfield, who loves Dora. But both of those make up our perceptions and not necessarily those of Dickens' hero.

What does Copperfield feel and think as his author portrays him? With respect to emotion, David describes his own sadness as accounting for his weeping spells. He seeks consolation from an understanding that will allow him to resign himself to the coming loss. But he notes that his own ability to grasp the idea of his Rosebud's demise simply fails him. The cognitive truth of her death is far away from his consciousness—"far from sure," in his words. He has not reached an understanding of the event that matches his feelings about it. Nor does he do so by the end of the scene: Dora dies, and all goes dark in his remembrance, which is to say in his memory of her death.

Dickens, a man who wrote many hundreds of thousands of words, here in a few elegant lines puts the process of Repression before us in one of his characters. Copperfield's feelings and his thoughts uncouple completely. Affect is present in his conscious perception of Rosebud's death, but cognition has gone dark.

The chapter ends, the next one begins, and as the book concludes we find that Dickens' hero seems to have resolved his Repression rather than become locked in the repetitive prison to which the Neurotic Domain adaptive mechanisms can fall prey. He goes on to marry Agnes, the woman whom the reader has known from the start will be his true love, and the book ends with David Copperfield singing her praises. Would that all such psychological adaptive mechanisms might reach such spontaneous resolution in all cases! Very frequently in the great world, they do not, as may be considered in the following instance.

THE HOSPITALIZED MAN: REPRESSION BECAUSE OF THE PAIN

The psychiatry consultation team receives a call from their internal medicine colleagues to see a 75-year-old Caucasian man admitted to hospital the night before with an infection requiring intravenous antibiotics. As they get to know him, the medicine team becomes concerned that he may be depressed. They notice, for example, that he has crying spells that appear out of the blue during their conversations with him on ward rounds. The ward nurses report this as well and note that he tells them he is unsure where he will live when he leaves the hospital. At interview, the psychiatry consultation resident collects further historical data.

About two days before coming to hospital, the patient had returned to the United States after living for three years in Costa Rica. He moved there because he heard that the cost of living was cheaper, and that his modest pension could support him and a future wife there. He had further heard that Costa Rican women are anxious to find a (relatively) rich American to marry.

When the resident inquired, the now hospitalized man related the history of his many years as one that included three divorces from women to whom he been married for varying lengths of time, as well as broken ties with three other women with whom he had long-term relationships but never married. He had no children from any of these relationships. He grew up in a home with a violent alcoholic father and then lived with his mother after she divorced his father, when the patient was a boy of about six years. He described his mother as always one who had little good to say about men, certainly about his father, and yet who entertained other men in their home from time to time. The patient himself left home to join the service at age 18 and saw his mother only intermittently after that. He related that he had always had difficulty trusting women and his history suggested that he fared little better with men in a work environment. He was a skilled carpenter and always earned a steady income but found it difficult to work in the same business establishment for more than two years.

He sat comfortably in his hospital bed in no apparent distress as he related his story to the resident. Then, like the shadow of a cloud sweeping over a wheat field on a summer day, his facial expression darkened to sadness. He became tearful and began to sob. The resident found a box of tissues for him and then sat quietly while the episode ran its course.

The resident then commented to the patient, "You seemed very sad just then." The patient acknowledged that he felt sad. After a little time, the resident again commented, "Perhaps you could tell me what you were feeling sad about." The patient surprised him when he said, "I can't put my finger on it, Doctor. I just feel sad." Although tempted to press on with further questioning around the sadness, the resident thought better of it. He had an inkling that somehow no further information about the sadness could be gotten with specific questions. As the crying spell dissipated and the patient composed himself, they explored the patient's understanding of his illness and then conducted a cognitive examination. The resident established that this gentleman had a very clear understanding of what was physically wrong with him, as well as the likely result of the antibiotic treatment versus no treatment. At the same time, he was able to perform a series of bedside tasks that allowed the resident to conclude that his thought processes were clear and appropriate.

As they brought the conversation back around to his present situation, the resident asked the patient what his plans were when the antibiotic treatment was completed and he no longer needed to be in hospital. The man explained that he had used up all of his money, mostly from the sale of his house in the United States before he went Costa Rica, and had no income other than his pension. He had met many women in Costa Rica but felt that he could not trust any of them. After three years away, he noted that his social networks had dwindled. "I'm almost 80 years old," he said, dry eyed and with perfect calm, "and I have no one and nowhere to live." When the resident asked whether this might have something to do with his feeling sad earlier in the interview, the patient replied, "Search me."

Like Copperfield, this man suffered crying spells.[1] And here again it may be easier for an outside observer, in this case the resident, to perceive the link between feeling and thought in this patient's history than it is for the patient himself. Both the patient's own independent perceptions, and the observer's apprehension of them, provide the key to recognizing the Neurotic Domain psychological adaptive mechanisms.

Following the algorithm, the stress in the case of this elderly man appears contained in his statement that he has nowhere to live. But as his history makes clear, after a long life of repeated difficulty with trusting relationships, especially where women are concerned, the deeper stress seems to lie in his statement that he has no one. As in the subtleties of the description that Dickens gives David Copperfield to utter, we hear the anxiety in this man's case in both statements taken together. His response includes both his recognition of the reality of his situation and his clear sense that his disconnectedness is his responsibility, no matter how incompetent he may feel to resolve it. As in the algorithm, he does not adapt with a Primitive or an Immature strategy, leading us to conclude that he is at least in the Neurotic Domain of psychological adaptive mechanisms.

Are thought and feeling in his case disparate, or are they integrated and working together? Very clearly, his crying spells demonstrate the immediate availability of his emotions to his conscious perceptions. As with David Copperfield, however, any conscious relation of this patient's emotions to their appropriate thought content has gone missing. The cognitive half of the cognitive/emotion partnership absents itself. Baldly stated, the painful thought would be something like "I have never been able to trust women and now have no one to care about me." With the feeling present in his perceptions and the thought content elsewhere, this patient uses Repression as his most effective adaptive strategy. As his history makes clear, it appears to have resulted in a lifetime of repeated attempts at resolving his trust of others, to no avail. The Neurotic Domain psychological adaptive mechanisms occur frequently in adult life, as in this patient's case, but they do not of themselves offer successful resolutions to the stresses we encounter.

Nonetheless, the Neurotic Domain mechanisms so frequently occur in "normal" adult life so as to be considered part of adult functioning. That is, they occur in independently functioning adults who have progressed through adolescence, who require neither hospitalization nor the intervention of others to correct inappropriate behavior, and who hold jobs, maintain addresses, and find things

1. Medically sophisticated readers may be aware that one of the differential diagnoses for crying spells in a person of this age, especially when the spells appear to be independent of any thought content, is the pathological expression of emotions following subtle brain injuries, such as pseudobulbar stroke. A differentiating point is often the fact that in pathological crying or laughing, the patient has no subjective sense of feeling sad or happy. Weeping or laughing simply occurs as if on its own. In the case of the hospitalized man, by contrast, weeping is accompanied by a subjective sense of sadness that is appropriate to it. It also occurs in the setting of cognitive clarity, as demonstrated by careful clinical testing. These points may clarify differentiation in most cases, but some, especially those in which the subjective affect does not appear to match the objective expression of it, deserve further evaluation, including imaging of the brain.

to enjoy in life. As with the Primitive and the Immature Domains, we ask the relevant question, when are the Neurotic Domain adaptive mechanisms normal? Perhaps our recurring character, the sleep-deprived intern, can offer us some insight.

INTERN RAMPANT: REPRESSION IN THE SERVICE OF CONTINUING ON

Suffering neither from the ravages of a Victorian wasting disease nor the terrorizing howls of ghostly fortune, our intern has nonetheless found no respite in sleep. The early hours of the morning have brought no letup in the acuity of illness among the patients in ICU or in the calls for assistance and decisions in support of the care of those hospitalized on the general medical ward. As if by some pernicious cosmic plan, the inevitable phone call arrives from the chief resident in the ER with yet another acutely ill patient on his way up to intensive care. The intern meets the team as the gurney carrying the patient pushes off the elevator and into the unit. The intern takes over from there and with compassion and thoughtfulness reassures the patient, a middle-aged woman in a diabetic crisis, while efficiently organizing and directing her medical care. Everything goes well and three-quarters of an hour later, she is resting comfortably and in no imminent medical danger.

With a measure of professional pride and a sense of accomplishment, the intern walks out of the unit and into the hallway. At that point, however, a sudden sense of wanting to exercise surprises him and he heads to a deserted stairwell. He begins running up the stairs two at a time and finds himself cursing along the way. After two flights, he turns around and comes back down two flights and then up again. He repeats this two or three times and finds that his cursing accelerates as he feels himself more and more angry. Finally, in a furious state, he jogs down the six flights to the ground floor and out to the ER. He finds the chief resident somewhat startled to see him.

"You look upset," the chief resident tells him.

"Upset?" The intern says. "I'm so furious I could chew through nails."

"What's on your mind?" the chief asks.

"I haven't got a clue," the intern responds, "and if I did I'd probably beat the crap out of it. The patients are all doing fine but I could scream my head off."

The chief resident looks at him quizzically and says, "I got a little nap earlier. It's 4 A.M. Why don't you go upstairs and get some sleep? I'll let the night staff know to call me for the next couple of hours."

The intern thanks him, jogs back to the stairwell and up two flights, then takes the elevator to the sixth floor and collapses on the bed in the on-call room.

When we compare the consequences of the intern's behavior here in the Neurotic Domain of psychological adaptation mechanisms with those following the behaviors in the same stressful situation when met with either Primitive Domain or Immature Domain adaptive mechanisms, some notable differences appear. For one, no one carts the intern off to a mental hospital or calls the police to put him in handcuffs. For another, he functions well enough in his normal duties to be able to care for and stabilize his patients before finding expression for his own internal emotional toil. His anger in this instance has gotten the better of him, but he handles it in a contained manner. The intern approaches his chief resident with his dilemma in a way that allows him to verbalize his emotions rather than act on them or project them in one way or another. His relationship with chief resident has the quality of an alliance rather than that of adversaries. And although the intern voices only his emotions, and cannot use words to ask for help, his chief resident perceives his dilemma in a way that allows the intern at least some relief, if not a resolution.

Viewed in this light, most would see the intern as functioning well within the bounds of the very wide range of adult behaviors that we think of when we use the word *normal*. He struggles with his emotions, especially when they occur in response to the anxiety from a stressful situation. Despite this, he continues to do his work, to care for those for whom he is responsible, and he finds a way to ally, rather than estrange, himself in relation to others. To a greater or lesser degree, this is true of the other characters in this chapter: the woman with ghosts who maintains a loving intimate relationship with her husband; David Copperfield, who sees his Rosebud through the final days of her life; and even the hospitalized man, who maintains himself with his work as long as he is physically able despite the emotional privations of his childhood that block the way to his finding the intimacy he craves. None of them, in adult life, uses the far less flexible and far more limiting psychological adaptive mechanisms seen normally in early childhood or in adolescence.

Yet none of them functions at an optimal level and the intern is no exception. Referring again to the recognition algorithm, he both recognizes the stress of overwork—lifting him above the Primitive Domain range—and he makes the perception of it his own—rising above the Immature Domain. He is clearly in touch with his anger, even though he translates it into physical exertion that exhausts him even more than before. As he speaks to the chief resident, he is fully aware of being angry—he can voice the emotional component of his adaptation—but the fact of his being unable to ask for help—the cognitive content of his adaptation—remains unavailable. He literally cannot find the words because, in this model of psychological adaptation, the concept of asking for help itself is not in his consciousness. As defined in this chapter, he, like the others, uses Repression as an adaptive mechanism: the feeling content of his response to the anxiety of the stress of overwork presents itself in dramatic fashion, while the thought content that might formulate the stress of overwork into a request for help exists separately with no recourse to his awareness.

In the culture of medicine, the intern is by definition in his first year of professional training after medical school. In this example, therefore, we have yet to learn whether the sequence of his exhaustion, anger, and inability to ask for help will become a pattern in the setting of his professional life. Should it do so, it would then take on the repetitive limitations, and repeating pain, of the behaviors that result from the Neurotic Domain psychological adaptive mechanisms. The behaviors may be regarded as normal in the sense of a Gaussian curve, plotting out behaviors around a mean found among adults, but they cannot be construed as optimal with regard to adult functioning. The same pattern of suboptimal functioning occurs in each of the other Neurotic Domain adaptation mechanisms, a characteristic we shall see in further mechanisms in the same Domain.

REFERENCE

Dickens, C. (1994). *David Copperfield.* London, Penguin Books.

Primitive
Immature
Neurotic

CHAPTER 13

Intellectualization, or Isolation of Affect

The alternate titles of this chapter point, from different angles, toward the same process in this psychological adaptive mechanism. To intellectualize, in popular speech, means to express concepts without feeling—thoughts without emotion. It carries with it the mildly negative connotation that intellectualized content in speech or conversation has no practical use and little to do with everyday life. The connotation suggests a harmlessness of abstract thought and therefore its only mildly negative valence: nobody much cares about intellectualized content since it only matters to the individual who is talking largely to himself about his subject, or to the participants in a conversation in which intellectual constructs are themselves the focus of the conversation. As examples, consider a botany professor whose hour-long lectures include intricate details of plant cellular and molecular physiology, all delivered with his eyes alternately fixed on the two, far upper corners at the back of the lecture hall ceiling. Or an erudite scholar of English literature with command of the words and syntax of several modern languages as well as classical Latin and Greek, whose detailed presentations he provides to the one chair at the seminar table in which no one sat. Sir Walter Scott had something similar in mind when he coined the surname Dryasdust, for a character who preferred the background historical information of novels to the novels themselves.

The alternate title—isolation of affect—at first may seem vague as it may be difficult to see just how affect, emotion, or feeling—all words with the same meaning that we have seen in Chapter 12—can be isolated as one might isolate bacterium, a single example, or an individual. The term *isolate* here is better thought to mean something like corralled, or sequestered, or even quarantined. These words suggest that there is something powerful afoot that needs to be controlled or it will very quickly leave its boundaries and become dangerous. The affect, therefore, must be isolated in the interest of maintaining some form of stability. This returns us to our model in which some stress has activated anxiety that must itself be isolated in some way. At the same time, use of the term implies that the feelings evoked in response to the stress must themselves be limited or put in isolation. Consider the following case.

THE ENGINEER

On a bright, inviting Sunday afternoon in early autumn, a petite woman in her early 30s, with straight dark hair and plain features, trudges into the ER of a university teaching hospital carrying two large, heavy textbooks, one under each arm. She asks to speak to a doctor about the contents of the textbooks and insists that only a physician will understand the questions she has to ask. When she agrees that any medical doctor will do, the triage physician adroitly refers her to "the best doctor we have for listening to questions," and contacts the psychiatrist on call, who is one of the senior residents and a woman about the same age as the patient.

The two sit in an interview room, the bright sun streaming through the window. As they talk, the psychiatrist learns that the patient is single and a trained electrical engineer with three advanced degrees. She works in the research and development department of a technology firm that specializes in the component parts of highly technical machines used in molecular research.

The psychiatrist then asks, "On such a beautiful sunny day as this, what brings you to the ER?"

"Well, you see doctor, it's like this. I spent the last two days in the medical library, and I can't seem to understand several points that seem to be at issue in much of what I've read. I've checked out two of the printed texts that I brought with me for reference. They let me check them out since I didn't want to purchase an electronic version. In this first, for example, a textbook of internal medicine, I've read that multiple sclerosis symptoms can change from time to time and in location from one part of the brain to the other. Whereas, in this neurology textbook," she says, pointing to the other tome, "they describe a consistent downhill course that may include some variations but is ultimately difficult treat. It isn't clear to me how they go about reaching these conclusions. I am sure they must use scientific method in order to collect and sort data and then apply it in some way, perhaps not too different from what we do in engineering, but there seem to be far more variables in medicine than there are in the electrical work I do. So my hope today is to get some perspective and try to understand somewhat further the methods of clinical medicine and how empirical observation can result in meanings that aren't necessarily clear to all who assessed the same data."

The psychiatrist has already felt a wince, a feeling of alertness, a notation, at the mention of multiple sclerosis. Contrary to the patient's matter-of-fact description of the contradictions in the two textbooks, the psychiatrist senses fearfulness behind the patient's words.

She asks, "Here we are on a beautiful Sunday afternoon. I wonder whether there might be some reason for your concern about sorting out the contradictions between these two sources that brings you in today."

The patient, with direct eye contact, says unemotionally and in a tone that she might use in taking a reading from one of her instruments, "Oh yes, Doctor. I should have mentioned. My doctor sent me to a neurologist whom I saw last Friday who said I had multiple sclerosis. Now, can we get back to my questions on data? I've marked some of the passages we might want to consider."

The psychiatrist listens carefully and then gently brings the conversation around to consider that "other people I've talked with who have heard similar diagnoses from their doctors sometimes find it a little frightening. When that happens, having someone to talk to about it often eases things."

They discuss this, at arm's length where the patient is concerned, and arrive at arranging an appointment for the patient to be seen the next day by a therapist in the psychiatry clinic.

Using the recognition algorithm, we begin by characterizing the stress that has brought this particular psychological adaptive mechanism forward into an observable behavior pattern. In this vignette, the engineer's recently diagnosed multiple sclerosis—a fearful illness of the brain and nervous system with changing, and often unpredictable symptoms—gives substance to that stress. The normal sense of anxiety from any diagnosis—a phenomenon that we defined earlier as the experience of an impending sense of disaster or doom—worsens in this case by the diagnosis of a condition that can result in actual personal and physical disaster.

Moving further along the algorithm, the observer next ascertains whether the person recognizes the stress. In this case, the engineer clearly does. Her behavior tells us that it has sent her to the medical library, a place she does not normally frequent, in order to learn more about her diagnosis from expert sources. The observer must then question whether, having recognized it, she casts it out of her conscious sense of herself as being someone else's responsibility to deal with. She answers this, too, by her behavior: she appears at the ER door loaded down with medical textbooks, asking for help in her understanding. Rather than putting off the people around her, she creates a sense of something heroic about her in the effort to understand her illness using the best means that she has available. This is her intellect, the biological basis of which suffers now under the threat of her illness. From the point of view of adaptive mechanism recognition, her response to the anxiety of the stress does not qualify for either the Primitive or Immature Domains.

The next criterion in characterizing the Neurotic psychological adaptive mechanisms with reference to Figure 12.1 asks whether the intellectual and the emotional contents of her perception of the stress appear disjoined or integrated: working together, or functioning independently of, and we might even say unchecked by, each other. Her behavior likewise answers this. We notice that she presents herself as though she were trying to solve a crossword puzzle. The vertical and the horizontal words don't match, however, and this in turn results in an even greater interest as to why they don't match and how people go about assessing the clues in a case like that. We don't learn of the stress until, at interview, the psychiatry resident asks why it is that she gives up an enjoyable Sunday afternoon to present her scientific conundrum to the ER. And she goes on at length in describing the summarized data on multiple sclerosis that she finds in the medical textbooks in a way that is reminiscent of Professor Dryasdust, feeling at home in the world of facts while completely estranged from the world of emotions. The observer reasonably concludes that her discussion in response to the stress and its anxiety fills the room with her cognitive processes, perhaps to the point of boredom for anyone listening passively, as she goes further and further into detail.

If it is clear to the observer that the information content is present, where can we find her feelings? If we go back a few paragraphs to the patient's account at the point where we learn of her multiple sclerosis, we may recall a sense of fright when first reading those words. If so, we have located, at least in part, the emotion of the situation: it is reflected in *our* feelings as we hear the story, similar to the experience of the "listening doctor." The psychiatry resident clearly tunes in when she notices her own "wince" during the interview. In both cases, the reader and the resident, we see examples of what in the clinical behavioral sciences is referred to as *transference*. One noted teacher in the author's experience defined it as "the patient's emotional baggage" that he or she hands to the interviewer.[1] The ability of the interviewer, and in this case of the reader, to sense the patient's emotional content in themselves at the time—that is, to recognize the patient's emotional baggage by paying attention to its reflection in their own feelings—refers to the transference reaction in that setting.[2]

In clinical situations, transference is a tool in common use in a number of different settings and models,[3] as well as in the psychological adaptive mechanism model used here. It finds a particular usefulness in considering Isolation of Affect/Intellectualization, however, because it makes clear that the person's emotional baggage lies well outside of her conscious experience. To the psychiatry resident, the patient's transference is her fear, and that is very far away from her conscious sense of herself. Another prominent teacher once described fear as that emotion against which we are most heavily defended—the one we least like to experience in comparison to other difficult emotions such as anger or sadness.[4] And yet we as readers can sense the engineer's fear in the above account, not necessarily as a clinical tool, but simply because of our human ability to sense the emotions of others. The words *sympathy* and *compassion*, the first derived from Greek and the second from Latin, both mean to "feel with" another person, that is, to share their emotion.

Returning to the algorithm with this human capacity for shared feeling in mind, we may therefore conclude that the cognition of receiving a serious diagnosis remains in the engineer's immediately conscious thought, while the accompanying emotion lives within those of us who hear or read of her experience rather than within her own conscious perception. We may therefore conclude as observers that emotion and thought by no means work together in this patient's adaptive style and that we are once again in the Neurotic Domain of psychological adaptive mechanisms.

Reflecting on Intellectualization, or Isolation of Affect, in this chapter, in comparison to Repression in the last, we can see that in many ways we are dealing with

---

1. The late Norman Zinberg, M.D., of Boston, Massachusetts, who taught at The Cambridge [City] Hospital.

2. This is sometimes erroneously referred to as *countertransference* rather than the *transference reaction*. By convention, *countertransference* refers to the interviewer's own emotional baggage in this dyad situation. It is vitally important to keep the two properly defined in the interest of keeping the interviewer's countertransference—his/her emotional baggage—out of the clinical encounter.

3. Freudian and later forms of psychoanalysis use the term *transference*. Sullivan's interpersonal psychiatry uses *parataxic distortion* to denote the same phenomenon in a different theoretical framework.

4. George Vaillant, M.D., who also taught at The Cambridge [City] Hospital.

two sides of the same coin. In Intellectualization, the stressful thought is present in consciousness and the associated painful feeling is miles away. In Repression, by contrast, the feeling content is clear and present in the person's consciousness but the associated thought content rests miles away. In dealing with thought and feeling disjoined in this manner, the object of psychotherapy in one or another of its forms entails assisting the patient to link the two in consciousness. This must occur in order for them to work together in moving toward a more effective, more flexible adaptation to the stress and its anxiety. In some instances this can be a very difficult task, while in others the two resolve in short order, as in the next example.

A CASE OF AUTOPSY: TRACKING THE ISOLATED AFFECT

Consider a man in his mid-30s who is gainfully employed in oil and gas exploration and has a family, but whose liver is failing as a result of a hepatitis virus infection. In the course of a routine psychiatric evaluation for a liver transplant procedure, the patient describes being unable to sleep. He finds it difficult to fall asleep and cannot sustain sleep for more than a few hours at a time. At first his insomnia appeared to be due to his liver failure, but this condition had remitted somewhat and doesn't account for it. His liver doctors then tried a series of sleep medications, none of which appeared to work. Finally, not sure what else to do, they referred him back to the psychiatrist, who requested, and was given, the patient's permission to do a video interview for teaching purposes. As the interview began, the psychiatrist asked the patient why he had come to the clinic.

The patient responded, "I found my skin a yellowish color one day and went to see my doctor. He evaluated it and, when they did an autopsy, they found that I had liver failure." Asked if he meant *biopsy* instead of *autopsy*, the patient chuckled nervously and said that he meant to say *biopsy*. The interviewer followed the trail that began with the word *autopsy* with a conversation about the man's possibly being worried about dying from his liver disease. At first, the patient's reaction was a list of how successful liver transplantation had become nowadays, as well as his enthusiasm for this life-saving form of treatment. But, through the course of the interview, he began to allow the idea that there might be some fear involved and agreed to a trial of six weekly sessions of psychotherapy focused on addressing this fear. After two sessions, he noted being able to sleep through the night, and after six, both he and his therapist concluded that both his cognition and emotion were now available to him.

Considering this case from the algorithm's point of view, we have no evidence for either the lack of recognition of the stress of liver failure as seen in Primitive Domain adaptive mechanisms or the suggestion that liver failure is someone else's problem, as would be consistent with Immature Domain mechanisms. This man clearly understood and could describe the thought content related to his liver failure and its treatment. But at first, his consciousness lived far away from the fears that came to haunt him at night. He had Isolated the Affect from the idea of a liver transplant, consistent with that adaptation mechanism. When this became clear to his caregivers, he made use of the assistance he needed in order to make his affect and his cognition partners for the purpose of adapting to his medical condition. This had the effect of lessening the anxiety that had kept him awake nights. In the propitious setting of psychotherapy and over a short space of time, this patient made use of the human capacity to grow into more adaptable styles. In other cases, this may be much more difficult and may not happen at all. As further examples of both adaptation and the ability of others to perceive painful feelings that we cannot perceive in ourselves, consider the following scene from Wallace Stegner's novel.

ALL THE LITTLE LIVE THINGS: SENSING THE ISOLATED AFFECT IN SOMEONE ELSE

The scene is a hot afternoon in California in the mid-1960s. Marian, in her late 20s, the wife of a young science professor, carries her first pregnancy, several months after treatment for breast cancer. She has just plodded up a hill to join a retired couple, Joe and his wife Ruth, on their garden patio. Joe tells the story:

> The haggard look which Marian had worn when she arrived was smoothing out, almost as if it had been only the effect of the heat and the hill. I looked for the scared or distressed or begging expression I thought I had caught earlier, and all I saw was her usual amused combativeness. She said to me, "Pain is a form of pleasure, don't you know that?"
>
> "You meant when it quits."
>
> "No, pain itself."
>
> "Only for sadists and masochists," I said. "For thee and me, pleasure extends only to the near edge of the uncomfortable."
>
> "But when it's summer don't you like it to be real *hot* old summer, and when its winter don't you like it to *freeze*? Pain makes things valuable. How would women feel if having babies was as easy as picking apples? Don't you get pleasure—satisfaction—no, pleasure it really is—out of all the rough, hot, cold, scratchy, hard, uncomfortable things?"
>
> "No." ...
>
> "You wouldn't have made this [garden] so beautiful if it didn't please you," Marian said, "and it wouldn't please you so much if it wasn't hot and dry all around.... What's an oasis without a desert around it? What's a garden if you don't come to it from a dirty street or a closed-in house?" ...
>
> I saw the slight awkward stiffness of her left arm.
>
> A cold finger was laid on my insides. I could not help appraising the false breast swelling above the real swelling of her pregnancy.... Would I have so doted on this girl if she had not been maimed and threatened? Was it to herself or to her danger that I responded with so much anxious solicitude? Talk about the need for contrast in a garden! She was herself, if one believed her thesis, the indispensable reminder of danger and pain to make this sanctuary blessed. She saw stars by daylight because she lived down a well, and she watched them with passion because any day the cover might go on and she might be bottled forever in the dark....

> I said angrily…"Pain is fine when you can turn it off. It may even be good for the soul in small quantities, the way strychnine in small quantities is good for sick hearts. But they don't arrange pain in this world so you can turn it off when you want.… Pain is poison! Don't go hunting for it. Never praise it. Avoid it all you can and bear it if you must, but never never never mistake it for something desirable!"…
>
> I met Marian's eyes. She smiled tentatively, willing at a hint to forget this awkward moment and go back to the playful heckling that was our minds' habitual disguise.
>
> (Stegner 1967, pp. 207–213)

Regarding this passage in terms of the adaptive recognition model, let us focus on Marian and her reaction to the advanced cancer, as well as the pain she experiences, both of which qualify for our definition of stresses that engender anxiety. She clearly recognizes their occurrence and the fact that the cancer is something she herself must adapt to, by definition therefore moving beyond Primitive Domain and Immature Domain mechanisms, respectively. She goes on to discuss the existential advantages of her cancer and its pain in terms that might apply to Chapter 16's discussion of Reaction Formation, another of the Neurotic Domain mechanisms in the adaptive model. As in this perspective-widening example, humans can deploy more than one psychological adaptive mechanism at a time and, viewed in respect to the adaptive mechanism that is our focus in this chapter, we may ask where Marian places her emotion as she describes the difficulties to which she must adapt. Neither in this vignette nor anywhere else in the novel does Marian voice any upset. The character who becomes emotionally perturbed and expressive isn't Marian but Joe. And he becomes infuriated. He not only senses his own reaction, but he voices it in a way that he finds embarrassing. Marian will not participate in it and distances herself from it, leaving Joe to pick up the pieces of his emotions on his own.

If we think of Joe's anger as an example of this compassion, the scene takes on at least a suggestion that he is reacting to Marian's anger as well. From that point of view, some aspect of Marian's adaptation includes isolating that angry affect in a way that Joe can perceive but in a way that she does not. We can construe, therefore, the disjunction between Marian's cognition and the location of her affect as fitting our model formulation of the Neurotic Domain mechanism of Isolation, or Intellectualization.

Clinically, like Stegner's fictional Marian and Joe, intellectualization may often show up in couples who seek help in their relationship, usually in a marriage. One of the couple may be good at Isolating Affect and the other, like Joe, good at sensing it. As this becomes a repeating pattern—recalling repetition as characteristic of the Neurotic Domain adaptive mechanisms—the intellectualizing partner regards the other as overly emotional and often distraught, and the emotional partner comes to regard the other as unbearably cold and insensitive. The current model suggests that part of a therapist's task in that instance includes assessing the consistent adaptive styles that each of the partners uses in respect to assisting both parties to change. Although psychotherapy itself, whether individual, for couples, or in some other format, is beyond the scope of this discussion, the model itself can offer practical usefulness in assessing both the present state of adaptive mechanisms and in recognizing changes to more mature adaptive styles—the goal of most psychotherapies in this model.

In practical use, therefore, appropriate adaptive mechanism recognition can provide one window for observing change as humans develop their adaptive abilities. Likewise, however, it can also indicate change when specific psychological adaptive mechanisms fail, as when the stress becomes so overwhelming as to render a specific mechanism ineffective or poorly effective. Let us see what our intern might have to teach us on the subject.

SHERLOCK INTERN: WHEN ANALYTIC THOUGHT IS NOT ENOUGH

"I am a brain, Watson. The rest of me is a mere appendix. Therefore, it is the brain I must consider."[5] The words of the great detective Sherlock Holmes comfort our overworked medical intern as they cycle through his thoughts in sleepless consciousness at 2:30 A.M. The world seems to him so full of pain and suffering. There are seven ill patients on the medicine ward and four more very ill patients in intensive care. What is there to do but understand their illnesses one by one and in great detail? It is only by understanding—using one's brain, Watson—that one can walk on the solid ground of an island in this sea of human misery. How precious was that understanding as he was growing up?[6] His mother, distant and cold, valued above all else the family's social reputation and their being perceived as something better than their lower-middle-class reality. His father avoided hours spent at home with his children as much as he could and when he was home preferred the company of his newspaper to theirs. It was important to do well in school and to find he could understand things and understand them easily. If not applause, at least recognition came at school from teacher after teacher who told him he did well, from friends who admired him for his understanding, and even from those he did not like, who complimented him with their jealousy. And now he finds that that same understanding would give him solid footing among the waves of people who came to him for his understanding and the promise that it would make their lives, if not easier or whole again, at least more bearable. His brain was on call and at their service. The rest was a mere appendix.

The night charge nurse in the ICU waves him to the phone. He takes the receiver from her and hears the voice of the chief resident in the ER describing the facts of a new admission coming to intensive care: a very ill man in his 70s who has had the first seizure of his life and is now showing signs of partial paralysis. "A diagnostic puzzle worthy of the brain," the intern thinks to himself, "a true challenge. One that

5. Doyle (2009, p. 7).

6. This version of the intern, our stalwart recurring character, finds part of its basis in the model of social phobia, that syndrome characterized by anxiety difficulties in relating to other people, a tendency toward isolative behavior, and recourse to intellectualized adaptive styles. It often occurs in the context of an adult's having experienced a bleak childhood with a limited range of interpersonal development.

I will meet and bring to bear on it the logic of modern science in parsing out the differential diagnoses, whether common or requiring more subtle differentiation."

As he puts down the receiver, the charge nurse becomes concerned. The intern looks ashen, and his eyes glaze over as though staring into distance. She worries that he is exhausted and at the end of his rope.

"Are you all right?" she asks.

He stares at her with a blank expression and mumbles some quotation about someone named Watson. He finds two sheets of paper and begins diagramming a series of circles with the names of various diagnostic entities written in each and connected by a series of lines, some with arrows, some without. He begins telling her that he has a terrible headache but intends to pursue the differential diagnosis for the patient coming up from the ER. She notes her worry changing into a vague combination of anger and sadness: there is something about him that makes her think he might be angry about the new admission but also something that suggests a terrific sadness in him reaching some kind of limit that he could not predict. She notices that as he continues to draw the circles and lines, they become less and less exact, and more and more as though they were written by someone experiencing muscle paralysis. Finally, the diagramming stops altogether and the intern lays his head on the desk with a quiet moan of pain from "a terrific headache." She phones the chief resident in the ER, who comes up to evaluate the situation. The chief calls in backup help and admits the intern to hospital for observation of his symptoms.

With further recourse to our model of psychological adaptive behavior, we begin the algorithm with the identification of the stress. In this case, the surface stress is clearly overwork with little rest. Does the intern perceive this as a stress? In his own characteristic way, he does when he translates it into a "challenge." Does he recognize it as a stress that he must face rather than ascribe the responsibility for the next patient and his overwork to others? He locates the stress and the anxiety within himself when he construes the oncoming diagnostic puzzle as a challenge to his intellect, one that he must meet. In the terms of the recognition algorithm, therefore, he functions above the Psychotic Domain and the Immature Domain adaptive ranges.

The algorithm next asks whether his emotions and thoughts are working together or apart. His intellect has served him well in helping him find safety in understanding the cold and uncaring world around him. The world of his experience is itself one of little feeling and less emotional warmth. And here, in what he perceives as an ocean of misery, he clings to his brain as to a lifeboat, his brain symbolizing that intellectual capability that has preserved him to this point. In his experience, he is cognitive content. The rest is a mere appendix.

To the charge nurse, however, he is a human being whose feelings appear to be overwhelming him, causing her to worry. It is she who perceives his anger and his sadness at feeling somehow unprepared to navigate the waves of human misery. From the point of view of the adaptive schema in Figure 12.1, his feelings are largely unavailable to him but can be apprehended by an outside observer, in this case the charge nurse. From the observer's point of view, there is a deeper stress than simply the workload late at night. The possibility of needing something more than just repeated solutions to intellectual puzzles—a requirement for some kind of kind of leavening to set the burden of responsibility for the lives of others in some workable perspective—and finding that ingredient missing, constitutes a far deeper stress. It strikes at the intern's conscious sense of himself as a functioning human being. Something is missing. There is no feeling that allows a sense of compassion, and therefore human connection, with those who suffer around him. The waves of suffering do not make up part of him, and therefore they threaten him. In the present model, the intern suffers a particularly severe disjunction between his cognitive apprehension of the situation and a constructive emotional experiencing of it. His feeling state remains unavailable to his consciousness, as it has been for much of his life. And, unlike our other examples, his ability to isolate that affect, to depend on intellectualized behavior to adapt to the world around him itself, loses its effectiveness. His characteristic adaptive mechanism is Intellectualization, and that is no longer serving him as it once did.

When adaptive mechanisms break down—when they lose their adaptive use whether through repetition or by increasing burdens of stress—the characteristics of both crisis and opportunity present themselves.[7] The crisis lies in the crumbling of the mechanism that is no longer as useful as it once was. The person must continue to adapt in some way, however, and this frequently results in a subjective sense of vulnerability that is usually, and often temporarily, managed by another adaptive mechanism, often one from the next lower Domain on the algorithm hierarchy. In this case, the intern develops a terrific headache: an adaptive bodily symptom as discussed in Chapter 9 on Hypochondriasis. His behavior, his headache, and his apparent difficulty in managing his intellectual diagrams lead to the charge nurse's recognition that he is in trouble. The charge nurse and the chief resident effectively remove him from the stress for his own good and that of those around him. They recognize that something must be done, even though they may not formulate their perceptions in the psychological adaptive mechanism model as we discuss it here.

Opportunity lies in the possibility of growth. If an individual has functioned at the level of the Neurotic Domain adaptive mechanisms, there is usually a high likelihood that they will be able to replace this functioning mechanism with a more flexible mechanism in the Mature Domain. As noted in other examples, this is not always the case, in part because the transition from one adaptation mechanism to the next—moving toward greater adaptive flexibility—may include a period of vulnerability when neither mechanism is in place and functioning at its best. As we shall discuss further in Chapter 22, the sense of vulnerability often presents with the mood symptoms that may look like depression: a subjective sense of lessened personal worth, of helplessness in moving forward, and of questionable hope that things will get better. The support of a careful psychotherapy and an active social system may act to assuage this form of mood change as the momentum of development moves forward in the natural course of growth toward more mature psychological adaptive mechanisms.

7. The Chinese alphabet reflects this when it combines the concepts of crisis and opportunity in a famous pictograph.

To summarize, the adaptive mechanism of Intellectualization, or Isolation of Affect, one of the Neurotic Domain mechanisms, cognition and affect are separate and do not work together. The painful thoughts present in consciousness, by definition, and the painful feeling does not. This mechanism's observable behaviors characteristically present a Dryasdust tone in response to stress anxiety. At the same time, the feeling tone is often noticed by someone nearby and, in this sense, seems to be outside the person who is using Intellectualization as a primary adaptive mechanism. While not an "externalizing" adaptive mechanism in the sense of the Immature Domain group, affect here remains nonetheless consciously unavailable. In this context, clinically, it is sometimes difficult to note that persons who isolate affect, who intellectualize, nonetheless often carry with them a sense of subjective discomfort or dysphoria at the continually repeating behaviors that seem to render them out of step with the people around them. Finding this and making use of it often requires considerable clinical open-mindedness along with the technical art of interview styles that allow the subjective discomfort to flower forth into useful conversation in a professional setting.

REFERENCE

Doyle, A. C. (2009). The Mazarin Stone. In *The Case-Book of Sherlock Holmes*. Oxford, Oxford University Press.

Stegner, W. (1967). *All Little Live Things*. New York, Viking.

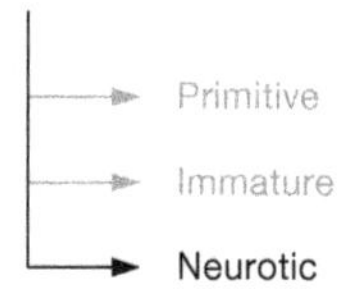

CHAPTER 14
Dissociation

In the model of psychological adaptive mechanisms, the respective approaches of Repression and Intellectualization use opposite strategies to handle the thought and feeling contents of a stressful perturbation to waking consciousness. In Repression, a person in waking consciousness experiences, and reports, the feeling content of the stress but cannot find the idea content related to it. By contrast, in Intellectualization, alternately termed Isolation of Affect, the conscious person fully perceives and usually understands the idea content of the stress but remains consciously out of touch with the emotions it calls forth.

In contrast to both of these, as Vaillant points out, Dissociation allows a form of psychological adaptation that sequesters, if only for a time, both the idea *and* the feeling contents of the perturbing stress in the interest of relieving the stress-generated anxiety.[1] Dissociation takes the person somewhere else in wakeful consciousness, leaving the painful thoughts and feelings behind.

Whether it does this as a strategy of adaptation in the Neurotic Domain, the Immature Domain, or the Primitive Domain speaks to one of the unique clinical aspects of Dissociation as an adaptive mechanism itself. If we may, with a bow to that wise and kind-hearted teacher, let us consider two instances of Vaillant's writings themselves as part of the phenomenology considered in the present discussion. In *Adaptation to Life*,[2] Dissociation appears as one of the Neurotic Domain adaptive mechanisms—the Neurotic ego defense mechanisms to use the psychoanalytic terminology. Sixteen years later, in *The Wisdom of the Ego*,[3] and again nine years after that in *Aging Well*,[4] he lists Dissociation among the Immature Domain mechanisms. Rather than an imprecision in description, we can best regard the changing character as a reflection of the phenomenon itself: Dissociation is the most protean,[5] that is, the most shape shifting, of all the adaptive styles discussed here. Considered in

1. Vaillant (1998a; first published in 1977); Vaillant (1998b, pp. 55–57; first published in 1993).
2. Vaillant (1998a, p. 385).
3. Vaillant (1998b, pp. 55–57).
4. Vaillant (2002, pp. 334–335).
5. Proteus, the Water God of ancient myth, could, like the water he personifies, change shape to fit any surface or container or boundary. His changes were both fluid and persistent.

the recognition algorithm from Chapter 3, at its best Dissociation can appear in the Neurotic Domain. It can also take on the characteristics of the adaptive styles in the Immature Domain. Although only the Mature Domain adaptive approach remains closed to it, in the present model Dissociation may even take on Primitive Domain characteristics as well. Consider the following example.

THE MAN WHO FORGOT HIMSELF: DISSOCIATION IN THE PRIMITIVE DOMAIN

A 35-year-old man hears of a famous hospital in a large New England city and goes there to seek help. On his arrival in the emergency department, the admitting clerk asks his name. Awake and alert, in a clear voice he states that he does not know his name. The clerk asks him to sit for a few minutes until it is his turn to be seen, and he complies. Hearing the story, the medical intern on duty consults with his resident, and they invite the assistance of the hospital security officers. They usher the man into an examination suite to which he goes willingly. He is cooperative but appears completely puzzled by his predicament. He knows where he is and what day of the week, month, and year it is, and otherwise looks fully cognizant of his surroundings. But he cannot remember his name. One of the security officers asks whether he has any identification documents such as a driver's license. The man hands the officer a wallet, saying that he has noticed there is a driver's license in it but that he does not recognize the name or the picture on the front. The officer notes that the picture on the driver's license appears to be that of the patient and excuses himself while asking the other officer to remain with the patient and doctors as they carry out their examination. With further questions and examination of his thought capabilities, they establish that he is thinking clearly, is not suffering from any delusions or hallucinations, and has no thoughts of hurting himself or anyone else. After a few minutes, the security officer reenters the suite and asks whether the doctors have found anything wrong with this patient that might require hospitalization. When they answer negatively, he asks the man to stand up, and he and the other officer place him in handcuffs as they read him his Miranda rights and advise him that they have received information that he is wanted for murder in a nearby state. He cooperates with them but still appears puzzled.

Using the recognition algorithm in this case, the stress involved appears to be the very significant one of having allegedly committed murder and being wanted for that crime. But the anxiety is nowhere to be seen, with a possible exception reflected in a mild degree of puzzlement. This patient does not otherwise present with symptoms of confusion or of the disorders of thought or perception that might characterize a major mental illness. Some psychological adaptation has occurred that has contained the anxiety such that it is barely noticeable to both the patient and his caretakers alike.

The algorithm next asks whether this emergency department patient recognizes the existence of the stress or the anxiety it generates. He clearly does not, even to the extent of recognizing neither his name nor his picture on his driver's license.

And yet he knows that something is wrong. He has come to seek help because of that. He does not, in the concrete use of our definitions in Chapters 4, 5, and 6, deny the existence of something being wrong, avoid the possibility, or blame it on some unreal cause such as advertisements in the subway trains. At the same time, his lack of recognition extends only to his personal identity, not to his other perceptions of the components of reality, such as his present location and time.

Consistent with one definition of Dissociation, he has lost complete cognizance of an inner reality, namely his identity as a person.[6] In addition, however, he has also lost complete cognizance of an outer reality, specifically his alleged involvement in a murder. In the view of the recognition algorithm, therefore, he presents both an adaptation at a Primitive level—having lost touch with reality—and fulfills the definition of a Dissociative adaptive strategy in losing touch with the inner reality of his personal identity. In this instance, he presents a form of Dissociation that is most consistent with that style used in the manner of the Primitive Domain psychological adaptive mechanisms: both inner and outer realities do not appear in his cognizance.

In this way, Dissociation can form a Primitive Domain adaptive style in the present recognition model for psychological adaptive mechanisms. Unlike some other forms of Dissociation at higher levels, however, Primitive Dissociation comes from an unconscious, rather than conscious, source: in this case, the intolerable stress and anxiety that can be handled only with the most basic adaptive strategies. Clinically, as in this case and in many others similar to it, this patient presents a dangerous situation. It is not clear whether his Dissociation emanates from his legal difficulties or from his own murderous impulses. Nor is it clear to what extent and for how long he may maintain the Dissociation as likely his last effective psychological adaptation against an overwhelming anxiety that could lead to his striking out at others or himself. In this case, the Dissociation indicates the need for a controlled setting that can assure the safety of everyone involved, especially the patient.

THE COLD: DISSOCIATION AMONG THE IMMATURE DOMAIN MECHANISMS

Less primitive and far less dramatic examples of Dissociation occur as its shape changes in moving up the levels of the recognition algorithm. In the next example, a vignette taken from John Williams' (1965) novel *Stoner*,[7] the reader learns the inner thoughts of an associate professor of English at a large midwestern university in the United States whose marriage brings only a passionless indifference. He has learned that his only child, his daughter, is the campus' easy make, and his job is a repetitive dead end with no hope of promotion. He looks out his window on a winter's evening.

---

6. In another model, one without reference to the inner reality of mental perception (DSM-IV-TR; American Psychiatric Association, 2000), this patient presents what can be considered a fugue state: a severe disconnection with outer reality in the setting of normal attention and cognition and without delusions or hallucinations.

7. Williams wrote the novel well before the word *stoner* came to mean a marijuana addict in common speech.

> Nothing moved upon the whiteness; it was a dead scene which seemed to pull at him, to suck his consciousness just as it pulled the sound from the air and buried it within a white softness. He felt himself pulled outward toward the whiteness, which spread as far as he could see, and which was a part of the darkness from which it glowed, of the clear and cloudless sky without height or depth. For an instant he felt himself go out of the body that sat motionless before the window; and as he felt himself slip away, everything—the flat whiteness, the trees, the tall columns, the night, the far stars—seemed incredibly tiny and far away, as if they were dwindling to a nothingness....
>
> During that year and especially in the winter months, he found himself returning more and more frequently to such a state of unreality;... he knew he ought to be troubled by it, but he was numb, and he could not convince himself that it mattered. He was forty-two years old, and he could see nothing before him that he wished to enjoy and little behind him that he cared to remember.
>
> (Williams 1965, pp. 180, 181)

When we apply the recognition algorithm to this vignette, we already know that the principal stress in this man's life comes from his sense of being trapped, both in his job and his marriage, as well as in his provincial college town and its closed community that looks down on him and his daughter; and all with no way out. A sense of doom—that is, his subjective perception of a psychological suffocation—rises from this. The next task on the algorithm pathway requires an assessment of whether or not he recognizes the stress and its anxiety. This passage offers no indication of his ignoring his outer reality through a Primitive denial that it exists, a distortion of his experience into something joyful, or a projection of it onto some unreality. He lives trapped in place not only socially but in time as well: he is acutely aware that he has nothing to look forward to and nothing he wants to remember. His adaptation uses something more than the Primitive Domain mechanisms.

The algorithm next assesses whether he identifies the stress as inside or outside himself. The writing is particularly interesting at this point because it describes the landscape that he sees through his window as somehow constituting a force greater than him. There is a de-realizing, if not haunting, aspect about it, especially in the whiteness of the snow against the dark night sky. It seems to suck all of his conscious energies, including his anxiety, out of his body and into the frozen landscape. The associate professor finds himself drifting out into the landscape and experiences this as being outside his body, moving ever higher as the landmarks grow smaller. His inner reality—the sense of doom at being trapped—does not live in consciousness when he lifts out of the window and above the landscape. He leaves that behind in his de-realized body. His inner reality, therefore, disappears from consciousness for a time while the outer circumstances of his life do not change.

His adaptation therefore is one in which he leaves behind both the cognitive content of his stressful circumstances and the emotional hopelessness he feels from being caught in them. His adaptive style is clearly that of Dissociation: moving his consciousness far away from both painful idea and painful feeling. In the second paragraph, however, the narrator describes the associate professor as first sensing that he ought not to indulge in his dissociative flights—the implied alternative being to remain and begin a resolution of his circumstance. But the English professor has become numb to any emotional energy that might propel him in that direction. He then goes on to make a pattern of his dissociative episodes as escapes from the loveless boredom of his everyday existence. The details of his adaptation, therefore, describe it as an external one in which he leaves the circumstances intermittently for brief periods, always to return but never including an indication of his taking responsibility for change. In this regard, therefore, according to our model of psychological adaptive mechanisms he uses Dissociation to locate his consciousness well outside of the range of the stressful situations that he does not face.

As with the other Immature Domain mechanisms, Dissociation here locates the stress and its anxiety outside consciousness, in a place where it cannot be addressed or resolved. In so doing, the protean adaptive style now conforms itself to the Immature Domain adaptive strategies. Interestingly, it does this in a manner opposite of that Neurotic Projection, in which the perceptions of unwanted thoughts and feelings locate themselves in the persons of others. Immature Domain Dissociation, by contrast, takes the person, in the form of consciousness, far away from the unwanted thoughts and feelings that remain behind.

When an individual utilizes Dissociation in its Immature Domain form to adapt to the anxiety-generating stresses, further development into the Neurotic Domain adaptive styles will require a shift from external to internal localization of active responsibility. Psychotherapeutic treatment, in that circumstance, takes on the same attributes as those needed for the other Immature Domain adaptive styles to move what other models term the *locus of control* into the conscious self from outside it.

As an adaptive style in the present model, Dissociation has a second unique characteristic that sometimes aids, rather than thwarts, the progression to more Mature Domain adaptive mechanisms. Among all of the adaptive styles, only Dissociation allows a conscious turning on of its use. This brings a measure of control within the bounds of conscious choice, although Dissociation may certainly spring up unconsciously as well, especially when supported in a pathologically repeated pattern of use as in the vignette just quoted from John Williams' novel. In other circumstances, however, Dissociation itself may take on the characteristics of the Neurotic Domain of psychological adaptive mechanisms and use its on/off switch capability to do so. This may allow circumstances in which Dissociation carries a more positive valence, rather than the negative ones discussed in the two instances above. To illustrate, let us consider the special circumstance in the following description.

HEARTS THAT FLOWER: DISSOCIATION AS A NEUROTIC DOMAIN MECHANISM

Intensive care units (ICUs) and cardiac monitoring came into practice in the 1960s in U.S. hospitals. Early cardiac monitors included a cardiac wave that ran across an oscilloscope as each heartbeat traced its electrical properties on the screen. No heartbeat, seen as a flat line, indicated cardiac arrest, and the term *flatlined* reached common speech as a euphemism for death. At the same time, the early monitors included a small noise signal, usually a beeping sound, triggered by the monitoring wave reflected on the screen, each time the heart contracted its major muscles—its ventricles. The patient lying in a hospital bed with cardiac leads connecting him or her to the monitor therefore heard a beep every time his or her heart beat. A regular beep from the monitor was a good sign, while a period of silence, as in a skipped or delayed heartbeat, became immediately obvious in the patient's awareness because of the monitor's silence. The beeping sounds went on day and night for as long as the patient stayed in the ICU. For some, the noise was a nuisance not entirely unrelated to torture because there was no escaping it. For others, however, it was "your guardian angel," as one creative ICU nurse put it, because it watched over the cardiac patient day and night.

This raised the question, was the continuous monitoring beeping a cause for anxiety or an occasion of reassurance? Investigators of the time noted that some people could block out the beeping noise by imagining themselves as being somewhere else, for example, in retracing the experiences of their last vacation to Florida, where the bright sun, warm water, and light reflecting beaches offered their enjoyment. Others, however, could not shut this out and appeared to live from moment to moment with each beat, waiting for the other shoe to drop, as an old joke has it, when the beeping stopped and the silence extended. Researchers of the time therefore devised a comparison study between those who could take their minds elsewhere while in ICU and those who could not (Hackett and Cassem 1975).

The first adaptive strategy employed Dissociation, as we use that term here referring to the Neurotic Domain of adaptive styles.[8] Applying the recognition algorithm, the stress in the situation came from the possibility of a heartbeat stopping, as might well occur to anyone hospitalized for a heart attack or heart failure. Next, those admitted to ICU for cardiac monitoring clearly recognized this stress as present in their lives, as opposed to Primitive adaptive mechanisms in which the stress is not acknowledged—it would be hard not to recognize it with a reminder beeping at 60 to 80 times or more a minute. And further, the ICU patients admitted to the study, while not specifically assessed in this manner, most likely perceived the anxiety of the cardiac monitor beeps as having to do with them rather than as some extraneous responsibility that belonged to someone else. In the adaptive style recognition model, this located them beyond the Immature range of adaptive mechanisms.

The researchers then followed the course of cardiac monitoring and treatment using two outcome measures: frequencies of discharge from the ICU, that is, survival, and of its opposite, namely death. At the conclusion of the study, the data showed unequivocally that those patients who could employ Dissociation while undergoing cardiac monitoring in the ICU had significantly higher survival rates than those who could not. The adaptive strategy itself did not include any particular effort at trying to reconcile the cognitive content of the stress—"My heart may stop beating"—with

8. In the original report, the researchers used the term *denial* rather than dissociation. Close reading, however, makes clear that their definition fits Dissociation rather that Primitive Domain Denial in the present model.

its emotional burden: fear. The study examined the natural history of ICU survivorship and made no attempt at reconciling the thought content related to the silence of the monitor as indicating an absence of heartbeat and the fright of recognizing that one's heart has stopped. Dissociation, considered in the Neurotic Domain, does not reconcile painful ideas and emotions as part of an adaptation response to the threat of the anxiety. Rather, it simply leaves both in place and goes somewhere else for a brief period.

The ability to do this in an acute situation, such as during monitoring after heart attack, has survival value in that it reduces the anxiety itself and quiets any contribution to the situation that may come from the neural responses that anxiety generates. In this case, for example, a heightened heart rate might raise the risk of irregular heart rhythms that can result in cardiac arrest and death.

Having gone somewhere else for a little while, Neurotic Domain Dissociation must always return to its starting point simply because the underlying disjunction between feeling and thought content doesn't allow the person to do otherwise when using this adaptive mechanism. Dissociation may be very helpful in surviving the ICU, but, following that crisis, it may not be particularly useful in coming to grips with cardiac rehabilitation programs and changes in lifestyle or medication that enhance cardiac health. In those settings, Dissociation may become more of a hindrance when planning and behavioral change require conscious attention.

The usefulness of "positive" Dissociation for brief periods often confers a relief from the anxiety that may apply in acute situations. Other examples of its active use, including active patient training in dissociative techniques, can be seen in healthcare settings that may include cancer chemotherapy, kidney dialysis, or other procedures in which patients remain conscious throughout. In those settings, they may learn to imagine themselves elsewhere during the course of the treatment, a positive step as compared to remaining on the edge of disaster—as we learned from the early studies of cardiac monitoring.

THE SLEEPY INTERN TAKES A VACATION: DISSOCIATION AS TEMPORARY RELIEF

Once again we find our sleepless intern surveilling the progress of the four patients in the unit as well as that of the eight patients in the regular medical ward. It is three in the morning, and while sitting in front of the computer screen writing notes and checking medical orders, the intern notices a recollection of his last vacation to a beach in South Florida coming to mind. It is a pleasant thought that recalls clear blue waters and gentle white waves heaving themselves up in graduated ranks in crescendo-decrescendo rhythms onto the shallow reaches in the curved lines that define the edges of the margin between land and sea and stretch off in the distance into the off-white color of the sand that gleams from a warming sun in a contrast to the stark white pillows of the thunderheads floating in a painfully bright blue sky. Somewhere from behind the palm trees that line the beach comes the gentle percussion of Jamaican steel drums that beat out the tinkling rhythm of the Caribbean over the pulse of bass guitar notes amplified and coursing through the trees close to the ground like alligators at a run. As if in time with the rhythm, the telephone rings.

It is the ER on the line and the night resident's voice on the phone. The rhythm sounds harsh and disturbing in the intern's ear. Another patient is on the way to the unit: an unconscious man in a diabetic crisis whose care will likely make sleep impossible through the rest of the shift. Will it never end? Will life ever reach some civility? Will it mean only admission after admission at all hours of the day or night? The intern acknowledges the admission and hangs up the phone, logs off the computer on the ward, and walks the long hallway to the ICU. After a few steps, he asks his memory for the rhythm of the steel drums and it returns. A lightness comes with it, that of a dance, a swaying in his steps as they lead down the hall, a Jamaican spring in his steps that stops as the intern enters the ICU door and takes charge of the new admission there.

Applying the recognition algorithm to the intern's reaction in the middle of the night in this vignette, the stress of the new admission aggravates an already ongoing perturbation: the intern is not happy with long hours and the lack of more balanced life despite his dedicated service to his patients. News of the impending admission causes him to voice his sense of despair at the possibility of being doomed to care for others at a great cost to himself. The recognition algorithm equates the sense of doom with anxiety resulting from the stress, in this case that of his overwork and with yet another obligation.

He voices his anxious concerns and their relationship to the stress clearly. He does not employ any of the Primitive Domain mechanisms to avoid or ignore the outward reality of his work life, nor does he project it onto some unreal cause such as a government plot to overwork him. Moving to the next level, the algorithm asks whether he locates the stress or its anxiety outside himself by dissociating himself from it and taking his own consciousness in flight from it, as in the example of the English professor in John Williams' fictional vignette mentioned earlier in this chapter. The intern does not do that: he remains in his body, he keeps his memories intact, and when the situation indicates it, he is ready to turn his attention to the task at hand: namely, taking care of the newest admission. His approach is therefore not that of the Immature Domain adaptive mechanisms.

At the next level of the algorithm, we must first identify both the cognitive and emotional contents, respectively, of the stress and its anxiety. As noted, the intern gives voice to both after hearing news of the next complicated medical admission that will ensure his remaining sleepless for the rest of the night. The painful idea content asks whether this continuously increasing load will ever end, and whether his life will ever again become *civil*, that is, with a sufficient balance between his professional and his personal lives, and allow him to connect meaningfully in social relations with other people. The anxious doom he feels reflects the stress's emotional content: a fear that he never will find that balance and that he has made a terrible choice.

Does the vignette provide any suggestion that he has integrated these two toward some resolution of the stress, or do they remain disjoined? The answer to this lies in the nature of his recollections of his last vacation to a South Florida beach. They take him away from the grueling work at hand for a brief respite that occurs without any deleterious effects on his work performance. In the first, he simply drifts away while looking at the computer screen, and in the second, he consciously transforms his steps into dance rhythms with the Jamaican music in his mind as he proceeds to his next task. He makes no effort here to resolve the thought content of his dilemma of overwork with the feeling content of fearing that he may have chosen the wrong profession. To an outside observer, he may well have chosen the wrong profession if he finds himself having difficulty maintaining his concentration on his work and drifting off to his last vacation, or he may have chosen the correct profession for him and needs to reconcile his worries with his work. The outside observer simply doesn't know one way or the other since the intern does not address integrating the two. Instead, characteristic of Dissociation at the level of the Neurotic Domain of adaptive mechanisms, he simply leaves both stressful cognition and affect to themselves and goes somewhere else in his mind for brief periods. He gains a certain distance, similar to taking a deep breath and backing up a step before continuing on, but this does not change, in either a positive or a negative direction, his relationship to the stress or its attributes. He dissociates this consciousness from the grueling experience at hand and then returns to work consciously and in response to its demands.

In this way, therefore, Dissociation may occur in ways (1) that ignore both inner and outer realities in the fashion of the Primitive Domain mechanisms, as in the example of the man who forgot his name, (2) that lead only to the inner reality, in the manner of the Immature Domain adaptive styles of de-realization that the English professor practiced, or (3) that recognize both inner and outer realities but fail to integrate the separated feelings and thoughts in the interest of leaving them for a time, as in the intern's use of Dissociation in a Neurotic Domain adaptation. With its protean nature in respect to the three lower categories in the adaptive mechanism model, Dissociation by definition never reaches to the Mature Domain level of psychological adaptive styles: its strategy aims at temporary absence from the stress, not at integrating the stress' idea and feeling contents. As noted in the above examples, this adaptive strategy can include both pathological and nonpathological uses. And, because it is unique among the adaptive mechanisms in conscious deployment, the positive uses remain available when needed in the style of the Neurotic Domain mechanisms. Pathology results when ongoing patterns develop in any of the three Domains, and especially in the lower two when continuing Dissociation results in impaired, rather than improved, functioning.

REFERENCES

American Psychiatric Association. (2000). *Diagnostic and Statistical Manual of Mental Disorders* (4th ed., Text. Rev.). Washington, DC, American Psychiatric Press.

Hackett, T. P., and N. H. Cassem. (1975). "Psychological management of the myocardial infarction patient." *J Human Stress 1*(3): 25–38.

Vaillant, G. E. (1998a). *Adaptation to Life*. Cambridge, Harvard University Press.

Vaillant, G. E. (1998b). *The Wisdom of the Ego*. Cambridge, Harvard University Press.

Vaillant, G. E. (2002). *Aging Well*. Boston, Little, Brown.

Williams, J. (1965). *Stoner*. Fayetteville, University of Arkansas Press.

Primitive
Immature
Neurotic

CHAPTER 15
Displacement

Sometimes anxiety is not to be borne, but not to be got rid of either. This frequently happens when one is in the company of other people and, in some behavioral models, refers to a sense of social anxiety. A person feels as if he or she is on display, and something about him or her causes others around the person to engage in a continuous process of harsh or negative judgment. This takes on the attributes of a stress as the person being judged feels more like a specimen viewed under a microscope, or an object hanging from a string held between thumb and forefinger and twirled around for inspection, than a competent human being no different from any other. The perception itself takes on a sense of social doom or disaster. One simply isn't up to scratch, and everyone knows it. The sense of social disaster increases and becomes intolerable. What to do?

One adaptive strategy aims it outward, rather than inward where it hurts. But this must be done carefully. Blaming someone else for one's own inner torment, as we have seen in Neurotic Projection, can bring further hurt and social isolation on oneself. And this defeats the purpose: it confirms other people's pejorative judgments. To be useful in this setting, the required adaptive mechanism must both mitigate the sense of social doom and provide some positive, redeeming perception of oneself, if at the expense of others.

LOVE AND LABOR: DISPLACING ANXIETY ON TO OTHERS

Shakespeare, one can argue, devotes an entire play, *Love's Labour's Lost*, one of his comedies, to an exploration of Displacement. We can make illustrative use of a passage, as quoted below. For ease of understanding, it needs both setting the scene and an explanation of some of the diction that Shakespeare used 400 years ago. Even then, it may require reading through a few times to perceive its insults at a gut level.

As the dialogue opens, a group of amateur actors have been engaged to entertain a group of young nobles by enacting scenes from classical mythology. Holofernes, a local schoolteacher with pretensions of learning, leads the group of actors. His pretensions are immediately obvious when, for example, he mixes the biblical story of Judas Maccabaeus with the classical Greek story of Hercules. At the same time, he frequently misuses archaic words such as *ycleped*—a very old word meaning "called," as in my dog is called Rover—giving it as "ycliped" instead. And he throws in Latin words as a mark of his learning when English would do better in the conversations.

Unbeknown to Holofernes, however, he and his actors are to entertain an audience that has its own purposes at work. The four young men of the play are trying their best to impress their four young women counterparts in the interests of love. The nobles are far better educated than poor Holofernes, and the men (Dumain, Biron, Boyet, and Longaville) sense this quickly. They recognize that here is an opportunity to show off their cleverness of wit in order to impress the ladies. They target Holofernes with the goal of exposing his pretentiousness and demonstrating their own wit. For the reader's benefit, unfamiliar words will include explanations in the right-hand margin. As the scene begins, Holofernes is sending off a fellow actor, Moth, who plays the part of Hercules:

Enter HOLOFERNES, for Judas; and MOTH, for Hercules

Holofernes:

Great Hercules is presented by this imp,
Whose club kill'd Cerberus, that three-headed *canis*; (dog)
And when he was a babe, a child, a shrimp,
Thus did he strangle serpents in his *manus*. (hand)
Quoniam he seemeth in minority, (since)
Ergo I come with this apology. (therefore)
Keep some state in thy exit, and vanish.

MOTH retires

Judas I am,—

Dumain:	A Judas!	
Holofernes:	Not Iscariot, sir.	
	Judas I am, *ycliped* Maccabaeus.	(spelled "ycleped": called)
Dumain:	Judas Maccabaeus *clipt* is plain Judas.	(clipped, shortened)
Biron:	A kissing traitor. How art thou proved Judas?	
Holofernes:	Judas I am,—	
Dumain:	The more shame for you, Judas.	
Holofernes:	What mean you, sir?	
Boyet:	To make Judas hang himself.	
Holofernes:	Begin, sir; you are my *elder*.	(higher in status)
Biron:	Well followed: Judas was hanged on an *elder*.	(a kind of tree)
Holofernes:	I will not be put out of *countenance*.	(meanings: 1. disposition, 2. face)
Biron:	Because thou hast no face.	
Holofernes:	What is this?	

Boyet:	A *cittern-head*.	(the peg head of a stringed instrument)
Dumain:	The *head of a bodkin*.	(the handle of a knife)
Biron:	A Death's face in a ring.	
Longaville:	The face of an old Roman coin, scarce seen.	
Boyet:	The *pommel* of Caesar's *falchion*.	(the handle of a Roman sword)
Dumain:	The carved-bone face on a flask.	
Biron:	Saint George's half-cheek in a brooch.	
Dumain:	Ay, and in a brooch of lead.	
Biron:	Ay, and worn in the cap of a tooth-drawer. And now forward; for we have put thee in *countenance*.	 (face)
Holofernes:	You have put me out of *countenance*.	(disposition)
Biron:	False; we have given thee faces.	
Holofernes:	But you have out-faced them all.	
Biron:	An thou wert a lion, we would do so.	
Boyet:	Therefore, as he is an ass, let him go. And so adieu, sweet Jude! nay, why dost thou stay?	
Dumain:	For the latter end of his name.	
Biron:	For the ass to the Jude; give it him:—Jud-as, away!	
Holofernes:	This is not generous, not gentle, not humble.	
Boyet:	A light for Monsieur Judas! it grows dark, he may stumble.	
Princess:	Alas! Poor Maccabaeus, how hath he been baited.	

(Shakespeare, *Love's Labour's Lost*, Act V, Scene 2, lines 589–632)

The young men make fierce and rapid fun of Holofernes, including his use of language, his knowledge of the characters he plays, and even his face. How, we may ask, does this resemble any adaptive response to a stress, and if so, in whose psyche? To answer this, we take recourse to our recognition algorithm. What stress may we identify as operating in this scene? The obvious one would be the derision that the young nobles mete out to Holofernes. But this is not Shakespeare's true mark as we might conclude from the play's title. It is not "The Trials of Holofernes"; it is *Love's Labour's Lost*. The play is about the young noblemen and women as they pursue in their dance of love. It is to them, therefore, that we must look for Shakespeare's location of the stress, the psychological tension, in the play. Focusing specifically on the men, their stress can be only the pursuit of the women whom, they hope, will find them each worthy swains. Anxiety emanating from whether or not each will eventually be found worthy serves to heighten the play's comedic potential, and Shakespeare makes the most of it.

For the purposes of this discussion on recognizing psychological adaptive mechanisms, however, we once again refer to the algorithm and ask whether the sharp-tongued heroes ignore the tensions in the play that occur between the genders, as one might expect in the Primitive Domain mechanisms. Shakespeare begins the play with the four of them swearing off women, as it were, in a group. This does not last, however, and the chase begins pell-mell within the terms of culture and breeding of their social set. They respond to the stress not by avoiding it or projecting it onto supernatural superstitions, as Shakespeare uses in some of his other plays. There are no witches, cauldrons, or ghosts, and the race is on to see who is the wittiest, or at least witty enough to win the fair maid. Primitive Domain mechanisms need not apply.

Next, the algorithm examines whether the four swains locate the anxiety as something to do with themselves personally or whether they regard it as someone else's problem. The dialogue makes it obvious, for example, that they do not blame Holofernes for their sense of impending disaster when it comes to affairs of the heart and the continuing possibility of hearts being broken. Nor do they find ways to act on the anxiety without thinking, to behave toward the women in a passive manner, or to use any of the other styles of adaptation we recognize as part of the Immature Domain. From the dialogue among the four men given in other parts of the play, each clearly regards the anxieties of love as part of their conscious lives and concerns, passing well beyond the portals of the Immature Domain psychological adaptive mechanisms.

To follow the algorithm to the level of the Neurotic Domain psychological adaptive mechanisms requires first the identification of the stress in its cognitive content and, at the same time, in its emotional characteristic. Will the woman of my dreams find me worthy?—is a fair statement of the painful idea involved. There is always the possibility that she will not. The associated emotions may include the fear of outright rejection, the sadness of feeling alone and unworthy, the anger at someone else's negative judgment of one's true worth as a suitor, or some combination of all of these. Such feelings are difficult to experience singly or in any combination, especially in the context of giving one's heart to another. Uncomfortable and impossible to deny, the tension between idea—Will I be found worthy?—and feeling—fear at rejection—leads to the question of whether or not they are integrated in responding to the stress of the situation.

Enter the unfortunate Holofernes. As the dialogue develops, all of the emotional tension, all of the sardonic dialogue in response to being thought worthy or unworthy in my lady's eye, cascades onto him like the arrows of distant archers falling on a prey. They compare him to Judas Iscariot, the disciple in the Christian metaphor who handed Jesus over for execution. They describe his face as the handle of a knife or the peg end of a lute. And to cap it all, they describe him as an ass, that is, a braying animal. In their zeal to be thought of as clever and intelligent by the women whom they are trying to impress, they assault Holofernes' dignity as a human being. And he finally says so, breaking through the social boundaries between the nobles and the yeomanry to describe them as not living up to the three virtues that should define persons of noble birth and education: they are not generous, gentle, or humble toward him. And the leader of the four women, the Princess, agrees with Holofernes in the last line of the passage when she says she recognizes how badly he has been baited, that is, insulted as if provoked. It is she who shows him some sense of compassion, in his pretensions, ill education, and all.

Shakespeare leaves little doubt that in the case of his four young noblemen, the idea of being found unworthy and the fearful emotion that it raises have little commerce with each other in the interest of adapting to the anxiety of the situation.

Aiming the intellectual and emotional tensions at Holofernes, when their source lies rightfully in the tension between the two genders, serves to offset, rather than resolve, the true difficulty of the situation, namely the quest for human affection. Rather than creating a sense of compassion, as one would expect were idea and feeling integrated, the opposite prevails, as the Princess notes. Aiming the anxiety, and its painful ideas and feelings, at a target that cannot hurt us defines Displacement. Insulting Holofernes, whose opinion doesn't matter, is far worse than risking witty insult of any of the women, whose opinions do matter. And yet the processes of love, both sweet and painful, when aimed at Holofernes, appear only painful. Integrating the two remains far away. The disjunction of thought and feeling resulting in the expression of the stress generated anxiety at the expense of others places Displacement in the Neurotic Domain of the psychological adaptive mechanisms.

Love's Labour's Lost proceeds to its predictable conclusion when each of the suitors finds acceptance by his lady love and all proceed to the happy ending that distinguishes a comedy from a tragedy. And as a consolation prize, Holofernes and his band of actors receive a mighty applause from the noble couples, now remarkably free of the tensions of who will be found worthy by whom.

This raises the question of the play's title: what is it that Shakespeare means when he says that some part of the labor of love has been lost? The answer charts the difference between the Neurotic and the Mature adaptive mechanisms in our present model. True love in any setting, whether romantic or simply that of human acceptance, creates compassion: a connection in which humans share both the painful or joyful thought contents as well as the joyful or painful feelings of their existence. The integration of thought and feeling creates an alliance on this common ground. Unintegrated thought and feeling from the pain of human existence does not serve compassion. A limitation of the Neurotic Domain psychological adaptive mechanisms is simply the preservation of the conscious equilibrium at the expense of fully connecting with those around us. The anxieties may be relieved for a time, but compassion, the ability of humans to relate to each other both intellectually and emotionally at the same time, does not occur.

LOOKING GOOD: DISPLACEMENT AS PROTECTIVE DURING STRESS

If this is true, how does our model of psychological adaptive mechanisms explain the next vignette taken from the *Histories* of Herodotus, circa 446 B.C.? In it, a Persian spy with excellent eyesight has crept to a vantage point near the mountain pass at Thermopylae in Greece. From there he can see the actions of the Spartans who are preparing to hold the narrow pass against attack from an overwhelmingly large Persian army, a force thwarted by the terrain. He cannot believe what he sees. He reports back to Xerxes, the Persian emperor, who then consults with Demaratus, a Spartan turncoat. Herodotus records the spy's experience:

> The scout approached the Greeks' camp and kept them under close surveillance.... [The Spartans] were posted outside, where their arms and armour lay in

> front of the wall, and he was able to take stock of them. He watched them in a variety of occupations, such as exercising naked and combing their hair; this surprised him, but he took careful note of their numbers and made his way back to Xerxes. . . . Xerxes listened to what the scout had to say, but he could not understand that in actual fact the Greeks were getting themselves ready to kill or be killed to the best of their ability. Their behaviour struck him as laughable. He sent for Demaratus [who told Xerxes] . . . "These men have come to fight us for the pass and they are getting ready to do just that. It is their custom to do their hair when they are about to risk their lives."
>
> (Herodotus 1998, 478–479)

At first glance the reader may be inclined to agree with Xerxes: is attention to personal grooming really the most appropriate preparation for a bloody battle? Application of the recognition algorithm, however, offers some further insight. First, to identify the stress: everyone on both sides knows that a terrible battle will soon begin. The Spartans, who are both the leaders and the mainstays of the Greek troops, understand that many, and potentially all, of their number will die in the conflict. The Spartan troops are professional warriors, raised in a warrior culture and trained from birth in the stamina and skills of hand-to-hand combat with spears, helmets, shields, and swords. Yet even they sense the potential of incipient disaster and the likelihood of personal doom. These, in the model of psychological adaptive mechanisms, constitute the definition of the anxiety that results from the stress of any situation that perturbs the psychological equilibrium humans know in conscious wakefulness.

Following the algorithm, do the Spartans in Herodotus' description give any evidence of deploying Primitive Domain mechanisms in order to rein in the anxiety? They do not stand listlessly around as if in the belief that this day is no different from any other and that no battle will occur or, if it does, that there will be no danger involved. Nor do they leave the pass in order to avoid any unpleasant difficulties. And they do not describe the Persians as a group of sorcerers against whom magic is a better defense than spears and swords. They perceive the reality of the oncoming battle and do not invoke any of the Primitive Domain adaptive mechanisms in relationship to it.

According to the algorithm, we next ask whether the Spartan warriors locate the anxiety of the oncoming battle as being someone else's problem or theirs. Just as they do not avoid the battle by physically running away from it, Herodotus gives us no indication that the Spartan troops blame the battle or the necessity of preparing for it on some other person or circumstance. No one engages in a Hypochondriasis response and claims physical debilitation, for example. Rather, some of them are exercising as if warming up before an athletic contest. The spy witnesses a group of warriors preparing for the battle rather than making excuses about it. Their behavior does not reflect any of the mechanisms in the Immature Domain of adaptive styles.

The next task in using the algorithm requires identification of the cognitive and emotional contents of the stress itself. Herodotus makes these clear: the fact that pain and death are on the way makes up the thought content, and the feeling content comes forward in an appropriate fear. But to a warrior about to enter a battle, Fear and its brother Panic are the intolerable luxuries of the spectator and clear dangers to the combatants, whose effectiveness and only chance of survival Fear and Panic severely compromise. For some in that or similar situations, fear cannot even be voiced: a famous American jet pilot, when asked if he was scared before flying dangerous missions, replied that he was "apprehensive," a euphemism that both acknowledges the emotional content and at the same time lessens the potential for panic. The Spartans' behavior seems to reflect something similar. They do not appear before us either frozen in their terror or running about in a frenzy of panic driven activity. At the same time, however, they do not bear their fear by sitting with it and actively examining its ramifications and nuances. Echoing the formula in the first sentence of this chapter, the fear generated by the specter of the oncoming battle can neither be borne as a sole occupation nor entirely gotten rid of until the battle is over.

The psyche can, however, displace it. To assess this, the algorithm asks whether the feeling and the idea contents of the stress—terror and the likelihood of incipient death, respectively—work together toward a common resolution or exist in the disjoined state that results in repetitive, if distracting, behavior. The Spartans' activities in combing their hair that the spy ascribes to them alone among the Greek warriors, that so puzzle Xerxes as occurring among a group of warriors who are about to die and deal death to others, and that Demaratus sees as typical of the Spartan culture do not reconcile the painful thoughts and feelings of the moment. Careful attention to the proper grooming of one's hair does not allow the Spartan warrior to make peace with his fate at Thermopylae. Rather, it acknowledges that all of the other preparations before a battle are in order, so as to allow attention to grooming and a focus on leaving this life both acting and looking one's best. The grooming is repetitive and in its way comforting: going into the battle at the top of one's game. It serves as the Displacement of the anxiety onto the lesser concerns of grooming and appearance during the apprehensive, anxiety-laden time of waiting before the battle begins. This manages the anxiety but does not resolve it, just as it manages the fear of the battle and the idea of its inevitability without resolving either of those. The Displacement of the anxiety that so puzzles Xerxes and his spy exemplifies the style of the Neurotic Domain of adaptive mechanisms.

The adaptive qualities of Displacement take on positive aspects for the defenders of the pass before the Persian army. Displacement promotes their function in avoiding a panic and in going about their soldierly duties in an effective manner. As Herodotus relates the battle, the Greek defenders blocked the Persian invasion for a considerable time until the discovery of an alternate route over the mountains allowed the Persians to get behind the Greek warriors, a circumstance that spelled their destruction.

But to return to the question of whether Displacement—or any of the Neurotic Domain adaptive mechanisms—foster compassion between people we must look again at Herodotus' description. All of the Spartan warriors prepare for the battle, some by exercising and some by grooming. Like most warrior groups, they share the cognitive knowledge of oncoming combat as well as the emotional apprehension—the euphemistic fear—that it brings. Demaratus, a native of the same culture, recognizes it as well when he says it is common behavior among the Spartans before a battle. This, however, resembles not so much a sharing of integrated thought and feeling that draws in others so much as it does a group of people all looking at the same thing at the same time, whether it is an oncoming battle or a pleasant sunset. Xerxes and his spy do not find the Spartans' behavior personally engaging so much as mystifying. The grooming behavior supports the Spartans' task of killing as many Persian warriors as possible, but it does not create the common ground for a compassionate alliance between Persians and Spartans. As with Holofernes and his tormentors, Displacement here again does not allow humans to rise to the level of compassionate understanding with those whom we find pretentious or whom we define as enemies. Like Dissociation, it may serve its purpose in managing anxiety for a time, but, because the anxiety never resolves, the Displacement must either be repeated or the person must advance into the Mature range of adaptive mechanisms. In some cases, as in the next vignette involving a fictional character, that maturity never takes place.

ALONE IN THE WUTHERING HEIGHTS: STUCK IN DISPLACEMENT

Heathcliff, Emily Brontë's troubled hero of *Wuthering Heights*, arrives at the Earnshaw family seat as a street urchin whose life has been one of neglect and abuse until Mr. Earnshaw, the family's head, rescues him. As children, Heathcliff and Earnshaw's daughter Cathy fall in love with each other. They grow to adulthood, and Cathy marries their neighbor, the landed Edgar Linton, over the penniless Heathcliff for reasons more to do with social status than with love. But Heathcliff will not rest. He learns that Linton's younger sister, Isabella, has a crush on him, and he decides to act on the information, as Emily Brontë puts him before us in the following scene. Mrs. Dean, the Earnshaw's faithful nurse who raised Cathy and now works in the Linton household, narrates the conversation that includes both her mistress and Heathcliff:

> "And would Mr. Linton approve of his sister marrying that man?" I inquired.
>
> "Mr. Linton should approve," returned my lady decisively.
>
> "He might spare himself the trouble," said Heathcliff, "I could do as well without his approbation—And, as to you, Catherine, I have a mind to speak a few words, now, while we are at it—I want you to be aware that I *know* you have treated me infernally—infernally! Do you hear? And, if you flatter yourself that I don't perceive that you are a fool—and if you think I can be consoled by sweet words you're an idiot—and if you fancy I'll suffer unrevenged, I'll convince you of the contrary, in a very little while! Meantime, thank you for telling me your sister-in-law's secret—I swear I'll make the most of it, and stand you aside!"
>
> "What new phase of his character is this?" exclaimed Mrs. Linton, in amazement. "I've treated you infernally—and you'll take revenge! How will you take it, ungrateful brute? How have I treated you infernally?"
>
> "I seek no revenge on you," replied Heathcliff less vehemently. "That's not the plan—the tyrant grinds down his slaves and they don't turn against him, they crush those beneath them—you are welcome to torture me to death for your amusement,

> only, allow me to amuse myself a little in the same style—and refrain from insult, as much as you are able. Having leveled my palace, don't erect a hovel and complacently admire your own charity in giving me that for a home. If I imagined you really wished me to marry Isabella, I'd cut my throat!"
>
> (Brontë 1998, p. 112)

Cathy's rejection of him by her marriage to Edgar Linton provides the stress that perturbs Heathcliff in waking consciousness: the starting point in the adaptation recognition algorithm. The anxiety resulting from it allows him no leeway: it is with him constantly. Another indication that life brings only pain and that trusting others brings the worst of it. Worse still, his love for Cathy drives him to his anger at her and he tells her plainly that she has treated him "infernally." She has doomed him to live without her in his Inferno, another word for Hell that the Christianity of Emily Brontë's time defined as the absence of one's beloved. She has sent him to Hell, in his view of it. Doomed and angry as he is, however, Heathcliff must adapt.

Does he rid himself of the circumstance by ignoring it, the algorithm asks? He does not leave the area to avoid it, he does not pretend that it has not happened, nor does he develop a system of delusions that might explain it away. Despite his neglectful upbringing, Heathcliff has no tendencies toward the Primitive Domain mechanisms or their expression in a psychosis.

Does he blame his anxiety in this state of affairs on others? To do so, according to the algorithm, would locate his adaptation in the Immature Domain of psychological mechanisms. But again Emily Brontë's portrayal does not include Heathcliff as acting without thinking, retreating into a fantasy, expressing his anger in a passive manner, suddenly developing a debilitating unexplainable illness, or insisting that Cathy and others have conspired to plan Cathy's marriage just in order to hurt him. He does not locate his adaptation outside himself and see it as the responsibility of others around him. In this regard, he does not serve the algorithm's definition of one who adapts by engaging the Immature Domain psychological mechanisms.

The recognition algorithm takes us then into the realm of the Neurotic Domain mechanisms, where the first task is to identify the cognitive and the emotional components of the stress that so torments him and the second is to ask whether he has combined them in such a way that they work together to resolve the stress or whether they remain separated from each other. Emily Brontë has provided us with the first answers: the painful idea that Heathcliff must live without Cathy and the painful feelings of an anger overlying a profound sorrow and disappointment. Heathcliff cannot get rid of the painful feelings and ideas; nor can he, like many in real life with neglectful childhoods that make it difficult to trust others, tolerate them. He must provide himself some relief, if only temporary and without resolution.

In this portrayal, Heathcliff will not turn against Cathy, to whom he refers as a tyrant, who tortures him and by implication is in a position to torture him even more. Tyrants, even those of the heart, can make life miserable for their "slaves," as Heathcliff describes himself. Rather, he will use his anger to "crush those beneath" him, in this instance Isabella, Cathy's sister-in-law. In these words Emily Brontë gives us the definition of Displacement: Heathcliff aims his anxiety, and his painful ideas and feelings, at someone who cannot hurt him. And he does it purely as an expression of his anger, for if it were otherwise—if Cathy truly thought he had any interest of love in Isabella—his Displacement in the service of his anger would have no usefulness. And the next alternative would be to cut his own throat—in our model of adaptive mechanisms a regressive downshifting from Displacing his anger onto another toward Acting it Out impulsively against himself.

Like Holofernes before the barrage of insults and like the hapless Persians who must face the Spartans' sharp-edged spears, Isabella becomes the target of Heathcliff's Displacement of the anger he would aim at Cathy, who does not even recognize it until his expression of injured fury surprises and amazes her. Until then she does not seem to apprehend Heathcliff's sensitivity as an issue, where by contrast he sees her power to hurt him even more. As in the other two examples, human compassion—the shared pain of the ideas and feelings—cannot occur and save the day so long as Displacement remains at work. This, at least at one level, is the point Emily Brontë leaves with us in her novel.

THE STYLISH PURSE: DISPLACEMENT CRUMBLES

Displacement need not always be aimed at a person. Inanimate objects, as well as other living beings, such as plants and animals, can serve as targets or surrogates for painful anxieties when returned fire at a powerful source can worsen matters. Katherine Anne Porter describes a down-and-out comedy writer who lives in a tiny apartment in New York City and comes home one evening in a rainstorm. She empties her expensive purse, one of the few possessions she values, and opens it out to dry. The next morning, while the woman is in the bathtub, the building janitress comes in to check the radiators, and then leaves. When woman comes out of the bathroom, she notices her purse missing. She goes down to the basement, where she finds the janitress shoveling coal into the building's furnace. She confronts the janitress, who denies ever having seen the purse, and she goes back up to her apartment. The janitress arrives a few minutes later and gives the purse back, asking the woman not tell on her. The woman addresses the janitress:

> She said: "I missed this because it was a present to me from someone . . ."
>
> The janitress said: "He'd get you another if you lost this one. My niece is young and needs pretty things. We ought to give the young ones a chance. She's got a young man after her maybe will want to marry her. She oughta have nice things. She needs them bad right now. You're a grown woman, you had your chance, you ought to know how it is!"
>
> She held the purse out to the janitress saying: "You don't know what you're talking about. Here, take it, I've changed my mind. I really don't want it."
>
> The janitress looked up at her with hatred and said: "I don't want it either now. My niece is young and pretty, she don't need fixing up to be pretty, she's young and pretty anyhow! I guess you need it worse than she does!"

> "It wasn't really yours in the first place," she said, turning away. "You mustn't talk as if I had stolen it from you."
>
> "It's not for me, it's from her you're stealing it," said the janitress, and went back downstairs.
>
> (Porter 1972, p. 65)

In practicing the recognition algorithm, we can focus on the behavior of the janitress in this passage. In a job held mostly by men of little sophistication or elegance, and one that involves stoking coal into a furnace—not the most ladylike of pastimes—she comes upon an elegant purse and steals it. The reader may infer that the purse symbolizes all things feminine that the janitress wishes to be but is not. This suggests the first step in our algorithm, namely describing the stress, in this case a forced conscious apprehension of the janitress's own lack of pleasing feminine attributes. But she behaves in such a way as to bring down on herself the owner's anger at the obvious theft. The expressed anxiety in the story belongs to the owner until we see the janitress bring the purse back to the woman who owns it, claiming that she stole it in order to provide her niece with nice things that will attract a man—a detail suggesting that the janitress herself is childless and likely spouseless. When the owner refuses the purse, the janitress shoves it back at her angrily, saying that her niece is pretty enough without it.

The algorithm asks, what anxiety belongs to the janitress? What is her sense of doom? The woman who lives in the apartment has received a stylish purse from "someone," and the janitress immediately assumes, probably with good reason, that it came from a man who would get her another one. Inferring from the story, the janitress herself has never received a gift to complement her femininity and likely never will. Her doom appears as her loneliness, and perhaps occurs from feeling cheated in respect to her fair share of femininity.

How does she adapt to this circumstance of her life? The algorithm first asks whether she uses Primitive Domain adaptive mechanisms. Does she ignore her circumstance by denying it exists? By ascribing it to devils living in the city sewer system? Or by avoiding it altogether? None of these Primitive Domain stratagems operate here. The janitress's awareness of the limits of her femininity comes through in the story by way of her description of her attractive young niece who has yet to have her chance in attracting men. The author leaves the implied meaning that there is no such chance for the janitress and that she knows it.

Moving to a consideration of the Immature Domain mechanisms addresses the janitress's location of the responsibility for her sense of being doomed to an unpleasing femininity. Does she blame it on others, or does she accept it as her own? The story does not give any evidence to suggest that she formulates her doom as belonging to everyone else. For example, she does not accuse the owner of the purse of thinking of her as ugly. She does not describe herself as suffering from an inexplicable illness, nor does she retreat into a world of fantasy. She does not use the Immature Domain adaptive strategy of locating her stress and its sense of doom outside of herself. She comes to work and she does her job, if not a traditionally feminine one.

Then one day she comes across a beautiful purse, the sort that stylish women carry with them in public to complement their clothes. As if in a mirror, she sees the reflection of all that she desires and all she does not have. The recognition algorithm requires an assessment of the idea and the feeling contents of her underlying stress. The first, by inference from the story, is something like "I am ugly and will never find happiness with a 'someone.'" The second might include "I don't deserve this. No one does. And it makes me very angry." The algorithm next asks whether the two components—the cognitive and the affective contents, respectively—work together in an integrated fashion. Had they done so, there would be no reason for her to steal the purse. She would have reached some other creative resolution of the dilemma more along the lines of the Mature Domain adaptive mechanisms such as finding gentle ways to laugh at herself with a sense of compassion or transmuting her pain into some idealistic work with children who don't feel very happy about themselves. Instead, she Acts Out in an instant and steals the purse in an Immature Domain fashion.

When the owner confronts her, she first denies it, regressing further, if only briefly, into the Primitive Domain and then realizes that neither Primitive Domain Denial nor Immature Domain Acting Out will work. She returns the purse—the symbol of her desired femininity and the mirror of her own lack of it—only to find that the owner, who is now angry, doesn't want the purse anymore. Metaphorically, the owner says in effect, "Keep your doom. I don't want it." At this point, the janitress replies in kind that she does not want this symbol of her doom either, adding the unlikely excuse that she stole it only to help her niece. It is as though the janitress can now neither tolerate the purse and its personal symbolism nor get rid of it. She has displaced much of her stress onto the purse as a symbol that does not relieve the underlying dilemma no matter how much it may distract her anxiety for a time. In this sense, she uses the Neurotic Domain mechanism of Displacement with the purse as its target. In the process she alienates the owner of the purse and devalues the inanimate object of her Displacement itself. The conversation devolves into mutual accusations and, like the barbed witticisms aimed at Holofernes' and Heathcliff's Displaced rage, leads only to a split between people. In the story, neither character finds common ground on which they might begin a sense of understanding and compassion. The janitress's Displacement becomes as inanimate as the object to which she aims it.[1] Other targets, however, may be more retributive.

THE INTERN AND THE NIGHT NURSE: THE LIMITED USEFULNESS OF DISPLACEMENT

Once again it is 3 A.M. on our beleaguered intern's night to cover the inpatient medical service. He has been scurrying back and forth between the medical ward, where

1. In "Theft," Katherine Ann Porter gives us a much more complex story than would be appropriate to discuss here beyond considering only the character of the janitress. The algorithm might suggest that the janitress's Displacement with respect to the purse may not be the only such psychological adaptive mechanism going on in the story, and perhaps not the only Displacement.

eight patients depend on him to keep track of their medicines and vital functions as they recover from a series of physical illnesses, and the ICU, where four other patients deserve close observation, two of which survive by breathing tubes and intravenous lines on a touch-and-go basis. Sitting in the ward station, with the two compromised ICU patients on his mind and writing the last of the orders to renew the medicines for those recovering on the ward, the night charge nurse motions him over to a phone and hands him the receiver. The chief resident's voice on the other end of the line informs him that another very ill person from emergency is on the way up to the ICU and will be there in a few minutes. The intern says a polite "Thank you. I appreciate the heads up," and then hangs up the phone. Casting his eye down to a list of orders on the computer screen, he notes that one of the medicines he ordered an hour before has not yet been given to the patient meant to receive it. He angrily stands up and begins demanding that the night shift charge nurse explain to him why this has not happened. She points out that they are short-staffed and that the medicine is on its way. He begins by telling her that that is not good enough, raising his voice and saying they all have to do the best they can with what they have. She says she agrees, but he continues on in a tirade, saying that it is unconscionable if not unethical to delay medicine administration like this and that he intends to report the incident to the nursing supervisor. With that, he stalks off to the ICU. For the next three months, until he completes his rotation at this hospital and moves to another in the program, this intern gets no sleep whatsoever during any of his night coverage call shifts. This puzzles him when he talks to his colleagues, who seem to be able to get some restful sleep most nights. They comment on how well the nurses both on the ward and in the ICU manage the patients so as to allow them a little rest.

Our hapless intern here uses a Displacement from the Domain of the Neurotic mechanisms. The stress, constant to all of our intern vignettes—another acutely ill patient admitted to the overworked and sleepless denizen of the hospital night shifts—raises a sense of inadequacy that feels like an impending disaster. But contrary to previous reactions, the intern does not employ Primitive Domain adaptive mechanisms that would, in very concrete fashion, have the effect of saying that the stress just does not exist. It clearly does, and the intern notices it. At the same time, the intern does not apply the Immature Domain psychological adaptive mechanisms in locating the responsibility for managing the stress of the new admission as outside of himself. He knows that it is his responsibility, and he begins moving to accept it as he walks angrily to the ICU.

But before doing so, he has found a target for his Displaced anger in the person of the night charge nurse whom he believes will not be in a position to hurt him, as compared to the chief resident who can send him more work. In order to tolerate his own intolerable anxiety in a stressful situation, he finds a minor reason to direct an angry tirade at her. Not recognizing his own Displacement, he continues the tirade despite her giving him alternative ways to cease and desist. In righteous indignation, he leaves the ward with threats to make an administrative issue out of his displeasure. In the fury of the moment, his calculation underestimates the night nurse's role as a member of the nursing team that staffs the ward and the ICU twenty-four hours a day, seven days a week. As a result, he gets far more nighttime phone calls from the nurses in both locales during his tenure at that hospital than do his colleagues, who have found more diplomatic ways to adjust to the stresses of the job. As in the other examples in this chapter, there is no alliance between the intern and the nurses with whom he must work. Displacement does not allow compassion. And this occurs with Displacement much more than any of the other Neurotic Domain psychological adaptive mechanisms as it continues to separate idea and feeling rather than facilitate their working together.

SLIPPING AND SLIDING: DISPLACEMENT IN CLINICAL TREATMENT

A previously successful man in his mid-40s arrives for a follow-up appointment in a specialized clinic that treats alcohol use disorders. He has been continuously abstinent from alcohol for 14 months and has slowly been reestablishing his social networks with his work colleagues and his estranged family. His social and personal devastation had accelerated in the five years just prior to his reaching sobriety; during that time he had "lost everything" because of his uncontrolled alcohol use.

Over the past two months, since reaching his one-year abstinence anniversary, he has become increasingly concerned that he is entering the early stages of dementia. He complains to the clinic doctor that he has noticed an inability to remember things that happened in the course of the day and of misplacing objects at home, such as his car keys and his wallet. He confides to the clinic psychiatrist with a sense of fright that he does not want "to end up like my mother," who died at 87 after two years in a demented state. The psychiatric physician tells him that dementia is highly unlikely for a man of his age but that some office testing and further neuropsychological evaluation will shed light on the matter.

Because the alcohol clinic staff watches for memory problems related to the Wernicke-Korsakoff Syndrome (Alcohol Amnestic Syndrome), the patient's record includes a series of four memory tests over the past year. The psychiatrist notes that the patient's working memory—the ability to establish and then retrieve new memories—has been excellent. During the interview, the doctor gives the man four unrelated objects to remember and asks him to repeat them out loud. Five minutes later, he asks him to recall the objects and finds that he remembers all four without error, consistent with the previous tests in the past year. Other office tests of cognitive ability likewise point only to normal function. The patient, however, remains distraught over the possibility of dementia and agrees to more formal neurocognitive testing.

When he returns to the clinic a month later, the psychiatrist mentions that the neuropsychological tests were all negative and that he did far better at them than most people his age. The patient replies that he finds little comfort in the test results because he himself knows that he is "slipping" no matter what the normed averages say. The psychiatrist adds that the two of them will keep a close eye on the matter. But in the meantime, he may also be experiencing something that other patients in the clinic mention from time to time: that when they become worried about a drinking "slip," they sometimes find themselves complaining of something else instead.

The patient at first says that nothing like that has happened to him, but then breaks into tears. He confesses that he has been thinking about a return to alcohol use since his anniversary and that this has become constant in his thoughts, both night and day with no relief, for the past two weeks. He says that he is at his wits' end.

Doctor and patient devise a plan aimed at giving him some relief from the constant crisis. First, they agree to increase his contacts with the clinic, adding in two more group sessions weekly along with spending volunteer time helping out in the day program, both in the interest of structuring his time. The physician, after checking the patient's liver status, adds monitored disulfiram taken three times weekly in the presence of the clinic nurse. This has the effect of the patient making the decision not to drink when he takes the disulfiram tablet and feeling relief from his ruminating thoughts until taking the next dose two to three days later.

A month after this extended treatment approach, with careful monitoring of his liver enzymes and no indication of disulfiram toxicity, they reduce the dose of the disulfiram. They stop it altogether a month later with no return of the acute anxiety in maintaining abstinence. The patient meanwhile continues with the clinic groups for five more months until all concerned believe his crisis has passed. Over the course of this work, he has come to notice and to value the fact of his feeling frightened from time to time about drinking as a signal. It is his indication to replace the time spent ruminating about drinking with time spent in the company of other people who don't drink, whether in the clinic or in self-help groups. He begins to regard his intermittent worry about a drinking slip as more than just an emotional phenomenon: it serves him both as a point of conversation with others in supporting his sobriety and as a source of energy in continuing his abstinence "One day at a time."

For the purpose of understanding psychological adaptive mechanisms, the stress in this man's case originates in his unresolved wish to drink alcohol as he relates the story to the clinic psychiatrist. The first anniversary of living alcohol free often brings with it a sense of futility: daily life itself has not become perfect or trouble free even though the drinking has stopped after a great deal of effort. This disappointment in the face of unrealistically high expectations can fuel the desire to drink again because abstinence does not seem all that it is cracked up to be. The other side of this ambivalence about drinking, however, recalls the personal destruction that the addictive alcohol use caused. The result is a conflict between the two that brings on anxiety as the sense of an impending disaster. The push toward resuming alcohol with certain loss of control grows increasingly strong as does the counterbalancing terror of falling off the cliff of sobriety.

Applying the recognition algorithm in this situation, the patient does not respond to his anxiety with Primitive Domain adaptive mechanisms. He does not ignore it, minimize it, or blame it on aliens who control his Alcoholics Anonymous (AA) meetings. Nor does he employ the Immature Domain mechanisms. He views the problem as something to do with him rather than as the province and responsibility of others.

But, interestingly, his first response to something being amiss in his newfound alcohol-free life takes the form of a new and irresolvable concern about dementia overtaking his brain. The psychiatrist takes the matter seriously but finds no clinical evidence to support the patient's worry. While brain disorders can present very subtly and may manifest themselves in a downward course over long periods, the differential diagnosis in the present instance shifts to psychological causes that might explain this patient's implacable concern about dementia.

One clue appears in the parapraxic use of the verb *slipping* when he describes his self-perceived lessening of cognitive abilities. The nominative form of the same word can refer to a return to alcoholic drinking, that is, to a *slip*. At the same time, the overwhelming body of evidence in this patient's case points to the difficulties of maintaining abstinence as the principal source of anxiety expressed in any form. The experienced psychiatrist recognizes the worry over dementia as a Displacement of the fear over returning to addictive alcohol use. In effect, this patient finds it easier to think that his brain is losing its faculties than to think of his attraction to drinking and the repulsion of losing his sobriety. A return to drinking may also seem to him "demented," considered symbolically and at a level somewhere below his waking consciousness.

If the concern over impending dementia is a Displacement, one of the Neurotic Domain adaptive mechanisms, the recognition algorithm asks the clinician to establish that a disjunction exists between painful thoughts and painful emotions, as is characteristic of that Domain. In the case vignette, both unintegrated emotion and cognition flood into the conversation. Interestingly, this occurs when the psychiatrist employs a clinical Displacement in the interview: he refers to "others" who have reported similar experiences and wonders whether the patient may have noticed something similar. This interpersonal interview stratagem allows the patient to talk both of his painful thoughts and of the terror of returning to drinking, along with not knowing what to do as the situation gets worse. The use of Displacement in the interview allows patient and doctor to look at the problem together: they both look at an *It*—namely the painful thoughts and feelings associated with losing clinical ground in the patient's struggle with alcoholism. The reader will notice that neither Displacement, whether the patient's own or that introduced into the conversation by the psychiatrist, resolves the underlying stress or integrates the patient's painful thoughts and feelings. But it does set the stage for further improvement.

Displacement, considered as an adaptive mechanism, allows both patient and doctor sufficient time and relief from the crisis to devise a plan of action. This limits the turmoil and puts the patient in an environment in which he can pursue the integration of thought and feeling. First, they limit the minute-by-minute anxiety crisis to once every two days by starting the monitored disulfiram. At the same time, they increase the group therapy exposure in which the patient can find a supportive environment wherein to work further toward resolution. The net effect is to take sobriety "One day at a time," a commonly used AA approach. This patient makes use of the temporary relief found in the Neurotic Domain adaptive mechanism to move forward toward a better integration of the emotions and cognitive content of this crisis.

As treatment unfolds, he depends less and less on the disulfiram for relief of the constant anxiety and he and his doctor stop it a few months later without incident. At the same time, he begins putting in place one of the Mature Domain psychological adaptive mechanisms, namely Anticipation, the strategy discussed in Chapter 18.

He begins to notice his feeling of anxious fear as a signal rather than as a burden. He finds that he can use it to engage others in the support groups that help him maintain his abstinence. Communicating with other people helps him to locate the painful stress in his drinking history rather than in concerns of impending dementia. This also provides him support in the steps of its resolution: he begins to integrate the painful thoughts and feelings as he moves to Anticipation.

Recognizing Displacement and bringing it into clinical consideration in this case served as a crucial psychotherapeutic maneuver to assist this patient's psychological growth. In some instances, however, it may be better to provide continuing support until the Displacement wanes on its own accord, as in the following case from another fear-filled setting.

RELIEF FROM THE MOMENT: DISPLACEMENT IN FACING CANCER

A woman in her mid-20s consults her primary care doctor about a concerning dimple in her left breast that she thinks may be related to a lump she thinks she feels in the same area but is not sure about. They arrange a timely consultation with an oncologist, who does an imaging test followed by a biopsy. Microscopic examination of the tissue sample confirms the diagnosis of breast cancer. As the young woman talks with the oncologist, she learns that she will need surgery to excise the tumor, followed by a course of radiation treatment to the area, and then several months of chemotherapy delivered first by intravenous infusion and then continuing anticancer coverage in tablet form. The course of treatment adds up to about a year, but she is more concerned about the surgery in the immediate term. She and her boyfriend had planned their engagement soon, but now she worries that the surgery may make her look mutilated and unattractive. Mentioning this to the oncologist, they review a series of anonymous before-and-after photos of women who had undergone the breast surgery procedure followed by cosmetic reconstructive surgery. After doing so, she comments to the oncologist in all seriousness, "You know, I've always wanted to have my ears pierced. Do you think they could do that at the same time?"

For many readers, this case may call to mind the scene from Herodotus, quoted in earlier this chapter, of the Spartan warriors paying special attention to their grooming in the face of oncoming destruction. Whether facing an overwhelming force in ancient battle or here-and-now breast cancer at an age when forming social relationships is all-important, style matters. The Displacement of painful thoughts and feelings into looking one's best, whether in hairstyle or in earrings, provides a distinct, if temporary, relief in the Neurotic Domain psychological adaptive mechanisms. It leads on, as in the case of the alcoholic businessman, to the Mature Domain mechanisms in which true psychological resolution of the stress occurs. Or it may serve as the best psychological adaptive mechanism that the individual person can deploy for long periods of time. In that case, as with the other Neurotic Domain mechanisms, the continuing lack of integration of painful feelings and thoughts cycles back to the unresolved anxiety, and from there into another round of painful feelings and thoughts, as schematized in Figure 12.1.

The young woman with the cancer diagnosis, for example, may develop a Mature Domain Altruism as she combines her emotional and cognitive discomfort in the constructive activity of raising money for breast cancer research. Or she may continue her Neurotic Domain Displacement as she moves through a series of sequential boyfriends, disappointed each time in their inability to think of her earrings without her cancer history. The repeating pattern signals the adaptive limitation of the Neurotic Domain psychological mechanisms. This in its own way can be as psychologically and socially debilitating, as growth limiting, as the mechanisms of the Primitive and Immature Domains, respectively. In the setting of healthy brain function, the Neurotic Domain mechanisms in adult life do not require central nervous system medicinal interventions as often must occur in treating the Primitive Domain mechanisms in one or another form of psychosis. Neither do they require the social extrusion of the person into treatment settings, or the constant attention of relocating adaptive responses from outside to inside that characterize the Immature Domain mechanisms in adulthood. Persons suffering from pain in the context of the Neurotic Domain psychological adaptive mechanisms in adulthood know that they suffer and often find their way to treatment because of it. It rests with clinicians to meet them there and to apply appropriate models, such as the one presented in this volume, in the interest of catalyzing more flexible, more successful psychological adaptation.

REFERENCES

Brontë, E. (1998). *Wuthering Heights*. New York, Oxford University Press.

Herodotus. (1998). *The Histories* (Robin Waterfield, Trans.). New York, Oxford University Press.

Porter, K. A. (1972). Theft. In *The Collected Stories of Katherine Anne Porter*. New York, Harcourt Brace Jovanovich.

Shakespeare, W. (1955). *Love's Labour's Lost*. In *The Complete Works of Shakespeare* (W. J. Craig, Ed.). New York, Oxford University Press.

Primitive
Immature
Neurotic

CHAPTER 16

Reaction Formation

Of the various adaptive styles in the human repertoire, Reaction Formation is often one of the most colorful. As a psychological adaptive mechanism in respect to stress, its expression can be engaging or off-putting to the persons in the general vicinity of those using it. Clinically, Vaillant offers us a key to recognition of the Reaction Formation style: when using it, the person defines what is normally good as bad and what is normally bad as good. In one of his training lectures many years ago, Vaillant described the example of a person who is afraid of heights taking up skydiving. Persons using this style may often say that they will "beat this thing on its own terms," referring to the stress that poses a threat to conscious psychological equilibrium. Some further examples illustrate this point.

THE HEART AND ITS HEROES: REACTION FORMATION AS A PLATFORM FOR HOPE

A pleasant appearing, middle-aged woman comes to the hospital in an ambulance, having lost consciousness while at work seated at her desk. Her breathing is fast and labored, her ankles have swollen with the backed up fluid that her heart no longer pumps efficiently, and she has regained consciousness, wide-eyed with fear, stoically silent, and sensing the impending doom that her caretakers in the ER are working hard to stave off. They are successful in their efforts in treating her cardiac system collapse, and the next day while in hospital, she is offered an opportunity to join a research study of a new drug that the clinical scientists of the medical center have developed. They hypothesize that it will allow her heart to function more efficiently than will the standard treatments for the same affliction, but they must prove this. If she elects to join the study, she will get either the new treatment or the standard treatment and will herself be blind to which she receives, as will her treating doctors. She agrees to do so, and both the research team and her clinical team independently establish that she is thinking properly and is capable of giving informed consent. After she signs a document to that effect, the team begins giving her the study drug in a blinded fashion, with a 50% chance of getting either the new medicine or the standard medicine.

Twenty-four hours later, her heart function has worsened considerably, and she is now bed bound. Another day later, she has suffered heart failure to such an extent that the study drug is discontinued and a team of specialists has convened to review her case. After their conference, a senior heart specialist on the team converses with her and informs her that her heart function is now so bad that she will not recover sufficiently to leave the hospital without first undergoing a heart transplant. She agrees to the doctor's offer to begin the process of evaluation for the grafting of a new heart, taken from a deceased donor whose family has given permission to do so.

As part of the transplant evaluation, the team's psychiatrist interviews her in the ICU. He asks her to review with him the events of the past few days leading up to their conversation, which she does faithfully and accurately. "You've been through a lot," the psychiatrist comments. She agrees, tearfully, and the psychiatrist waits until her mood eases before continuing the conversation again. Then, with an empathic demeanor, he comments, "If I were in your shoes and came into the hospital with a serious heart problem and found myself feeling better with treatment, only to be so much worse after an experimental treatment, I believe I might find it difficult to have much faith in my doctors." At this, her face brightens, and she smiles in a reserved manner. With barely enough strength to lift her head from her pillow, she says "Oh no, Doctor. My doctors here are the very best in the world. I have absolute faith in them, day and night."

As we apply the adaptive style identification algorithm to this woman's case, our first task of recognizing the stress to her well-being appears obvious. It is clearly the acute heart failure that robs her of strength and breath, and triggers her anxiety with respect to whether she will live or die. Her condition improved with the first round of standard treatment, only to worsen with the experimental treatment that, in this scenario, removed any chance of recovery for her native heart. Her only choice now is a heart transplant. Her emotions flow forth when she contemplates the situation with the psychiatrist. It is clear that she understands and recognizes the anxiety, regards it as related to herself and her condition, and must find a way to face it. In first recognizing the stress and then regarding it as involving her health and requiring her own decisions, she passes beyond the first two levels of the recognition algorithm: Primitive Domain and Immature Domain psychological adaptive mechanisms, respectively.

Unexpectedly, however, her adaptation is to smile and sing the praises of the same doctors who put her on the experimental protocol to begin with. The discordant presentation between her tearful emotions on reviewing the sharp decline in her health and the smiling praises aimed at her doctors gives evidence of the lack of an integration of her emotions with the cognitive understanding of her condition. Whereas a detached observer, in this case the psychiatrist, might feel a sense of upset at the course of matters, she instead can only praise those who both played a role in her worsened physical state and on whom she now depends to provide the transplant and continue her life. Her doctors, rather than being objects of concern or at least questioning, stand as the unequivocal heroes in her life. She defines their judgment as good—possibly perfect—even though the results in her case could be considered less than that. Like the person afraid of heights, she too has leapt out of the aircraft cabin at 10,000 feet, depending on the parachute personified by her medical team for her safe landing. Although her sadness is available to her, and she expresses it, even mild forms of anger at the situation can nowhere be found. Her adaptive mechanism has separated any irritated or angry emotion from her thoughts in the characteristic manner of a Neurotic Domain style mechanism. Her overcompensation in describing her doctors as being, in her mind, the best anywhere, exemplifies a Reaction Formation.

The separation of thought and feeling in this way on the one hand projects a sense of surface heroism—the woman smiling and praising her doctors in the face of danger—but leaves a lingering sense of unresolved anger to be addressed another day. The psychiatrist makes no attempt at questioning her coping mechanism and merely notes it as her doing the best that she can in adapting to a very difficult circumstance. In her case, the Reaction Formation, so long as it remains intact—and this adaptive mechanism can be a brittle one, as we shall see—can serve her as a useful psychological mechanism for getting through the dangerous thicket of terminal heart failure and a cardiac transplant procedure. So long as the Reaction Formation remains intact, she may never, in fact, have to come to grips with her own anger at what has happened to her. Or, in the characteristic course of Neurotic Domain adaptive mechanisms, she may find that she becomes inexplicably angry on those occasions that remind her of her heart failure experience or even on those occasions in which she merely consults a physician for some other medical problem. As noted before, because the integration of thought and feeling in relation to a stress remains unresolved, their unsettled separation often provokes a human tendency to repeat the same Neurotic Domain behaviors until resolution occurs.

WAR AND "THOU SHALT NOT KILL": THE USE OF REACTION FORMATION IN COMBAT

One of the most obvious examples of Reaction Formation, and one of the most frequent in Western cultures, occurs in the setting of armed combat when military units—or indeed the public at large—face an opposing power labeled as the enemy. In most Western cultures that are influenced by Judeo-Christian ethics, killing another human being is defined as bad. According to the biblical tradition, the fifth commandment that Moses brought down from his visit to Mt. Sinai forbids killing outright. Further, and earlier in its cultural history, Western civilization affirmed a prior overarching principle, one first recorded symbolically 30,000 years ago in the cave paintings of the Neolithic hunters. It proclaimed the autonomous importance of the individual. "We hold these truths to be self-evident," states the Declaration of Independence, "that all men are created equal."

If these concepts apply to humans, they apply to all men and women. If that is true, they apply to the enemy as well as to us. The obvious syllogism concludes that the enemy too is human and we have no business killing other humans. The conclusion may further state that the enemy too is an individual or collection of them and that their lives, and their rights to them, are held as sacred for them as they are for our side. It is a very old observation that when wars are fought by young adults and overseen by their elders, combat troops often find themselves in the position of having to act against the cultural values that have been ingrained in their personalities since childhood.

The process of military training offsets much of the anxiety from this dilemma in two ways. First, the training of ordinary combat soldiers aims at the individual's membership in, and sacrifice to, the combat group and one's fellow soldiers. This occurs at a very intense emotional level as described by none other than Leo Tolstoy when he wrote, "The Regiment was a home, too, and a home as interchangeably dear and precious as the parental home."[1] But by itself, mere group membership does not actually address the conflict between home cultural values and behaviors that run counter to them in a combat situation. A second stratagem of dealing with anxiety occurs much more frequently both in ordinary troops and their officers, the latter group of whom must function more independently and take responsibility for the lives of their own men as well as for the destruction of the enemy soldiers. That is simply the stratagem of defining good as bad and bad as good. In this case, the enemy is defined as, if not inhuman, less than human or less than a perfect human whose values are not the same as ours. Because of their values, the enemy strikes at us with the aim of taking our lives and we therefore are eminently justified in taking enough enemy lives to preserve our own. Killing, therefore, reaches the definition of the good in that it saves our lives and the lives of those we care about. The enemy, who in other circumstances we would consider as good, by the same stratagem now turns into something qualitatively different: that which we would consider bad or evil. It is far easier to kill something less than human than it is to take the life of a person who is no less human than you or me. This general process, from the point of view of our model of psychological adaptive strategies, fits the definition of the Reaction Formation. We have successfully turned our perception of good into one of evil and our perception of evil into one of good. By analogy, we have taken our fear of a cultural evil, held our breaths and leaped headlong into the empty air at 10,000 feet with our limbs spread-eagled against the onrush of the life-negating values that upbringing taught us to oppose, while placing all of our faith in our nylon parachutes made of Reaction Formation.

Examples of this strategy stand in bold relief in a setting such as that of World War II, the least controversial of America's armed conflicts. The great majority of commentators, historians and ordinary people alike, agree in a very large consensus that America had to fight that war, that America did not enter it unprovoked, and that the forces of militarism in the Pacific and totalitarianism in Europe truly carried a direct threat to the personal liberty that is both the flower and the bedrock of Western civilization. Once unleashed, however, the dogs of war nonetheless effected a characteristic dehumanization of the enemy, whether "the Japs" or "the Krauts," two of the terms of the time, along with the process of turning them into subhuman demons. Citing one example, the late scholar of mythology Joseph Campbell related

1. Tolstoy (1994, p. 443).

an instance in which the *New York Times* published pictures of the monsters that served as entry statues to the garden of Nara wherein the famous statue of the Buddha sits. Its writers of that era commented in paraphrase that "the Japs worship such gods as these." Campbell, a world authority on comparative religions, knew better. The gods of the Buddhist culture make neither wrathful nor merciful judgments in respect to humans. That is characteristic only of the gods of the different biblical traditions. As an adaptive mechanism, however, the journalists at *The New York Times* had not only misinterpreted an Eastern culture but also had created a fine example of a Reaction Formation.

WHITHER COMPASSION? ONE LIMIT OF REACTION FORMATION

One correlative that we can observe here and use in considering clinical presentations in patients asking for help states that with deployment of Reaction Formation comes a necessary narrowing of vision. When this adaptive mechanism is at work, the enemy is always and everywhere the enemy. To consider otherwise is to begin to loosen the adaptive effect of this particular mechanism. As with all of the Neurotic Domain mechanisms, the result is a characteristic ruling out of compassion—of the shared feelings that unite humans with one another. As an example, in 1966 as part of a college group visiting Paris, I had heard that the Red (Communist) Chinese had an embassy there and was curious to see what it looked like and possibly even to talk with a person from that country. Thinking that someone at the U.S. embassy might know where this was located, I visited on a weekend day and found only a Marine sergeant in dress blue uniform, a young man perhaps a few years older than myself, at the desk. When I asked him where I could find the Red Chinese Embassy, his face darkened and he hammered out the response, "I don't know nothing about the Red Chinese. I don't want to know nothing about the Red Chinese." Having grown up as a military dependent myself, I recognized this as standard boot camp language, with its implied question of my loyalty to my country. This occurred in the particularly striking context of the Vietnam War of the time, one that was to expand even further than it had at that point. And I recognize it now as an adaptive response designed to keep a Reaction Formation in place. Ironically, only a few years later, the United States government itself pursued a similar, if less symbolic, path to the Red Chinese embassy, one that opened communications with China. Although I wished him all the best, I have always wondered what became of that Marine sergeant and how well his adaptive mechanism served him—and for how long.

PATTON: THE MOVIE AND THE MAN

The same mechanism, Reaction Formation, may take on different appearances among officers who must lead men, that is, among the men who must send other men into battle. A scene in the famous film *Patton* provides an introductory glimmer of understanding. In that scene, the title character and an aide drive through the area of a recent battle, a gentle plain littered with the wreckage of tanks and other war machines as well as the dead lying about the field. The general orders his aide to stop the jeep, and he gets out and walks about, encountering an exhausted and wounded soldier sitting on the ground, propped up against the wheel of a wrecked truck. Patton kneels next to him as if in fervent prayer, saying nothing, and after a few moments kisses the soldier on the forehead. The soldier appears dazed and too exhausted to notice, and the general moves on to look over other parts of the battlefield.

Referring again to the diagnostic algorithm, we can identify the stress in this scene as the general coming on the fruits of those decisions he had made that sent young men to their deaths, foreshortening their lives and affecting the lives of countless others. In the film the emotion is one of overwhelming sadness that Patton transmutes into a form of a religious experience. We do not learn his thoughts, but we do see him acting as though in prayer. We do not learn whether Patton feels (1) more than sadness and something akin to guilt for his role in the carnage, (2) a religious sense of the gratitude for the sacrifice of young lives in the cause, (3) admiration for the bravery of those who faced the fury and storm with their lives in the balance, or (4) some or all of these and perhaps others besides.

Because Patton does not express sadness outright, we do not know whether, in fact, that feeling has joined with or is disassociated from the carnage on the battlefield. This is a crucial distinction in differentiating the Neurotic Domain adaptive mechanisms. Finding a religious experience among the corpses where most might find a sense of horror or revulsion, and kissing one of the soldiers in an act that is outside the normal range of generalship, raises the possibility that what is normally considered improper Patton now defines as proper in this situation.

Consistent with the definition of a Reaction Formation, the real Patton was well known for slapping a soldier who suffered from battle fatigue—what we now call posttraumatic stress disorder (PTSD)—because he felt the man was a coward and insulted the other brave soldiers who had given their lives under his command. The same General Patton reputedly once said that he would take his military objectives even if he had to "send dog tags back home by the truckload." The energizing emotion that comes through in these two vignettes is one of anger that again appears unintegrated with a general's role in commanding troops in a battle situation. Patton's actions—uncharacteristically slapping a soldier for which he later had to apologize publicly and was relieved of his command, along with his high casualty rates that likewise are not necessarily a point of pride among generals[2]—suggest the reversal of the valences of good and bad that characterizes Reaction Formation. Patton's continuing course of brilliant and highly effective military maneuvers along with public relations and leadership failures suggests the repetitive nature of the unresolved adaptive mechanisms that characterize the Neurotic Domain as we have defined it.

---

2. Douglas MacArthur, by contrast, had relatively low casualty rates among U.S. generals during World War II.

FRIABILITY: THE DIFFICULTY IN RECONSTITUTING REACTION FORMATION ONCE BROKEN

The scene is an airfield in the South Pacific during World War II. The commanding general of the air forces in the Pacific theater of war, George C. Kenney, a man in his mid-50s, and his top fighter pilot, Major Richard Bong, 25 years old and credited with 40 enemy planes shot down, have just arrived when Japanese planes attack the base. The local American fighters intercept them at 15,000 feet directly over the airfield. The American squadron commander sets the lead Japanese ship on fire. General Kenney describes the action:

> The Jap leader pilot, unable to stand the flames,[3] jumped overboard. The Nips didn't wear parachutes . . . so the plunge meant certain death.
> The Jap pilot hit flat on the steel planking of the airdrome about a hundred feet from where Dick and I were standing. . . . I watched for Bong's reaction. I had predicted a long while ago that if he ever found out that he was not shooting at clay pigeons, I would have to take him out of combat. This was a nice kid. He was no killer and his pet peeve against the newspapermen was that they kept referring to him as the "pilot with the most kills." As he watched the . . . death, I believe it was the first time he realized that he, Dick Bong, had been responsible for many similar occurrences. He walked over to some bushes at the edge of the field and for the next five minutes was violently ill.
> . . . He was no longer the happy-go-lucky, snub-nosed, country boy. He had definitely aged in the last few minutes. This was a rough dirty game that he had been playing, and I instinctively sensed that he didn't want any more of it.
>
> (Kenney 1960, p. 111)

General Kenney rightly removed Major Bong from any further combat operations.[4] His description leaves the impression that the trauma of watching another man die violently called forth a sudden and permanent change in his fighter ace's personality. The comment of another of his fellow pilots, Colonel William T. Coleman, however,

3. Death by fire is a constant fear for all pilots. Major Mannock referred to it as "flamerinos." Captain Eddie Rickenbacker, America's top air ace in World War I records the death of his mentor, Major Raoul Lufbery, who jumped from his flaming plane at altitude rather than burn alive in it (Rickenbacker 1919). Fire claimed the lives of the three Apollo I crew members in 1967 during a test procedure on the launch pad.

4. Major Richard I. Bong remains to this day the highest scoring of any American fighter pilot in any of the nation's armed conflicts. This designation is likely to last for a very long time, and very probably for all time, because air combat itself has become so increasingly technological as to have all but dispensed with the large-scale manned air battles of the wars of the 20th century. Like the Royal Flying Corps' Mick Mannock in WWI, the U.S. Army Air Corps' Dick Bong in WWII reputedly underestimated the total number of enemy planes he actually shot down. In the words of one of his fellow pilots, "That was the official number, 40. I sincerely believe that his actual score was at least half again that many aircraft. Dick was a factual man. Not simplistic, but simply honest to the point of painfulness" (Col. Robert DeHaven, quoted in Bong, 1991, p. 477).

offers further perspective on this description. Referring to the same time period, but apparently before the incident General Kenney describes, he comments as follows:

> It was during this period that I began to notice a change in Dick. Before he was outgoing and easy to engage in conversation. He didn't withdraw, but when he would come into the tent where we are playing cards or just a bull session, he would just listen and not say much.
>
> When a fighter pilot gets like that you get concerned about him and I remember myself saying that General Kenney oughta send Dick home. He had done far more than was ever asked of him.
>
> (Bong 1991, p. 443)

General Kenney's description gives us a picture of a Reaction Formation where Major Bong is concerned. He did not set out to become a fighter pilot. His brother documents that, like most aircraft pilots, Richard Bong simply wanted to fly airplanes and joined the Army to learn to do that before World War II had started. At one point, he had to list his preference for aircraft type and chose multiengine, rather than the more glamorous single seat/single engine "pursuit" planes of the period, suggesting that he would have been as happy flying the least glamorous transports. The P-38 fighter had two engines, and that may have explained his assignment to that aircraft. He was nevertheless an exceptional pilot with exceptional eyesight who could pick out the faraway dots or flashes in the horizon that indicated opposing aircraft in the days before radar.

Like many caught between duty[5] and the Fifth Commandment, however, Major Bong did not like the epithet of "kills" or that of "killer." In the general's view, he was shooting at aircraft, not men—what General Kenney refers to as clay pigeons—and was remarkably good at downing them because of his skills as a pilot. He found, for example, that he could turn the P-38 "as if on a pivot" by manipulating its two engines rather than using the aircraft's flight controls, a remarkably useful characteristic when aiming the guns in the nose of the aircraft. In his general's view, the apparently sudden realization that he was killing men, rather than simply destroying aircraft, brought on by the enemy pilot's death in front of them, meant that the means by which Major Bong had adapted to combat situations had very suddenly and permanently broken.

In applying the recognition algorithm, we first note that the stress of shooting at others while being shot at oneself during aerial combat easily results in a credible sense of disaster or doom, that is, the anxiety of the situation. In a fast-paced, life-or-death-environment, anxiety itself can be dangerous insofar as it detracts from the skills needed to adapt to the situation successfully. Using Primitive Domain adaptive mechanisms, as in ignoring the danger posed by a lethal opponent, or Immature Domain adaptation, as in waiting for someone else to handle the threat or in drifting off into a dream world, increases the likelihood of personal danger. Neither Domain's adaptive responses manage the anxiety in ways that allow effective action.

---

5. Arguably, preventing the attacking planes from reaching his own ground troops saved many more lives than may have been lost among the attackers.

Reaction Formation, among the Neurotic Domain psychological adaptive mechanisms, by contrast, offers adaptation to both the intellectual content of the situation, paraphrased here as "I could be killed," and the affective content, stated as "I hate the fact that to survive this I must become a killer." Reaction Formation states "I can survive if I become a better killer" and "I do not hate anyone. I target planes, not people" to address the thought and feeling contents, respectively. This follows the reversal of values in which killing changes from bad to good and the enemy transforms from human beings to impersonal aircraft.

But this adaptive mechanism does not solve the ultimate dilemma stated as "Killing stands against everything I have learned as good, and my emotions toward others are those of love rather than of hate." The two do not meet until the Reaction Formation crumbles. General Kenney believed that he witnessed the collapse of this adaptive strategy in Major Bong in a single incident. In Colonel Coleman's recollection, by contrast, the process appeared to have been wearing on for some time. In our view with respect to adaptive styles, both may be possible because Reaction Formation only temporizes rather than reach a permanent resolution. To his credit, however, General Kenney's conclusion that this adaptive style, once broken, could not be reconstituted reflected a prescient knowledge of the friability of Reaction Formation as an adaptive strategy. The decision to send Major Bong home fits the situation. Clinically, a broken Reaction Formation can create a remarkably dangerous situation, as illustrated in the next case.

SLASH AND BURN: REACTION FORMATION FAILURE AS A SUICIDE RISK

A busy, well-educated, business executive had risen to the top of his profession because of his ability to turn the failing companies that his corporation acquired into profitable ventures in record time. He did this by cutting overhead costs, and that meant firing the people who worked there, some after many years of loyalty to the businesses. In his view, however, he fired only those whose "bloated" salaries reflected seniority rather than ability in the marketplace. He took no notice of any personal impact of his actions either among those whom he discharged or those he retained. Over time, he became known as the best "hatchet man" in the corporate world, a reputation that he did not talk about with others because of its negative social connotations, but in which he took a measure of pride. As his success grew in making profits in a number of difficult business environments, he developed a thick hide for the negative comments of others along with a growing confidence in his own rightness of judgment.

This continued to develop for several years, leading him to take on more and more difficult challenges in order to keep his "perfect score" intact and increase his reputation for turning businesses around. In part, his sense of never having to contemplate failure led him to take on a failing financial operation that was located in the downtown section of a very troubled and volatile inner city. After working late one night, he went out to his car in the parking facility, where he was assaulted, beaten, and robbed. Although the police found the culprits, a gang of youths with histories of drug use and no connections to anyone in the business concern, the executive found that he could no longer return to work. With no prior history of depression, he withdrew into a sense of hopelessness and steadily decreasing self-esteem, along with the firm belief that no one could help him. His family and business colleagues brought him to a famous medical center, where he entered the hospital with suicidal concerns and received an antidepressant medication. Discharged 10 days later, he returned home to continue outpatient treatment. A month after that, and after what his outpatient psychiatrist described as a good response to the antidepressant, his wife came home from work to find to their two children at their neighbor's house and her husband's automobile running in the closed garage. He had been dead for some hours and had left a note that said simply "I am no good and must act."

Applying the recognition algorithm in this "psychological autopsy," the stress to this man's conscious sense of his own well-being had to do with his long-standing pattern of inflicting pain on others whom he had fired in the interest of economic gain. He had made no working human alliances with any of them, something he could not afford to do if he was to fire them the next day. In this respect, relationships in the workplace became more and more attenuated as others realized that he equated cutting overhead ruthlessly with good, and human relationships with bad. This, in turn, led to a necessary sense of self-reliance at all costs. His sense of personal competence and well-being depended on it. The assault, in which he found himself at the complete mercy of others, beaten with no defense, and robbed of his possessions, put him in an analogous position to some of those he had fired for the good of the corporation. Symbolically speaking, that clay pigeon shattered before him at the hands of criminals who did not fit in his world. Bereft of the ability to see good as bad and bad as good, his Reaction Formation no longer in working order, he shifted downward from a Neurotic Domain adaptation to those of the Immature Domain. Notably he withdrew from others into a private world resembling Schizoid Fantasy, and finally resorted to Acting Out his suicide, rather than tolerating the continued anxiety of thinking of himself as incompetent and bad rather than competent and good.

Clinically, this case, like that of General Kenney's view of Major Bong after the incident at the airfield, reflects the remarkable property of Reaction Formation to appear as hard as a cue ball smacking against the other billiard balls for long periods of time, only to shatter irreparably. In the case of his fighter ace, George Kenney could remove Richard Bong from the immediate situation to which he had had to adapt, knowing that the stress of feeling like a killer would likely not result in personal devastation anywhere other than in combat. Stateside, Major Bong could function normally doing what he did best: flying airplanes. We will meet him again in Chapter 19.

But the business executive, by contrast, had nowhere to go. The only combat, so to speak, was that which he generated. It became the source of his self-esteem and sense of competence in dealing with the rough-and-tumble marketplace. But his slash-and-burn management techniques did not lead to a resolution of the self-hatred and inaction that made themselves apparent once the Reaction Formation no longer served with effect. From the point of view of clinicians seeing patients, situations of this kind deserve consideration as potentially lethal. They may require intensive treatment—interpersonal and perhaps medicinal—in order to allow for the careful construction of psychological adaptive mechanisms in the Mature Domain range that are new to the person. Until that can occur, a sense of personal vulnerability akin to depression can pervade almost the totality of a person's experience and easily result in the loss of perspective and even hope. Interpersonal therapeutic alliances remain the best known method for stabilizing situations of this kind. As of this writing, the author is unaware of any controlled trials of antidepressant or other medicinal interventions aimed at improving psychological adaptation after the acute loss of Reaction Formation adaptations of this sort.

ONE SOCIETY AWAY: GROWING BEYOND REACTION FORMATION

Leaving Reaction Formation behind does not necessarily require a crashing through of some cataclysmic psychological trauma or a descent into depression. As in other forms of adaptive behaviors in relation to age appropriate growth and development, the Neurotic Domain mechanisms—Reaction Formation included—can simply be grown through and replaced by the more flexible, more creative, more compassionate Mature Domain mechanisms. Nathaniel Fick has given us a recollection of his experiences in commanding a Marine reconnaissance platoon in Afghanistan and Iraq (Fick 2005). In a touching moment at the end of his book, he states that he left his commission as a Marine captain when it became clear to him that he could no longer adapt in a constructive way (my paraphrase) to spending the capital that he and every other knowledgeable combat officer values highest: the lives of their men. He had completed two combat tours—first in Afghanistan and a second in Iraq—during which none of the men in his platoon had died. In his words,

> I left the Corps because I had become a reluctant warrior. Many Marines reminded me of gladiators. They had that mysterious quality that allows some men to strap on greaves and a breastplate and wade into the gore. I respected, admired, and emulated them, but I could never be like them. I could kill when killing was called for, and I got hooked on the rush of combat as much as any man did. But I couldn't make the conscious choice to put myself in that position again and again throughout my professional life. Great Marine commanders, like all great warriors, are able to kill that which they love most—their men. It's a fundamental law of warfare. Twice I had cheated it. I couldn't tempt fate again.
>
> (Fick 2005, p. 364)

In the context of this chapter, we may suppose that "that mysterious quality" to which Captain Fick refers may have something to do with using Reaction Formation as a style of adapting to the extreme circumstance of putting one's soldiers in harm's way. "Kill[ing] that which they love most" sounds intrinsically like a reversal of bad as good. In the ordinary experience of living, most humans act to preserve those whom they love most. In Captain Fick's case, the Reaction Formation did not apply. He could see through it, and he tells us that for him it had no use.

In the film portrayal of General Patton, the commander's love of the bravery of his men is second to none. But, in contrast to Captain Fick, the real Patton also saw himself as a child of destiny who would lead great armies victoriously into battle. The destiny of his men, therefore, affected his own destiny and would serve it. In our present model of adaptive styles, an effective Reaction Formation in Patton's case required that the deaths of many thousands of those whom he commanded would have to be defined as good. Similarly, the destiny of a single man served by those deaths required definition as good, contrary to the more common constructions of self-serving "destiny" as bad. Whether this was true of the real General Patton, the historians may decide. For the purpose of understanding Reaction Formation and how it fits into our diagnostic scheme, it is sufficient to raise the question as a matter of comparison. The most famous Confederate commander of the American Civil War, Robert E. Lee, reputedly said that it is well that war is so horrible. Otherwise we would come to love it. Reaction Formation in which the horror is defined as bravery or as heroism can provide some combatants with a way to love it in despite.

PSEUDO-ALTRUISM: A REACTION FORMATION TO KEEP HOPELESSNESS AT BAY

Bravery and heroism sound remarkably altruistic. And in many cases they are, as we shall see in Chapter 19. But oftentimes what looks like the Mature Domain adaptive mechanism of Altruism on closer examination appears truly as another form of Reaction Formation. A remarkable description of this comes from an unlikely source: a late Georgian/early Victorian English novelist writing about her heroine, an orphaned governess who must make her way through the social complexities of her time and place (Brontë 2000). Toward the end of *Jane Eyre*, Charlotte Brontë introduces us to the character of Mr. St. John Rivers, the young Anglican curate of a small village in rural England during the first half of the 19th century. Jane, who narrates the book, describes him:

> Zealous in his ministerial labors, blameless in his life and habits, he yet did not appear to enjoy that mental serenity, that inward content, which should be the reward of every sincere Christian and practical philanthropist. Often, of an evening, when he sat at the window, his desk and papers before him, he would cease reading or writing, rest his chin on his hand, and deliver himself up to I know not what course of thought: but that it was perturbed and exciting might be seen in the frequent flash and changeful dilation of his eye.
>
> (Brontë 2000, p. 351)

A few paragraphs on, she takes us into his church and describes a sermon that he delivers:

> It began calm—and indeed, as far as delivery and pitch of voice went, it was calm to the end: an earnestly felt, yet strictly restrained zeal breathed soon in the distinct

accents, and prompted the nervous language. This grew to force—compressed, condensed, controlled. The heart was thrilled, the mind astonished, by the power of the preacher: neither was softened. Throughout there was a strange bitterness; an absence of consolatory gentleness; stern allusions to the Calvinistic doctrines—election, predestination, reprobation—were frequent; and each reference to these points sounded like a sentence pronounced for doom. When he had done, instead of feeling better, calmer, more enlightened by his discourse, I experienced an inexpressible sadness; for it seemed to me—I know not whether equally so to others—that the eloquence to which I had been listening had sprung from a depth where lay turbid dregs of disappointment—where moved troubling impulses of insatiate yearnings and disquieting aspirations. I was sure St. John Rivers—pure lived, conscientious, zealous as he was—had not yet found that peace of God which passeth all understanding.

(p. 352)

In the next chapter, we hear from Reverend Rivers himself on the subject of how he came to his vocation, his calling to be a minister of God:

A year ago, I was myself intensely miserable because I had thought I had made a mistake in entering ministry: its uniform duties wearied me to death. I burnt for the more active life of the world—for the more exciting toils of the literary career—for the destiny of an artist, author, orator; anything rather than that of a priest: yes, the heart of a politician, of a soldier, of a votary of glory, a lover of renown, a luster after power, beat under my curate's surplice. I considered; my life was so wretched, it must be changed, or I must die. After a season of darkness and struggling, light broke and relief fell: my cramped existence all at once spread out to a plane without bounds—my powers heard a call from heaven to rise, gather their full strength, spread their wings and mount beyond ken. God had an errand for me; to bear which afar, to deliver it well, skill and strength, courage and eloquence, the best qualifications of the soldier, statesman, and orator, were all needed: for these all centre in the good missionary.

A missionary I resolved to be. From that moment my state of mind changed; the fetters dissolved and dropped from every faculty, leaving nothing of bondage but its galling soreness—which time only can heal.

(pp. 361–362)

We learn that Mr. Rivers' late father did not think the missionary idea a good one. Jane comes to that conclusion as well when she meets Miss Rosamond Oliver, a wealthy young woman of the area who is in love with St. John Rivers. He explains to Jane in the next chapter, however, that Miss Oliver will never make a good missionary's wife because of the necessary privations involved. Implying that love is more important than a religious cause, Jane says to him, "But you need not be a missionary. You might relinquish that scheme." To which he responds with a torrent of words:

Relinquish! What! My vocation? My great work? My foundation laid on earth for a mansion in heaven? My hopes of being numbered in the band who have merged all ambitions in the glorious one of bettering their race—of carrying knowledge into the realms of ignorance—of substituting peace for war—freedom for bondage—religion for superstition—the hope of heaven for the fear of hell? Must I relinquish that? It is dearer than the blood in my veins. It is what I have to look forward to, and to live for.

(p. 374)

Following the recognition algorithm's path through Charlotte Brontë's description of Mr. Rivers, we begin by establishing the nature of the perturbation to his conscious self that we call the stress in the model of psychological adaptation. We see it described in the first three passages: (1) Jane notices his animation when it interrupts his humdrum work as a curate, (2) she notices his sermon as a technically brilliant production that is completely unconvincing, sensing instead the deep sadness of a minister of God who has not found God's peace,[6] and (3) St. John Rivers describes the changes that came over him a year before when he found himself caged in a dead-end profession, one that "wearied (him) to death," as the character states. Unlike the other cases discussed in this chapter, St. John Rivers' perturbation comes from his own inner psychological turmoil rather than some outside circumstance such as heart disease, physical assault, or combat. Locked in humdrum while desiring power and glory, he finds himself facing the sense of doom that our psychological adaptation model defines as the anxiety resulting from the stress: he states plainly that his state a year previously required that he must either have changed his life or died.

Interestingly, he does not change his life, that is, he does not change his profession. Instead, recalling from Chapter 1 the words of Charlotte Brontë's contemporary Edgar Allan Poe, St. John Rivers engages in "that half-pleasurable, because poetic, sentiment with which the mind usually receives even the sternest natural images of the desolate and terrible." That is, he changes his own perception of the harsh reality he both recognizes and feels as a way of dealing with his sense of doom or personal disaster. The recognition algorithm next asks whether he does this by using a Primitive Domain adaptive mechanism that would allow him to ignore his own inner turmoil. His portrayal gives no evidence of this, nor does it suggest the presence of an Immature Domain adaptive style in which he blames his own inner torment on some external cause. As Charlotte Brontë portrays him, he recognizes both that his difficulties exist and that they lie within him.

The next step in the recognition algorithm requires a statement of both the cognitive and the emotional contents of Reverend Rivers' distress. The idea can be

---

6. Charlotte Brontë here precociously describes what modern models of clinical psychiatric interaction in the doctor-patient relationship later formulated as *transference* in Sigmund Freud's psychoanalytic model and *parataxic distortion* in Harry Stack Sullivan's interpersonal model. Using a phrase put forth in Chapter 13, *transference* refers to the person's emotional baggage—in this case, St. John Rivers' sadness that Jane finds reflected in her own mood during the sermon—and *parataxic distortion* has to do with the way that emotion changes the person's view of others—in this case Reverend Rivers' view of God as a punishing rather than a compassionate deity and Miss Oliver's love as a hindrance rather than a good, as Jane comments.

formulated as "I have chosen a life that I do not want," and the feeling as "I am stuck in quicksand with no hope of living the life I want to." The algorithm used in the present recognition model then asks whether the idea and the affective contents, respectively, work together or are separate phenomena disconnected from each other. Charlotte Brontë gives us no reason to suggest that they are working together. One clue lies in her character Jane finding only sadness in St. John Rivers' predicament that results in her pitying him, rather than a feeling of compassion that draws her into a sense of friendship or commonality.

But perhaps of the greatest importance, St. John Rivers does not resolve his difficulty of being stuck in the ministry. He merely redefines its terms, paraphrased as follows: the missionary ministry is good and the other worldly occupations that excite my soul are bad. He will become a missionary in order to take part in the characteristics of the now bad worldly occupations and he will use them to define his ministry as good. In this regard, his adaptive strategy fulfills the definition of a Neurotic Domain psychological adaptive mechanism in failing to come to grips with his own painful ideas and feelings in a way that resolves them. Rather than use the discordant feeling to change his profession for one that he likes and would find more satisfying, he will attack both the cognitive and the affective aspects of the stress he feels on its own terms and become a "super minister," so to speak, in the form of a missionary. The character's specific adaptive strategy is that of Reaction Formation, whereby he has now defined his previously bad choice of his ministerial profession as good and the professions he found personally stimulating, rather than humdrum, as bad.

Charlotte Brontë's description of the psychological process that transforms bad to good in the third passage quoted above allows us to draw the conclusions she wishes merely from the details she presents, a remarkable piece of writing indeed. But she is not finished with Mr. Rivers, nor with us. In the last passage quoted above, we learn that character will forgo not only a healthy change in professions but also the possibility of genuine love in the form of Miss Oliver. When Jane suggests the alternative of giving up becoming a missionary/super minister, he reacts with outrage. In his view, she does not realize that she is asking him to give up the love of others who will see the light of truth from his ministering as well as his own glory in earning his place in Heaven. From her point of view, both his love needs and his narcissistic gratification have wrapped themselves up in the cloak of his identity as a missionary. The options for real love and for a more satisfying work life cannot permeate it.

Clinically, this point differentiates true Altruism from the pseudo-altruism of Reaction Formation. Specifically, the continuing pseudo-altruism serves either or both the love needs and the narcissistic needs for the person using that adaptive strategy. The test lies in whether the particular activity, when given up, results in a return of the sadness and hopelessness that this adaptive mechanism has kept at bay, rather than resolved. Charlotte Brontë makes it clear that beneath St. John Rivers' zeal for missionary work lies a profound sadness—the emotion that Jane senses during his sermon—into which he would descend were his plans as a missionary—that is, his Reaction Formation—torn asunder. Deploying true Altruism, as we shall see in Chapter 19, offers a positive adaptation that does not serve as a patch for unrepaired love or narcissistic injury, the test being that one altruistic activity can be stopped or even substituted easily for another without retreat into depression. The view of pseudo-altruism as a form of Reaction Formation underscores the brittle nature of this psychological adaptive mechanism. There is no reconstituting it, and this, as we have observed before in the case of the business executive, may result in very dangerous and potentially lethal situations.

THE SLEEPY INTERN CHANGES JOBS: A POSITIVE OUTCOME OF BROKEN REACTION FORMATION

This does not occur, however, in the case of our overworked intern who, as always, is awake in the small hours of the morning with a heavy load of patients in intensive care as well as on the medicine floor. This chapter's intern chose medicine as a profession because it would allow him to keep other people alive. He studied hard and acquired a detailed knowledge of the intricacies and nuances of clinical medicine, all aimed at serving the same purpose. Now, in the third month of his internship, he has been pleased to note that his knowledge has paid off: no patient has died while on his watch. At 3 A.M., however, he receives an urgent call from the ICU about a person admitted there before his shift began. The patient suffers from a particularly malignant form of high blood pressure that has begun to spike to dangerously high levels. The intensive care nurses are afraid that he may develop a stroke—bleeding into his brain—if his condition is not controlled. The intern appears as requested and begins a timely and methodical progression through the medical treatments that will bring the blood pressure down. At first this seems to be working, and then the treatments appear to wear off for no apparent reason. He progresses through several levels of more and more aggressive treatment that include incrementally higher risks for side effects. Again the patient seems to respond for brief time and then worsens. Finally, after three hours, the patient suffers a massive stroke and expires 30 minutes later. Shaken by the experience, the intern very carefully goes around visiting each of the other patients under his care for that shift, assiduously reviewing their clinical state and their medication orders. In the morning, as the day staff comes on, he asks to speak to the chief resident and informs him that he has decided he can no longer function as an internal medicine intern. Reviewing this with the attending staff and chief of the service does not change his decision. They ask them to take the day off and talk with them again in 24 hours. When he appears the next day, he informs them that his decision is final and that he has arranged to transfer to a pathology residency in a hospital in another city. He apologizes to them for leaving the "program in a lurch" and then follows through with his plans to move and develop a career as a pathologist.

Following the recognition algorithm takes us first to the source of the stress, in this case the death of the intern's patient despite his methodical and scientifically based treatment, delivered in a timely manner and in accord with the best medical practice. The man died anyway, leaving the intern face-to-face with the limits of medicine as a profession: people die. Knowledge and compassion can ease suffering and can extend lives that might have been foreshortened otherwise. But people still die. And this death makes the intern anxious. At first bolstered by his luck in not encountering the death of a patient during his first few months as a physician, after the death of this patient he becomes extraordinarily focused on the details of the care of all the other patients for whom he is responsible, redoubling his efforts to make sure that none of them die during the same shift. One cataclysmic disaster is enough.

Following the clinical algorithm to its first plateau, the intern does not present any evidence to suggest a Primitive Domain adaptation to the death of his charge. He does not avoid acknowledgment of the fact, deny its existence, or refer it to a delusional belief in some evil power pervading the hospital ventilation system. Similarly, moving to the algorithm's next decision point with respect to Immature Domain adaptive strategies, the intern does not blame the occurrence on others by citing the incompetence of the admission team or accusing the nursing staff of improper care. Nor does he withdraw into a fantasy on some other topic, punch out the door to the ICU, or otherwise behave in a manner that locates his response to this stress as outside his control. He uses neither Primitive nor Immature Domain psychological adaptive strategies.

Recognition of a Neurotic Domain psychological adaptive mechanism requires first identification of the respective contents of the painful thought and feeling that the intern experiences as a result of the stress. The cognitive content can be stated in the first person as "I could not keep this man from dying." In this case, a corollary to this can be phrased as "I too will die." The associated emotional content comes forth as fear, if not terror. The algorithm next asks, in the intern's case, do the idea of death and the terrified feeling work together in some way that allows the intern to adapt with a Mature Domain approach, or do they remain separate? The answer lies in the rigidity of his response: he informs his supervisors that he cannot continue to take on the responsibility for other people's lives. He has first walked a very anxious line in ensuring that none of the other patients on his service will die and then removed himself from their proximity, relocating to a specialty in which he can remain in clinical science without that responsibility. His primary adaptive mechanism, one that we can state as "beating death on its own terms by overwhelming it with scientific understanding," has fallen apart. Proper scientific understanding served as his parachute when at 10,000 feet, he jumped out of the airplane to test death, only to find that the parachute contained a number of clinical holes. His adaptive strategy, a Reaction Formation, held that a career that took on the jaws of death was good, and putting scientific knowledge in a more realistic perspective was bad. Compare this to a more balanced Mature Domain approach, such as Suppression, discussed in the next chapter, that allows working through the painful thoughts and feelings incrementally, leading to their true resolution. In this case, however, as in General Kenney's view of his top P-38 pilot, the context must change to account for the friability of an adaptive style that no longer works.

From time immemorial, humans have had to adapt to the same difficult reality—human mortality—that led our intern into, and then out of, direct care clinical medicine. Humanity has often adapted, in different eras and across different cultures around the globe, by defining death as a passage to a new and better form of life rather than as a final ending. This has as its object, if not redefining death as entirely good, at least defining it as somewhat less bad. As a Reaction Formation, however, this strategy still falls prey to its own brittle nature when the basics of human idea and feeling have not cooperated to reach a resolution. As we shall see in some of the subsequent chapters, humanity has likewise found ways in which such painful feelings and ideas can be shared, understood, and brought to some resolution—when ideas remain accessible to feelings, and feelings to ideas.

REFERENCES

Bong, C. (1991). *Dear Mom So We Have a War*. Minneapolis, Burgess.
Brontë, C. (2000). *Jane Eyre*. New York, Oxford University Press.
Fick, N. (2005). *One Bullet Away, the Making of a Marine Officer*. Boston, Houghton Mifflin.
Kenney, G. C. (1960). *Dick Bong, Ace of Aces*. New York, Popular Library.
Rickenbacker, E. V. (1919). *Fighting the Flying Circus*. New York, Frederick A. Stokes.
Tolstoy, L. (1994). *War and Peace*. New York, Modern Library.

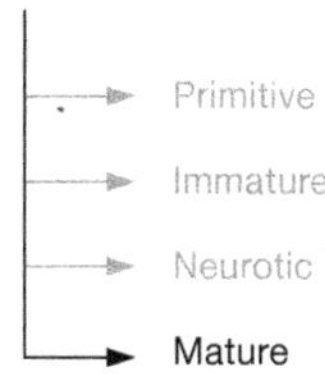

CHAPTER 17

Suppression

With Suppression we begin consideration of the Mature Domain of psychological adaptive mechanisms. We have come a long way. Beginning with the Primitive Domain mechanisms and their strategy of treating a perturbing stress and its resulting anxiety as not there—that is, that it doesn't exist—we first began the exercise of establishing the presence of the stress that perturbs conscious perception. Whether derived from conscious experience or unconscious thought, it serves to raise anxiety—that sense of disaster or doom—in waking awareness.

Moving on to the Immature Domain psychological adaptive mechanisms, we noted that at this level of psychological adaptation the person's own perceptions in wakeful consciousness recognize the existence of the stress. The adaptive strategy at this level, however, places the stress outside the psychological entity of the person and describes adaptation to it—the work of addressing anxiety—as belonging to other people.

In the last five chapters, exploring the Neurotic Domain psychological adaptive mechanisms, we noticed that the location of responsibility for adapting to the stress and its anxiety has shifted inside—within the psychological bounds of the person—where it can be addressed far more effectively than in the lower two domains of adaptive functioning. But in the Neurotic Domain, the two ingredients of the stress—its cognitive or idea or thought content, and its affective or emotional or feeling content—do not connect with each other. Their disjunction results in behaviors that repeat over and over again with no hope of a solution until the thoughts and feelings can reach a state of working together.

We notice, however, that each level moves the person's psychological adaptive mechanisms incrementally closer to an adaptive strategy that will address the stressful perturbation and resolve the anxiety it causes. So it is that in a developmental recapitulation of the adaptive stages from early childhood to adult life, the person moves from recognizing the existence of the stress and anxiety, to perceiving them as one's own, to finding that the thought and feeling contents involved make up the ingredients of their psychological resolution.

So, too, we find parallels in this hierarchical model of adaptive behaviors in models that describe psychological pathology such as those listed in the current diagnostic and statistical manuals indigenous either to the United States or Europe.[1] The Primitive Domain adaptive mechanisms find echoes in psychotic disorders or borderline personality diagnostic criteria. The Immature Domain psychological adaptive styles have analogs in the character/personality disorder diagnoses. And those of the Neurotic Domain most resemble pathological adjustment reactions. The present model of adaptive psychological mechanisms, like those models of diagnostic criteria, bases its recognition process on observable behavior. But unlike them, it seeks to recognize, understand, and make use of the dynamic interrelationship among stress, anxiety, and the ingredients of adaptation. As we shall see in Chapter 22, this model carries treatment as well as diagnostic implications.

In considering the Mature Domain psychological mechanisms of adaptation, however, our discussion leaves all references to pathology behind. Models of psychological pathology—whether listed as disorders, reactions, or illnesses—now no longer pertain. Instead, the discussion proceeds into the realm of the consideration of the highest forms of human functioning. That is to say, the model characterizes the most effective and flexible and creative ways that humans have of adapting to the stresses and anxieties of their lives in the human condition. Where before we walked in the realm of fear and frustration, now we converse with the just, the uplifting, and the courageous. Where before the psychological adaptive mechanisms pushed people apart from one another, now they provide the connections that bring us together. Where the sense of shared feeling with other human beings went unfulfilled before, now human compassion makes its entrance and acts to its full potential. Where before the observer felt puzzled or appalled, now he or she admires others and finds a sense of belonging to the human tumult.

With this sense of uplift, even of inspiration, in considering the Mature Domain methods of adapting to psychological pain, it may seem ironic to begin with Suppression, the most stoic and, along with Anticipation, the least given to poetry of the Mature styles. Yet its relative simplicity recommends it as a good place to begin. Like the jumbo jetliners of our day, it is the adaptive mechanism that lifts the most people off the ground: it is very likely the most frequently used of the Mature Domain mechanisms in everyday life. To introduce Suppression and the Mature Domain, consider a brief passage, about 3000 years old, from *The Odyssey*, Homer's picaresque tale of Odysseus' nine years of wandering as he returns from the 10-year siege of Troy. Toward the end of what some describe as the greatest single poem ever written, we come upon Homer's trickster hero as he once again sets foot in his own kingdom.

NOW OR LATER? SUPPRESSION IN THE INTEREST OF EFFECTIVE ACTION

Odysseus comes ashore near his home at Ithaca but does so disguised as a swineherd. No one has seen him in 19 years, and, wary of the circumstances into which he returns, he uses his disguise to reconnoiter and understand the changes that have taken place. He subsequently learns that his palace has been invaded by a group of

1. The DSM series and the ICD series.

greedy suitors who try to convince his patient wife, Queen Penelope, who still awaits him, that he is dead and that she should marry one of them. On his way toward the palace, he meets Melanthios, a goatherd and a lackey of the suitors. Melanthios ridicules the swineherd without knowledge of his true identity. After a long diatribe, he adds to his verbal abuse of the disguised Odysseus, to whom he refers as "he" in the first four lines of the passage:

> "But I tell you this straight out and it will be a thing accomplished.
> If he ever comes near the house of god-like Odysseus,
> his ribs and head will feel the weight of plenty of footstools
> flung at him all over the house by the hands of heroes."
> So he spoke, and as he went by recklessly lashed out
> with his heel to the hip, but failed to knock him out of the pathway,
> for Odysseus stood it, unshaken, while he pondered within him
> whether to go for him with his cudgel, and take the life from him,
> or pick him up like a jug and break his head on the ground. Yet
> still he stood him and kept it all inside him.
>
> (Homer, *The Odyssey*, Book XVII, lines 230–238)

Once again bringing the algorithm to bear for purposes of recognition, the stress that perturbs Odysseus comes from his tormentor's verbal abuse and his attempt to kick him out of the way. Faced with verbal and physical assault, we can infer Odysseus' anxiety rising in response. Homer implies as much when he says that Odysseus "stood," that is, endured, both the assault and his own reaction to it. Recognizing both the stress from the personal threat as well as the associated anxiety, the algorithm next asks whether he recognizes them or ignores them.

Homer leaves us in no doubt that Odysseus notices the threat Melanthios poses, inept though it may be, and does not respond by denying its existence, retreating elsewhere, or blaming it on some bad-tempered Greek deity. He does not employ a Primitive Domain adaptive mechanism, and this moves us further through the algorithm into consideration of his response as perhaps that of the Immature Domain mechanisms. But Homer does not portray his hero as blaming this misfortune on someone else. Odysseus does not bow to Melanthios and apologize for getting in the way of his foot, as one might expect were Passive Aggression at work. Nor does he withdraw into some fantasy state of mind as a way of escaping from the situation. In the passage, Homer makes it clear that Odysseus locates the resolution of the situation nowhere else but in himself. The Immature Domain adaptive mechanisms, like the Primitive, are not at work here.

To characterize his response as belonging to the Neurotic Domain of adaptive styles, the algorithm asks the observer to identify the cognitive content as well as the emotional content of the stress that Odysseus notices consciously in Melanthios' treatment of him. Cognitively, the physical and verbal assaults standout: "This man is trying to hurt me," we might paraphrase. This vignette, of the lowlife herder of goats trying to lord it over a herder of pigs, leaves little doubt about the emotional content: anger. Melanthios will let his inferiors know who they are, a stance reminiscent of the Neurotic Projection described in Chapter 11. But in respect to Odysseus, the algorithm asks whether thought and feeling contents appear disparate or well integrated: are they separate, or do they work together? If separate, we would expect to see either the thought immediately present and emotion far away, as in Intellectualization, or the reverse, as in Repression when emotion is at hand and its idea content somewhere else. Neither of those represents the case in this vignette.

Instead, Odysseus remains in touch with feeling and idea simultaneously in a way that allows the observer to know that he has integrated them, that is, that they are working together. With what Roman philosophers later referred to as stoicism, he endures the experience: he stands it, as Homer says. From the point of view of the adaptive model, he puts a lid on the anxiety and the anger, as it were, and coolly considers his options as to when to deal with this man who threatens him and tries to hurt him. Should he destroy him using his hardwood cudgel with a blow to the head? Should he pick him up and crack his skull against the ground? Or should he wait and not call attention to himself? He chooses the last of these actions. There is no passivity here as in the Immature Domain mechanisms. It is a matter of leaving the lid on the emotional energy until, in an appropriate circumstance, it can be taken off and the energy harnessed to a resolution of the dilemma.

Figure 17.1 presents the process of the Mature Domain psychological adaptive mechanisms in response to stress. Notice that in comparison to the previous schematics for the Primitive, Immature, and Neurotic Domains, respectively, the Mature Domain mechanisms complete the circle that begins with the stress and ends with its resolution. The Mature Domain adaptive mechanisms respond to the anxiety and provide for the integration of the cognitive and emotional contents that the stress

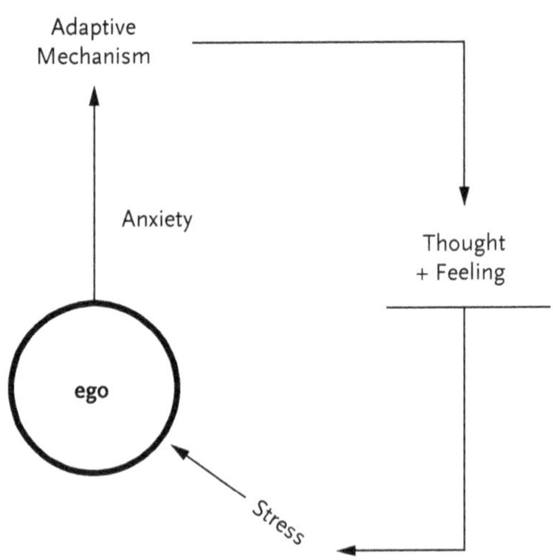

Figure 17.1
The Mature Domain strategies recognize the stress in waking consciousness, own it as belonging to the person involved, and call forth the Mature Domain psychological adaptive mechanisms. These include the appropriate integration of painful thoughts and painful feelings occasioned by the stress, resulting in the most flexible, and often most creative, adaptive behaviors. These allow the person to resolve the stress.

generates. So it is that in the case of Suppression, Mature Domain adaptation allows sufficient flexibility as to provide for patience, calculation, and emotional accounting in providing an appropriate response. In this case, Odysseus successfully limits his response in the context of the dangers of his return. He realizes that he must deal with many more dangerous people than Melanthios in displacing the suitors who would take over his kingdom.

As Homer's story unfolds, Odysseus finds bigger fish to fry, so to speak, and his attention to the use of surprise plays an important part in his return to Penelope and to the helm of his kingdom. From the algorithm's point of view, Homer's wandering hero finds that idea and feeling arrive simultaneously in waking consciousness, and work together. Odysseus' consciousness manages them until he can use them to their greatest effect to resolve both the stress and its anxiety as he regains his home. The story, as Homer passes it on to us, ends happily from the point of view of the adventure's principal character.

SUPPRESSION IGNORED: THE FATE OF ANCIENT TROY

In Homer, however, a character's consistent use of a Mature Domain adaptive mechanism does not necessarily result in a happy ending, as it does in *The Odyssey*. We return once more to *The Iliad*, in whose lines we have already met the furious Achilles (Achilleus), passively leaving his fellow Greeks to their bloody fate as a measure of his anger toward Agamemnon. We have met his opposite number, Hector of the shining helmet, who cannot tolerate his anxieties and acts on them, leading to his death. From the point of view of the psychological adaptation model, Homer presents both Achilles and Hector locked into their own Immature Domain adaptive styles, Passive Aggression and Acting Out, respectively. Neither character changes, or grows as we might say, and each proceeds without deviation to his respective destiny—to his fate as determined by the fatal flaws in the personality, according to the model the ancient Greeks used. The classic "fatal flaws" of character in that model were impervious to change as compared to adaptive styles in the present model.

But Homer presents his Trojan warriors with another option, one often overlooked in popular readings of the tale perhaps because it does not involve battle, but its opposite. A mention of *The Iliad* in conversation today brings to mind Achilles and Hector. Homer, however, gives us another Trojan warrior named Poulydamas, one whom the reader of this book has likely never heard unless he or she has spent time in a careful reading of Homer's war poem. He arrives late in the story and at a precise moment: just after Achilles has taken the field in his return to the battle but just before Hector, in a storm of ill-considered *machismo*, goes out to fight. Poulydamas rises to speak as the Trojans meet on their side of the battlefield. With their backs to their city walls, they find the Greeks inspired now by brave Achilles' angry return to the fighting:

> They stood on their feet in assembly, nor did any man have the patience
> to sit down, but the terror was on them all, seeing that Achilleus

had appeared, after he had stayed so long from the difficult fighting.
First among them to speak was the careful Poulydamas. . . .
"Now take careful thought, dear friends; for I myself urge you
to go back into the city and not wait for the divine dawn
in the plain beside the ships. We are too far from the wall now.
While this man was still angry with great Agamemnon,
for all that time the Achaians were easier men to fight with. . . .
With him, the fight will be for the sake of our city and our women. . . .
If all of us will do as I say, though it hurts us to do it,
this night we will hold our strength in the market place, and the great walls
and the gateways, and the long, smooth-planed, close-joined gate timbers
that close to fit them shall defend our city.

(Homer, *The Iliad*, Book 18, lines 246 and subsequent)

As if he had written recognition algorithm, Homer makes plain to us what constitutes the stress of the situation when he says that Achilles has returned to the battlefield: the equation that has deadlocked the two armies for a very long time has now changed. It has not changed in the Trojans' favor, a fact that is obvious to everyone. From this arises the anxiety: in Homer's words, "the terror was on them all." Their sense of disaster delivers the perception of a threat of such magnitude that they cannot even sit down. The story's interest, both to the audiences of Homer's time and to us, lies in what they do with this looming sense of disaster. We have already seen that the assembly has forgone any Primitive Domain adaptive effort at ignoring the change in the battle environment. An examination of immediately subsequent passages in Chapter 7 establishes that Hector and the great majority of the Trojan warriors will respond to their anxiety by trying to get rid of it through immediate action, that is, by Acting Out, one of the Immature Domain psychological adaptive mechanisms.

To pursue the alternative that Poulydamas, whom Homer portrays as the first to speak, offers returns us to the recognition algorithm, this time to assess the characteristics of his response to the stress and its anxiety from the view of the Neurotic Domain adaptive mechanisms. We start by articulating the idea and the feeling contents of the stress: the first can be paraphrased as, "We are now in danger for our lives where before we were not," and the second following Homer's description, "We are terrified." For Poulydamas, these two ingredients work together as an integrated whole. He does not speak to only to the terror or only to the logical change in the battlefield equation, as might be expected in Repression and Intellectualization, respectively: he talks of both simultaneously instead.

He tells the other warriors that they are overextended—too far out on the battle plain from their own walls—and, in modern terms, that they are outgunned now that the Greeks' best warrior has taken the field against them. He counsels the immediate action of retreat—rather than Hector's foolhardy alternative of immediate attack—for the purpose of withdrawing to a position of safety within the city that they have made impervious to direct assault from the Greeks. There, Homer implies, they will analyze the change in the situation and prepare an effective plan to counterbalance Achilles' return. Besides this intellectual response to the change in the battle, he simultaneously addresses the affective content of that change—the principal empirical characteristic of the Mature Domain psychological adaptive mechanisms—when he counsels retreat even though "it will hurt us to do it." He knows that an inglorious retreat will fly in the face of the warriors who view battle as an opportunity for glory and that their hurt will be the injured narcissism of appearing to run from a fight. Poulydamas balances this when he says that the battle is now to save and defend their city and their women, implying that concerns of personal glory no longer have relevance to the task at hand. His advice to the gathering is, in essence, to take their anxieties into the safety of the city and then look at the difficulties in a more controlled environment in which they will not need to respond from a sense of desperation. According to the clinical recognition method, therefore, Poulydamas himself exemplifies the adaptive response of Suppression. He argues that they must take control of their anxiety and put a cap on it until they can get to a safe place and begin to examine it in careful increments aimed at a solution to the stress itself that will solve the affective dilemma as well. In the story, as we have seen, the other warriors ignore him completely, an action that Homer calls foolish, and rush on to their destruction. In our present model, Homer portrays this state of affairs as a mob preferring the emotional release of instant action over tolerating their anxiety and approaching idea and feeling in a careful manner that attends to both.

Although the present model will have more to say on the clashes between the Immature or Neurotic Domain mechanisms and the Mature Domain strategies in social or interpersonal situations, the task of this chapter remains to define Suppression as observed in the individual. This focus returns us to settings in which individuals must function with relative independence in difficult situations. In this regard, the discussion calls forth, for the second of three appearances, an exemplar from an earlier chapter: Major Edward "Mick" Mannock of the Royal Flying Corps.

WING WALKER: SUPPRESSION IN A CRISIS

The aircraft of the First World War were largely constructed of wood, wire, and fabric with an engine attached. Although aircraft designers and builders had only begun to understand the similarities between the physical characteristics of air and fluid dynamics, popular imagination made the short leap by calling them airships. The sails of ships made up their rigging, and those who managed the sails became known as riggers. The same term described what we would now call the mechanics who kept in good order the wings, fuselage, and control surfaces of the biplanes that had both upper and lower wings—referred to as *planes* in the language of physics or mathematics. Consider then the following two descriptions of the same incident early in Edward Mannock's flying career, in France in near the front lines but well before he fired a shot in the defense of his country. He himself provides the first description in his diary shortly after it occurred. The second records that of his rigger.

> On the 19th (April, 1917) did some gun practice and in one dive from two thousand my right bottom plane [lower right wing on the Nieuport Scout] broke and fell clean away. Managed to right the machine after desperate efforts with the "joy stick" and landed slowly and safely about half a mile away from aerodrome. Such a thing has never happened before where the pilot has not been killed or injured by the fall.
>
> (Mannock 1966, pp. 45–47)

> According to Sergeant W. Bovett, who was in charge of aircraft rigging in Mannock's flight: "His bottom plane came off in the air, while diving vertically at the ground target. By skillful piloting he managed to get the machine down safely, but crashed it in the ploughed field without being hurt. It was a splendid effort. When his rigger reached the crash, Mannock scared the life out of him by asking him what he meant by it, but seeing the rigger's faced dropped to 40 below zero, he burst out laughing and cheered him up by showing him the defective strut socket which had broken."
>
> (Mannock 1966, p. 153, note 31)

Steering a broken airplane is no time for Primitive or Immature Domain adaptive mechanisms.[2] Had the pilot ignored the danger of the broken wing and the tumbling aircraft (Primitive) or recognized it but waited for someone else to take care of it (Immature), he likely would have died on the spot and we would have no account of it to read today. Similarly, the unintegrated split between emotion—in this case, fear—and cognitive content—here something like, "My lower right wing has fallen off"—that characterizes the Neurotic Domain psychological adaptive mechanisms can delay or interrupt the prompt and accurate apprehension of the situation as well as actions to remedy it. To experience the fear without considering its cause, as in Repression, is to render a solution impossible. To apprehend the cause of the aircraft gyrations while missing half of its lower weighting without sensing the fear, as in Isolation of Affect, is to lose a sense of urgency that may mean the difference between life and death. And to attack the situation on its own terms, as in Reaction Formation, is to risk a blind overcontrolling of the aircraft rather than a careful and precise assessment and response, if an instantaneous one. The Neurotic Domain mechanisms here serve only to increase the risk.

Edward Mannock's own laconic description puts both thought and feeling together when he first describes the bottom wing falling "clean away" and then regaining control of the aircraft after "desperate" efforts with the control stick. Here the word *desperate* implies anxiety as the sense of imminent disaster along with the fearfulness that disaster will occur. But he keeps the anxiety at bay in order to pursue reasserting control over the aircraft's motion. Capping the anxiety, along with an integrated use of idea and feeling in response to stress, defines the characteristics of Suppression. Only after some time has passed can the pilot sit down in a quiet environment, write

2. The reader may wonder why, then, Lieutenant Mannock didn't simply jump out of the aircraft and pull the rip cord of his parachute. The British pilots of the era were refused parachutes as a policy of their own war ministry, one that Mannock and most others fought against.

out the experience, and review it, adding the comment that no other pilot has ever survived losing a wing. And it is only after he has landed the aircraft that he can permit a certain release from the anxiety: sharing a joke about it with someone else, in this case his rigger. We will find this same release in another instance with another airplane and another pilot, 50 years later, in the next example.

SEVENTEEN TONS: SUPPRESSION AND PRESENCE OF MIND

Compared to the wood-fabric-and-wire aircraft of 1917, the sleek, supersonic, two engine, two-seat F-4 of 1967 was a thing of beauty. Reputedly, its designers originally drew up plans for a very fast, very stable flying aircraft, only to find it much less maneuverable than they had hoped. In order to provide the pilot greater range of motion when flying it, they made the original design less stable aerodynamically. This had the effect of making it a more challenging aircraft to fly through different aerobatic maneuvers, such as recovering from a stall—a condition in which the plane loses its forward momentum and then begins spinning rapidly in a free fall toward the ground. To recover control in a simple aircraft, the pilot pushes the control stick forward and the nose of the plane down along with moving the plane's rudder opposite the direction of the spin. But because of its complexity, however, putting the F-4 into a stall and spin carried more danger for plane and pilot in those first learning to fly the aircraft. Following our focus on individual adaptation to stressful circumstances, consider the description of one such spinning F-4, from the point of view of its pilot, Colonel Robin Olds. He encounters this situation high above the very unforgiving Arizona desert with a more experienced F-4 pilot in the backseat:

> The nose of the F-4 swerved left opposite my aileron input, sliced right, left again, then right, and tucked under violently. The ground spun around, stopped, and then spun the other way. The nose pitched up above the horizon then slammed under again, the earth spun and my shoulder harness bit me hard. A few years' worth of accumulated dust and dirt flew up over my head and lodged on the canopy. We seemed in an inverted tumble. I had seen spins in a lot of airplanes but this was something else. I worked furiously at the controls, but nothing seemed to have any effect. Then both engines flamed out.
>
> We were gyrating like a falling leaf in the wind storm when Bill hollered, "Get out the RAT (ram air turbine)—the engines are gone!"
>
> At least one of us knew what was going on. I found the handle on the console by my hip and extended the ram air turbine. I heard the small doors open as the fan device popped out into the air stream to run the hydraulics for flight controls. We continued tumbling crazily straight down, down, down; sky overhead, and then under, the ground appeared, then disappeared, negative G forces sucked at us, and the slam of positive, down we went. Thirty thousand, 20,000, 18,000, the altimeter unwinding. The bird tumbled, the earth spun, the horizon went crazy and I kept feeling out all the controls, trying to break the violent stall.
>
> "Okay, Colonel," Bill yelled, "14,000, we better get out!"

"No, no, wait!" I called back. "I think I've got it. Just one more turn!" As the nose went straight down and paused in its gyrations I slammed the stick full forward, ailerons with the turn, and full opposite rudder. The aircraft hesitated, then kicked farther forward in a wings-level dive. I immediately relaxed forward pressure and went neutral on the ailerons and rudder.

By God, that did it! I was back in control; the airspeed was building. I pulled gently out of our dive. We leveled out at 8000 feet above the deck, and with Bill's help, I restarted both engines. Whew! I could hear Bill gulping huge deep breaths in the backseat.

"Holy mackerel, Bill. That was fun! Let's go do that again!"

I laughed when Bill shouted, "Not on your life, sir!"

(Olds 2010, p. 250)

Considering this passage from the point of view of the adaptive mechanism recognition algorithm, the stress appears much the same as that Major Mannock describes when the wing falls off of his aircraft. Like him, Colonel Olds must regain control of an aircraft falling through an airspace. Unlike his earlier forbear, however, he has two advantages: he has much more experience as a pilot than Edward Mannock had in the earlier circumstance, and he has the option of an ejection seat and a parachute. Even with an escape route, however, his plane falls rapidly in little more than a few seconds while he tries to understand the plane's unique spin characteristics and respond to them. Colonel Olds has taken the aircraft near the edge of the safety zone and his copilot/instructor radios that the time has come to exit the aircraft, corroborating the apprehension that disaster is at hand—and articulating the anxiety of the situation.

Once again there is no indication of Primitive Domain adaptive mechanisms at work when to deny or distort the situation would have resulted in certain death. Clearly that does not occur, since Colonel Olds lives to tell the tale. Similarly, while he recognizes the difficulty of regaining control of the spinning aircraft, he does not blame the circumstance on the other pilot or wait for him to rectify the situation. The Immature Domain adaptive mechanisms that disclaim response to the stress and look for external factors to relieve the situation do not apply.

When considering whether this F-4 pilot uses Neurotic Domain adaptive mechanisms in this instance, the algorithm first notes that the cognitive and emotional contents, respectively, include an out-of-control aircraft and terror—the same as in the previous vignette of the World War I Nieuport pilot. And, like Mick Mannock, Robin Olds does not separate idea and feeling in the situation: he does not intellectualize about the problem or ignore the urgency of the situation, nor is he paralyzed by the overwhelming terror of falling rapidly to the ground. Similarly, there is no evidence of his slamming hard at the controls in an effort to "beat this thing on its own terms."

Rather, he too uses the adaptive mechanism of Suppression: he realizes the urgency but limits the anxiety that flows from it and at the same time begins to recognize the pattern in the aircraft's movement that allows him to construct a specific, and effective, response whereby he regains control of his 17-ton aircraft, restarts its engines, and returns to level flight. This is all well and good, but Suppression itself seems better at limiting—putting a lid on—the anxiety than it does at dispersing it, at least immediately. That, both in Major Mannock's and Colonel Olds' cases, requires something more, namely, the use of Humor. Rather than gripe about the aircraft's defective construction, Mannock makes a silly joke about himself as possibly the target of his rigger, something they both laugh about. Similarly, Olds indulges in the silly statement about what fun that was and let's do it again. He and his copilot can share both laughter and release. Humor, as we shall see in Chapter 21, serves this and other purposes far and wide in human society. In part, this may be due to the fact that Suppression, a ubiquitous Mature Domain adaptive mechanism, helps us through the challenges of the marketplace, of work responsibilities, of raising children, and through the many other stresses—"the thousand natural shocks / That flesh is heir to"[3]—in the incremental process of first capping the sense of doom or disaster and then releasing that same sense in manageable doses as we go about resolving it. We can take pride in the results, but if we want a sense of distance, we will laugh at it, and at ourselves. As in the next example, we can also cry.

THE INTERN'S BAD NEWS

Once again our intern, stalwart and true, lives as a denizen of the night, prowling, in the wee hours of the morning, the halls of the ICU and the general medical ward, with four acutely ill patients in the former and eight more out on the floor. A few minutes ago the intensive care nursing staff summoned him: two of the patients seem to have worsened, one with changes in his heart rhythm and the other with a worsening of her diabetic state. Shuttling back and forth between the two rooms, in constant touch with the nursing staff, the intern manages to stabilize both patients in their conditions, at least for now. But they demand constant attention and monitoring, and the intern keeps a careful eye on both, with an ear ready in the direction of the other 10 patients who depend on her (in this instance the night rotation has fallen to a female intern) for their health.

While watching the thin trace line on the monitor of the cardiac patient, the charge nurse gently taps the intern on the shoulder and says that she has a personal phone call waiting at the unit desk. "Be right there," the intern says, as she watches the cardiac monitor for a few more seconds before moving to the desk to take the phone call. She picks up the phone and finds her mother on the other end of the line: "I wanted to let you know that your Uncle Ned passed away a few minutes ago," she hears her mother's soft voice saying. The two of them talk for a few minutes—Ned was the intern's favorite uncle—until the intensive care nurse waves to her from the doorway of the diabetic patient's room. The intern apologizes to her mother, says that she can't talk any longer right now, but could she call tomorrow in the late afternoon before she goes on shift again? The two of them agree on a time and end the conversation. The intern continues through the rest of the night and goes home

3. Shakespeare, *Hamlet*, Act III, Scene 1.

the next day for some needed sleep. When she wakes, she phones her mother, and they talk for an hour about Uncle Ned, the family, and the funeral services. They feel sad and commiserate together.

By now the reader will be aware enough of the contrast in the recurring character of our intern beset with challenges in the middle of the night to know, as if using the recognition algorithm by second nature, that the intern has not here responded with any of the Primitive or Immature Domain psychological adaptive mechanisms. There is no ignoring the circumstance of the phone call from her mother or lack of personal attribution to the painful thought and feeling it raises. Similarly, the Neurotic Domain adaptive mechanisms do not obtain either: the painful loss of a favorite uncle and the deep sadness it causes do not separate themselves, one from the other.

Rather, here in the Domain of the Mature adaptive strategies, painful feeling and thought work together in the interest of the human process we know as mourning, through which we come to grips with—and even grow from—both the cognition and the affect of human loss. While this process is important, other processes are also important, for example paying attention to the health and well-being of those in our charge. Suppression provides particular usefulness in a situation when matters require prioritization. This chapter's intern recognizes that she cannot properly care for her ill patients and at the same time mourn her favorite uncle. Suppression allows her to put the mourning process in abeyance until such time as she can give it its due properly and with compassion. It is in this regard that she first asks her mother for a time to talk later, and then remembers to do so, listening to and voicing the sorrow in an appropriate manner. If flesh is heir to a thousand natural shocks, Suppression allows us to attend to them one at a time.

EVERYDAY EXAMPLES OF SUPPRESSION

As noted in Chapter 3, the Mature Domain psychological adaptive mechanisms are, by definition, never pathological. That is, their deployment does not result in impaired function. Rather, the Mature Domain psychological adaptive mechanisms improve function and raise it to the highest levels of which humans remain capable. As a result, providing "clinical" examples in the present discussion creates a misnomer: the Mature Domain mechanisms are never clinical in the sense of requiring diagnosis and treatment. Instead, they serve more often to allow observers to stand up and cheer at courage and creativity in the face of adverse circumstances, whether the Mature mechanisms occur in a clinical setting or any other context of human activity. Consider a few brief examples:

- A woman in her mid-40s works as the chief executive officer of a company that manages offshore government relations for U.S. businesses. She arrives at work one Monday morning and quickly learns that government A has rescinded its tax incentives for one client, that government B has defaulted on its loans to another, and that government C has decided to prolong their yearlong negotiations to finance a new enterprise with a third client after having given their final approval in the previous week. The executive calls her staff together to review each crisis, focusing on the specific points at issue with respect to the impact of timing on their clients. From this she devises a list of tasks prioritized by the order of their urgency. She and her team then go about tending to these problems by priority.

- A single man in his early 30s, a well-respected technical expert on information systems, loses consciousness at work and wakes up in a hospital. His doctors inform him that he has a rare form of leukemia for which there is no known effective treatment. They regard his condition as advanced and think that he may live no more than another 24 hours. They want to airlift him immediately to a major national center that specializes in this disease. There, a team of experts will review the diagnosis and consider the possibility of beginning an experimental treatment. They ask whether he would like to call his family members, but he says that he prefers to wait until he hears the second opinion at the research hospital. The next day, he learns that his condition is severe but not as acute as originally thought, and they recommend that he begin experimental treatment immediately before his condition grows worse. He acknowledges his understanding of their opinion, agrees to treatment, and then asks to contact his family to inform them of the events.
- The manager of a fast food restaurant, a woman in her late 20s, receives warning from a local Department of Agriculture representative that the restaurant's hamburger supply appears to be tainted and cannot be used. She learns from her regional manager that there is no hope of being resupplied for two days. Rather than close down the restaurant, she maintains their offerings of non-hamburger foods and gives each customer a coupon for two free hamburgers at the next available opportunity. Two days later, with a new supply on hand, her franchise begins redeeming the coupons, and she finds that the daily gross income doubles over the next month.
- The president of a local plumbers and pipefitters union has been engaged in a difficult negotiation with the contractor of a new multistory, high-rise building for the past week. This man in his 50s then learns that his reelection as president of his union, for which he was running unopposed, has now been challenged by a group of younger members whose campaign focuses on what they regard as his incompetence as a negotiator. The election is two weeks away, and he realizes that the present negotiation may not be concluded by that time. He considers carefully the implications of the negotiation with regard to the economic well-being of his membership, as well as the likelihood of his continuing contributions to the union effort in this community. He decides to continue both the negotiations and the reelection campaign, but sets the negotiation as his first priority. He enlists other union members to assist him in the election activity, recognizing that his time will be limited and must be used most effectively.

Common to all of these examples, the recognition algorithm points to the stresses involved, in each case during one or another form of crisis. Each of the protagonists, in his or her own way and own setting, identifies the stress and proceeds to use Mature Domain Suppression as a way of managing the stress-generated anxiety.

Each, in turn, revisits the respective crisis in a way that allows him or her to gain more information, and consider further options carefully, in the manner of Homer's Poulydamas when he recommends the same course to the Trojan warriors. With careful thought, and conscious apprehension of the emotions involved, each protagonist provides effective action in meeting a crisis.

These and many more examples come to us through the course of daily life. As human observers, we can identify the examples as they occur in those around us, as well as, with careful reflection, within ourselves. Suppression remains one of the most commonly used of the Mature Domain adaptive styles simply because of the frequency of present-day crises and the need to respond to them. Like Anticipation in Chapter 18, Suppression allows leeway to consider complex problems and find the best, often most creative, and most timely, solutions. Suppression does this after the ego senses perturbation in its waking consciousness and provides a response. Anticipation, as we shall see next, engages the same process before a crisis.

REFERENCES

Homer. (1951). *The Iliad of Homer* (R. Lattimore, Trans.). Chicago, University of Chicago.
Homer. (1967). *The Odyssey of Homer* (R. Lattimore, Trans.). New York, Harper and Row.
Mannock, M. E. (1966). *The Personal Diary of Major Edward Mannock*. London, Neville Spearman.
Olds, R., with C. Olds and E. Rasimus. (2010). *Fighter Pilot*. New York, St. Martin's Press.
Shakespeare, W. (1955). *Hamlet*. In *The Oxford Shakespeare* (W. J. Craig, Ed.). Oxford, Oxford University Press.

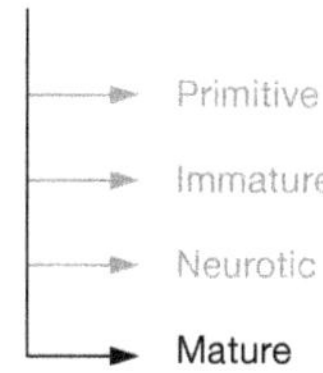

CHAPTER 18

Anticipation

We have set the other psychological adaptive mechanisms considered in this discussion in the context of a response to a crisis, whether the sleepy intern with yet another admission in the middle of the night or any of the historical or literary figures we have discussed as they face difficulties that upset their sense of conscious equilibrium. For Anticipation to be considered as a psychological adaptive mechanism, however, the discussion requires a new frame of reference.

Aeschylus, the Greek dramatist of the ancients, tells something of the nature of this psychological adaptive mechanism when he presents his dramatic character Cassandra in *Agamemnon*. In the story, she has been favored by the god Apollo with the gift of foreseeing events that no one else can. While this can be regarded as an advantage—just think how much money one could make in the stock market with a supernatural foresight—in Cassandra's case it does not destine her to a happy life. Because of it, she foresees horror after horror, only to find that no one believes her.[1] For one, she foretells the destruction of her home, Troy (Ilium), and the Greek victory. She foretells too that many of the Greeks will die in one way or another on the way home or shortly thereafter. In this passage, she recounts her predictions and talks about her own destiny:

> Since once I saw the citadel of Ilium
> die as it died, and those who broke the city, doomed
> by the gods, fare as they have fared accordingly,
> I will go through with it. I too will take my fate.
>
> (Aeschylus, 1953, p. 76)

For another, she is taken to Greece against her will as Agamemnon's mistress, a spoil of war. She is forced to live in a household with Agamemnon's wife Clytemnestra

1. According to one version of the myth, Cassandra is the most beautiful princess of the House of Troy. Infatuated with her, the god Apollo gives her the ability to foresee the future when she promises him her sexual favors in return. But Cassandra, a fickle princess according to the legend, breaks her word and refuses him. He cannot rescind her predictive powers—a bargain is a bargain from his point of view apparently—but he adds the curse that no one will believe what she says.

and her lover Aegisthus, who are conspiring to murder Agamemnon and will murder Cassandra as well. Despite all of her foresight, Cassandra is powerless to change anything,[2] and as a result finds that her prophesying only irritates those around her in a classic case of confusing the message with the messenger. She goes to her fate, if not happily, at least philosophically:

> Alas, poor men, their destiny. When all goes well
> a shadow will overthrow it. If it be unkind
> one stroke of a wet sponge wipes all the picture out;
> and that is far the most unhappy thing of all.
>
> (p. 78)

In contrast to Cassandra's prophesying as Aeschylus' symbol of destiny itself, Anticipation as a psychological adaptive mechanism includes not only seeing ahead but the opportunity to act, that is, to adapt. By definition, when humans anticipate a crisis, they foresee it and act to prevent it rather than waiting for it to occur and then acting in response to it. In a sense this is still a response to a stress—in this case an oncoming, rather than a present, circumstance of a troubling nature, or at least of a different nature from what has gone before. But it is not an immediate reaction to a stress that has already occurred. By one or another process of forethought, conscious perception has identified the oncoming crisis, and, because of this, the process remains amenable to assessment with the recognition algorithm. That is, the prospect of an oncoming stress still raises the anxiety that allows humans to recognize that something in their immediate experience must be dealt with in order to prevent some worse occurrence.

All of clinical medicine, for example, serves this mechanism of Anticipation when it considers prognosis: the empirical basis of signs, symptoms, risk and protective factors, and natural history that, when taken together, allow a reasonable prediction of the course of illness and the ability of treatment to alter that course. This approach to predicting future course can be very useful in day-to-day life, but it is not necessarily the stuff of fiction. Emily Brontë, in *Wuthering Heights*, gives her readers a memorable description of Heathcliff's love for Cathy and the excruciating pain he endures because of it. She does not describe his recognition of an oncoming crisis, such as Cathy's marriage to Edgar Linton, and the steps Heathcliff takes to prevent or even ameliorate his own emotional turmoil in response to it. He does not foresee; he reacts. We see him in his crucible, as with other good fictional characters who find their humanity in the experience of their pain. By contrast, a fictional character whose forethought prevents crisis after crisis, obviates stress after stress, might stand high in the running for the Most Boring Fictional Personality of all time.

Anticipation, however, can hold a fascination for us that is equal to no other in fact rather than in fiction. Which of us would not happily obviate pain rather than

2. In summary:
Here lies Cassandra,
Dead without doubt.
What she ruled in
She always ruled out.

experience it? How to do that often places us in the realm of history rather than creative imagination. The following example, from Mark Twain's recounting his *Life on the Mississippi*, rather than the fictionalized *The Adventures of Huckleberry Finn* published one year later, serves to illustrate.[3]

WHEN POETRY LEFT THE RIVER: ANTICIPATION AND LEARNING

The scene in this vignette occurs in the pilot house on the highest deck of a paddle-wheel steamboat working its way down the great south flowing river in the middle years of the 19th century, just before the American Civil War. The expert steamer pilot, a man named Horace Bixby, guides his cub pilot, Samuel Langhorne Clemens before he became Mark Twain, as they navigate the great boat through the treacheries that the river has in store for them. The cub spots a ripple in the waters immediately ahead and is afraid they are going to hit a submerged reef that the ripple signifies. He says that they must change course, but his teacher says no and tells him to steer straight through it. Fearing for his safety and that of all the passengers on the boat, the cub nonetheless obeys his teacher's direction and keeps a steady hand on the tiller. As they pass over the ripple without incident, Mr. Bixby speaks to his cub pilot:

> "Now don't you see the difference? It wasn't anything but a *wind* reef. The wind does that."
>
> "So I see. But it is exactly like a bluff reef. How am I ever going to tell them apart?"
>
> "I can't tell you. It is an instinct. By and by you will just naturally KNOW one from the other, but you never will be able to explain why or how you know them apart."
>
> It turned out to be true. The face of the water, in time, became a wonderful book—a book that was a dead language to the uneducated passenger, but which told its mind to me without reserve, delivering its most cherished secrets as clearly as if it uttered them with a voice.
>
> (Twain 1961, p. 66)

Anticipating danger is very important, Horace Bixby seems to tell young Sam, but learning when to use it and when not to may not be as easy as it looks. Twain goes on to say that it is an ongoing effort, one that does not end so long as the pilot guides a boat down the river. The pilot works at perceiving the river's patterns, and the river never rests in its propensity to change its face. But working with, and on, the great

3. Though mentioning two of Twain's books (and no pun intended), I do not wish to say that one of them is any better than the other, any more than to say that apples are better than cherries when baking a pie. The two have different characteristics that lead to different finished products. Fiction allows Twain to play with ideas, feelings, and the writing techniques that bring them forth, far more liberally in *The Adventures of Huckleberry Finn* than he can in his description of real experiences on the river. This results in *Huckleberry Finn* as Twain's fiction masterpiece and one of the great novels of literature written in English. Both books serve as explorations of human experience but use their respective methods in doing so.

river might even be fun just because of the changes in perception and the undercurrent of danger:

> And it was not a book to be read once and thrown aside, for it had a new story to tell every day. Throughout the long twelve hundred miles there was never a page that was void of interest, never one that you could leave unread without loss, never one that you would want to skip, thinking you could find higher enjoyment in some other thing. There never was so wonderful a book written by man; never one whose interest was so absorbing, so unflagging, so sparkingly renewed with every reperusal.
>
> (p. 67)

But the process of learning, in this case as in most technical disciplines, moves from the romantic to the mundane, and purposefully so. Danger is romantic. Safety is mundane. In piloting a steamboat, mundane is better:

> I still keep in mind a certain wonderful sunset which I witnessed when steamboating was new to me.... There were graceful curves, reflected images, woody heights, soft distances; and over the whole scene, far and near, the dissolving lights drifted steadily, enriching it, every passing moment, with new marvels of coloring.
> ... But as I have said, a day came when I began to cease from noting the glories and the charms which the moon and the sun and the twilight wrought upon the river's face; another day came when I ceased altogether to note them.
> ... No, the romance and the beauty were all gone from the river. All the value any feature of it had for me now was the amount of usefulness it could furnish toward compassing the safe piloting of a steamboat.
>
> (pp. 67–68)

Does the recognition algorithm apply to this vignette? And if so, in what way? Following the algorithm's path, we first ask, what stress is evident in the description that perturbs waking consciousness, and second, does it raise anxiety? Twain provides a very sharp description of his fear, as a novice river pilot, of the dangers of the river "that could tear the life out of the strongest vessel that ever floated" and end the lives of its passengers in the fast flowing currents. His anxiety comes from his inability to recognize safety from danger as he steers the many tonned vessel as a man might feel his clumsy way down a darkened hall with no light whatsoever among the many chairs, tables, and other pieces of furniture between him and the end of it.

Does the cub riverboat pilot recognize the stress, or does he ignore it in the characteristically concrete fashion of the Primitive Domain mechanisms? In Twain's description, he not only recognizes it, he studies it. Does he locate his anxiety in the river as a phenomenon that man was never meant to understand or to navigate—something beyond his powers—as might be the case in an Immature Domain mechanism? The answer again is *no*. Coming to grips with the river and its ways lies within him. He can learn them, and Horace Bixby is there to teach him. Young Sam Clemens may not understand the processes of learning any more than he understands how he can tell a wind ripple from a reef ripple just by looking at it, but he believes his teacher's words that he will come to learn it, and he makes the effort to do so. His adaptive style is well beyond those in the Immature Domain range of adaptive mechanisms.

The next task from the algorithm is to identify both the feeling and the thought contents of the stress, and then to ask whether they work together or exist in an uneasy, disjointed relationship. To do this, we must consider Twain's passage in its entirety, well beyond the interchange at the beginning between young Sam Clemens and his teacher Horace Bixby when Sam asks how on earth he is going to tell one ripple from another. Twain describes the learning process itself as the "face of the water" becoming "a wonderful book" that teaches him to master the recognition of the various signs along the river. Later in the same paragraph (not quoted here), he compares his knowledge as a river-educated pilot to that of a passenger who cannot read from the same book. In one difference, the passenger does not sense the cognitive content that young Sam does when he apprehends the dangers before him on the surface of the river. The passenger sees only "pretty pictures." In another, the passenger does not feel the fear or sense of impending disaster—that is to say, the anxiety—that Sam feels when his understanding tells him that danger lurks at hand. Stated briefly, learning the river means recognizing both the river's danger signs and the fearfulness of the shipwreck that they might occasion.

In the book, Mark Twain paints a picture—one of the most engagingly beautiful paragraphs anywhere in his writings[4]—of the great river at sunset from a time before he learned to look beyond the water's surface radiance and into its patterns. In the bright reflecting light at the end of the day—the black outline of a floating tree trunk against the red gold of the water, as one detail—holds him "like one bewitched." But then the thought content that he acquires from learning to read from the river's book begins to take over his relationship with the water. Besides the river's beauty, he recognizes its points of danger and their emotional meaning. This ripple means you can wreck the boat, and your fear advises to stay clear of it, we may paraphrase as one example. In this respect, as he goes through his list of the various signs and their cognitive as well as emotional meanings, Twain provides us with a description of adapting to the river in a way that integrates both thought and feeling. His last sentence adds an epilogue for his development as a riverboat pilot: what he once saw as beauty in the surface of the river, he now sees as information; what he once felt as fright, he now feels as an ongoing concern for safety. The

4. "I still keep in mind a certain wonderful sunset which I witnessed when steamboating was new to me. A broad expanse of the river was turned to blood; in the middle distance the red hue brightened into gold, through which a solitary log came floating, black and conspicuous; in one place a long, slanting mark lay sparkling upon the water; in another the surface was broken by boiling, tumbling rings, that were as many-tinted as an opal; where the ruddy flush was faintest, was a smooth spot that was covered with graceful circles and radiating lines, ever so delicately traced; the shore on our left was densely wooded, and the sombre shadow that fell from this forest was broken in one place by a long, ruffled trail that shone like silver; and high above the forest wall a clean-stemmed dead tree waved a single leafy bough that glowed like a flame in the unobstructed splendor that was flowing from the sun. There were graceful curves, reflected images, woody heights, soft distances; and over the whole scene, far and near, the dissolving lights drifted steadily, enriching it, every passing moment, with new marvels of coloring." p. 67

cub pilot has both thought and emotion working together in the here and now as he practices his steamboat piloting. He has learned to foresee the dangers that the river puts it his way and can take steps to avoid them. He has learned Anticipation, the Mature Domain mechanism of psychological adaptation that scans the horizon of experience, not to project feelings or ideas either onto others or move them out of conscious thought, but to integrate them into useful action. Viewed in the model of psychological adaptive mechanisms, we might consider seeing the river only as a very beautiful surface phenomenon without regard for its hidden dangers as an example of the Primitive Domain mechanism of Distortion. That, however, is now replaced by the Mature adaptive mechanism of Anticipation that can include both an observable cognitive content and a controlled fearfulness in the interest of using the anxiety rather than just trying to get rid of it. In this context, the "poetry" leaving the river, analogous to the wind ripple over which the cub pilot steers the boat, indicates a healthy growth rather than a submerged hazard.[5]

Those more hazardous ripples that come our way in life may also offer opportunities for growth, especially when they engage Mature Domain Anticipation in adapting to them. The opportunities are as ubiquitous as the stresses that each of us may learn to recognize in their early stages, such as those in the next case that is derived from a clinical setting.

---

5. Twain goes on in the descriptions quoted above to make a characteristically Romantic comment in the late 19th-century Victorian style about his sense of a lost "poetry" in learning the river. He says,

> Now when I had mastered the language of this water and had come to know every trifling feature that bordered the great river as familiarly as I knew the letters of the alphabet, I had made a valuable acquisition. But I had lost something, too. I had lost something which could never be restored to me while I lived. All the grace, the beauty, the poetry had gone out of the majestic river! (1961, p. 67)

And at the end of the passage,

> Since those days, I have pitied doctors from my heart. What does the lovely flush in a beauty's cheek mean to a doctor but a "break" that ripples above some deadly disease? Are not all her visible charms sown thick with what are to him the signs and symbols of hidden decay? Does he ever see her beauty at all, or doesn't he simply view her professionally, and comment upon her unwholesome condition all to himself? And doesn't he sometimes wonder whether he has gained most or lost most by learning his trade? (pp. 68–69)

While these are admirable sentiments of the time, someone writing from another point of view, say Zen philosophy, might say that Twain's learning the ways of the river beyond its surface appearances actually puts him in touch with a much greater poetry that is found in the dynamic forces of the universe. With respect to his second paragraph, from my own experience, I would disagree and say that one can still see both the concerns over illness and the beauty, and the personal heroism, in the sufferer. Science asks us to understand symptoms and signs in the interest of treating an illness, and compassion keeps us in touch in a professional alliance with the sufferer's personhood.

ANTICIPATION IN GRIEF: WORKING IT THROUGH AHEAD OF TIME

An 87-year-old woman's health has been failing. Her steady downhill course began four months earlier, when she had lost consciousness briefly at a social gathering. Her daughter, her middle child with whom she felt closest, had called the paramedics and gone with her to the hospital. There she learned that her mother had developed a cardiac valve abnormality that was inoperable because of her age and that would likely grow worse. Hearing the news, her mother bore matters stoically, using Suppression as her primary adaptive mechanism in saying, "I'll just take it one day at a time." In the course of the next few days, however, her daughter began noticing scenes from her own childhood that appeared periodically in her daydreams, as though she were reviewing old home movie reels. She could see her mother as a young woman with small children about her, all of them in a kitchen standing or sitting on chairs around the kitchen table making a fine mess with flour, water, and dough as they "helped" make pumpkin pies for a Thanksgiving dinner. In another reverie some days later, she recalled an incident at a later time, when she first asked her mother about trying on makeup. Instances of this kind continued over the months as she seemed to relive much of the past with her mother for whom she had great affection. Each time the recollections appeared, pleasant though they were in content, she noticed too a profound sense of sorrow. This seemed to wash over her like a great wave, causing her to cry quietly to herself, and then departing quickly as it washed away, leaving her with a sense of quiet as one might feel in recovering energy after an exercise session. Her mother would appear occasionally in her night dreams as well, with one repeating theme in which she would take her daughter by the hand and the two of them would walk.

After four months, her mother had become unsteady on her feet and came to live with her daughter at the latter's insistence. Two months later, the mother once again lost consciousness but continued to breathe well and maintain a pulse. The daughter called an ambulance and brought her to the ER. Two days later, the mother passed away in the hospital with her daughter at her side. The daughter notified her two siblings and arranged for the funeral. At the wake three days following, she talked with her older brother, an obsessive sort who seemed to her to keep his feelings at arm's length until they crashed in upon him. He looked ashen and hadn't slept well. He commented to her that he did not understand how she could be so composed, even-tempered, and rational with the loss of their mother so close at hand. She patted his shoulder and said that proximity was a gift. It had allowed her to let their mother go a little at a time over the past six months.

This daughter's case illustrates the clinical phenomenon of anticipatory grief. Viewed in the psychological adaptive mechanism model, it too exemplifies Anticipation, one of the Mature Domain group. Following the recognition algorithm, the stress the daughter perceives is her mother's worsening health. Initially, it raises the daughter's anxiety acutely in recognizing the transient loss of consciousness as a possible impending medical crisis that necessitates a call to the paramedics. With the progression of events, the stress of her mother's failing health continues to activate the daughter's adaptive processes in dealing with the increasingly likely occurrence of her mother's death. In the context of the stepwise algorithm, she does not engage the Primitive Domain mechanisms—by ignoring the whole situation—nor those of the Immature Domain—by looking to someone else to take care of her mother as her health fails. Similarly, the Neurotic Domain mechanisms do not apply—she is not burden down by repetitively sad affect that does not seem related to any rational cause on the one hand, nor does she consider only the rational causes of her mother's failing health in the absence of painfully sad feelings.

Rather, the daughter experiences both the painful thoughts and feelings involved in her mother's ill health simultaneously. They make up the integrated parts of her own grieving process: they surface into waking consciousness as she relives the memories in her daydreams and as she consciously retrieves the memories of her dreams during the night. In this way, she works through the emotions of her grief a little at a time over the six months leading to her mother's death. From her brother's point of view in the throes of acute grief at the funeral, she appears somewhat distant and rational. As is often the case, he mistakes this is as a lack of feeling, and she corrects him appropriately by noting all of the work she has done to resolve her painful thoughts and feelings in advance of their mother's departure. The two of them come to grips with the death of their mother in two different adaptive styles: hers by Anticipation and his by engaging Suppression in the face of the acute grief that he will resolve in smaller doses over the next six months or so. The grief must be worked through in these or some other adaptive style if the mourners are to avoid pathological reactions to it that may occur in using any of the three lower Domains on the recognition algorithm. From our point of view, the difference between Anticipation and Suppression in this setting is simply one of timing.

Anticipation as it may occur in the setting of clinical medicine does not limit itself just to grief processes. Common uses include prenatal preparation for parenthood in the well-defined nine-month term of human pregnancy and parturition, in adjusting to the necessities of ongoing monitoring and treatment as in the case of long-term conditions such as diabetes or high blood pressure, or in recognizing and effecting the changes in living brought on by cancer treatment. Mature Domain adaptation of this kind usually results in a sense of awe among medical and surgical practitioners in the face of their patients' adaptive capabilities rather than a search for the pathological. Awe and admiration are just as important in clinical work as any of the other transference feelings that physicians sense in themselves in the presence of their patients.

Nor is Anticipation by any means limited to medical patients or riverboat pilots. Major Edward Mannock could write down his Fifteen Rules for engaging the enemy derived from his own experience and teach them to his new pilots as a way of using Anticipation to limit the dangers of aerial combat. And marketplaces, both ancient and modern, provide daily examples of trying to anticipate the changes in the psychological or economic forces that will result in monetary gain or loss. Common to all such examples remains the elegant integration of both idea and feeling in the interest of looking over the horizon, toward those oncoming conditions that might be predicted and then dealt with.

THE RADAR OF THE SUCCESSFUL INTERN: ANTICIPATION AND BEING IN TUNE

For another view of anticipation, let us leave Twain's Mississippi and the sorrow of the grieving daughter and journey back to a virtual hospital. It is, again, the wee hours of the morning, say 3:30 A.M. or so, and our intern, this one often mistaken for a nurse, has had little sleep. She is a busy intern, fielding calls about the four very ill patients in the intensive care unit and the other eight people under her care hospitalized on the general medicine ward. With her diligence and economy of motion, she has slowly whittled down the long list of tasks that began the evening. The patients in the unit are stable, and there have been no calls in the last hour. Once more she ticks down the list of those on the medical floor. She has seen them all, and they all seem to be in good order. But, even though she has gone through the list, there remains some source of discomfort in her awareness that she cannot put her finger on. Something still doesn't seem quite right. To double-check, she asks the charge nurse on the medical ward if se can think of any problems, and the reply is *no*, everyone seems stable. This is welcome news, and yet something still seems out of place. She looks back through her notes, and, turning one page over to the writing on the back, she remembers from a notation there that she has one other patient on a surgical ward, admitted to that location because the regular medicine ward was full. She goes down to that floor and checks in with the charge nurse on duty. "What timing!" the nurse says to her. "I was just about to call you. We need the IV orders rewritten on that patient and his heart medicines reevaluated." The intern tends to the tasks, adjusting the medicines and rewriting orders for the intravenous fluids, and does both in a way that continues the care of the patient seamlessly.

At its most subtle, Anticipation can alert us to oncoming crises or dangers and can do so in very practical ways in everyday life. To examine how this might occur in the context of our model for psychological adaptive mechanisms, we look through the lens of the clinical recognition algorithm focused on our sleepy intern in the above vignette. First, identifying a stress that results in increased anxiety, we take note that the anxiety appears *before* the recognition of the stress in this instance. The otherwise conscientious intern is beset by a sense of discomfort that announces itself to her consciousness but does not go away. In this regard, part of the work of Anticipation may simply be to sort out where the anxiety is coming from as a way of identifying the specific stress. In the case of our intern late at night, she carefully examines and then reexamines all the possible sources of stress, namely the patients for whom she is caring through her duty hours. None of them, however, accounts for the discomfort, or, perhaps more significantly, consideration of them one by one does not serve to relieve it. The discomfort continues on, in an almost palpable way.

Contrary to the approach of the Primitive Domain adaptive mechanisms, it cannot be ignored or avoided. Similarly, the intern does not locate the stress anywhere but within herself. She does not project the discomfort onto other people as being their fault or otherwise located beyond her capacity to address it. According to the algorithm, therefore, her adaptive approach has risen above the Immature Domain mechanisms.

At this point, the algorithm asks us to define both the cognitive and emotional contents of the stress involved. In the intern's progression of behaviors, however, we can describe the emotional state only as a nagging sense of something wrong. Clearly the cognitive content of the stress has something to do with the intern's work at hand, but what that may be is not specifically clear. In this instance and others of the same type, we still ask, however, whether the relevant thought and feeling contents of the stress are working in tandem or are disjoined. In this case, the intern identifies her task as an effort to sort out the sources for both the feeling of discomfort and its causative reason, together, as she goes about the work of recognition. In her perception, both are linked—the emotional discomfort in this instance serving as a source of motivation for finding the appropriate cognitive basis that might explain it.

Finally, as she recalls the existence of another patient on another ward, a perception that falls outside the usual frame of reference as to where medical patients are generally housed in her hospital, the idea content makes itself clear. She recognizes the stress as simply the existence of that other patient to which she must attend. When this realization arrives in consciousness, the anxiety and its emotional discomfort drop away: a demonstration that thought and feeling link together in her response to the anxiety and stress. When she solves the puzzle of recognition and adjusts the clinical care for her patient on the other ward, she resolves the cognitive content of the stress and with it the emotional discomfort. In this respect she uses the Mature Domain adaptive mechanism of Anticipation.

The experience of emotional discomfort as the first indicator of a problem requiring conscious recognition suggests the flexibility of Anticipation as an adaptive mechanism that can unfold in different ways in order to address an oncoming stress. The thought content may precede emotional perception, as in Sam Clemens' learning the river. Conversely, the affective content may precede conscious apprehension of the stressful thought content, as in the intern locating the last patient as the source of her discomfort. Or they may appear simultaneously, as in the daughter who begins her grief work with the sad news of her mother's illness. Of special note, our intern arrives on the scene of the overlooked patient in a timely manner, something that the charge nurse recognizes and compliments. Owing to the very subtle properties of her Anticipation, she provides care for her patient on time, before any lapse in medicine or fluid administration can bring on a medical crisis. Anticipation aims to prevent crisis.

This very subtle sense of timeliness both demonstrates and characterizes Anticipation's adaptive strategy as one of flexibility in response both to the perceived anxiety and distress behind it. The brain, or the psyche, depending on the model used, carries with it the ability to perceive oncoming crises at a subconscious level that generally yields a sense of emotional discomfort. The relationship of that perceived discomfort to the timeliness of providing an appropriate—and conscious—response does not occur by accident. The neural mechanisms for the ways in which a human being's perception of time, and that perception's link to both the cognitive and emotional contents of stresses, has not yet received appropriate definition. Its complexity, however, suggests the involvement of several systems that include perceiving time, linking the flow of perceptions together serially such that we can monitor time internally, and the integration of this with those systems that mediate both cognition and emotion. How the time sense integrates with adaptation offers a creative area of inquiry that may have application into our abilities to obviate pain rather than react to it.

REFERENCES

Aeschylus. (1953). *Oresteia* (R. Lattimore, Trans.). Chicago, University of Chicago Press.
Twain, M. (1961). *Life on the Mississippi*. New York, New American Library (Signet Classics).

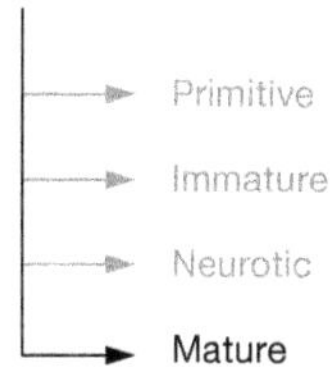

CHAPTER 19
Altruism

In 1840, on the occasion of its "not [having been] awarded a prize by the Royal Danish Society of Scientific Studies," Arthur Schopenhauer published an essay that has been translated as "On the Basis of Morality."[1] In it he asks, how is it that the suffering or the best interests of another can so move us as individuals as to put that other person's interests above our own? He answers that this is due to a particular ingredient in the nature of human beings:

> It is the everyday phenomenon of compassion, of the immediate participation, independent of all ulterior considerations, primarily in the suffering of another, and thus in the prevention or elimination of it; for all satisfaction and all well-being and happiness consists in this. It is simply and solely this compassion that is the real basis of all voluntary justice and genuine loving-kindness. Only insofar as an action has sprung from compassion does it have moral values; and every action resulting from any other motive has none.[2]

Schopenhauer goes on to explain this further by noting that when one person develops compassion for another, the two people will seem more alike than different. In a much longer and more famous work, *The World as Will and Idea*, he ascribes human alike-ness to the idea that all individuals share in the great energy of life that he describes as nature's force, or will. In his model, we all share in the conditions of being, and no more so than when we share both the painful and joyful feelings of others, even when that requires effort or self-sacrifice. To regard this phenomenon in the current model of psychological adaptive mechanisms, consider the following historical example.

---

1. Alternatively: "On the Foundations of Morality" or "On the Foundations of Ethics."
2. "Thus, how is it possible for another's weal and woe to become directly my motive, and this sometimes to such a degree that I more or less subordinate them to my own weal and woe, normally the sole source of my motives?" Schopenhauer (2005, p. 204). The sentence was one of the favorites of Joseph Campbell, who quoted it both in his books on comparative mythology and in a series of celebrated television interviews with Bill Moyers.

MAJOR BONG'S LAST FLIGHT: ALTRUISM TO SAVE OTHERS

On August 6, 1945, the same day the first atom bomb exploded over Hiroshima, Japan, Major Harold Gray, who would retire as an U.S. Air Force colonel, visited with Major Richard Bong, America's top-scoring fighter pilot, some of whose experiences we explored in Chapter 16. They met at the Lockheed Company's airfield in Burbank, California, a populous suburb of Los Angeles. Richard Bong had been assigned there as a test pilot for Lockheed's new jet fighter, the P-80, and Harold Gray was on his way to a new assignment after having served as a combat pilot in the South Pacific. Both had flown Lockheed's two-engine propeller-driven fighter, the P-38. Many years later, Colonel Gray wrote to Richard Bong's brother Carl describing his recollection of the events of that day:

> We visited for a while and, as it turned out, he had to run off a test flight on a P-80. I had to go to Santa Anna and check-in and we were to get together that evening and have dinner together. I had plenty of time, so I wandered out onto the flight strip. While I was looking around, Dick came out to run off his flight test, so I decided to watch. On his take-off run, there were a number of puffs of black smoke coming out of the tailpipe. It looked like something was haywire to me. He got into the air maybe three or four hundred feet, but the thing still was not operating right. All of a sudden, he started to get out of it and was out of the cockpit and then he got back in, turned it and started to get out again and the plane rolled on him and that was the last I saw of him.
>
> (Bong 1991, pp. 441–442)

Evaluating the evidence of this incident, Carl Bong writes further:

> Judging from all the evidence available, Dick was airborne for about 30 to 40 seconds. The plane crashed about a mile and a half from the point of liftoff. It would seem that he may have had enough altitude to survive a bailout attempt. According to Major Gray, he did get out of the airplane at the apex of his altitude, but then got back into the cockpit. One can only speculate as to the reason that Dick re-entered the plane. Maybe he saw a chance to guide the plane away from the houses below and crashed the plane within the right-of-way boundaries of the Pacific Gas & Electric power Company's transmission lines. The rolling of the plane would support that theory. Be that the case, the move certainly cost Dick his chance to save his life, as there was no longer enough time to get out of the plane and still have the parachute function. Maybe he saw a chance of trying to crash land in the right-of-way, but the plane had lost flying speed and stalled out on him. Again, leaving him no time to bail out.
>
> (p. 510)

As with other historical vignettes, in applying the recognition algorithm, we do not work from the window into the person's consciousness that autobiography or fictional narrative allow the reader. Instead, we work from descriptions that record behavior—not what a person said, but what they actually did. In this case, the stress of the situation appears with immediate clarity: Major Richard Bong must decide whether to abandon his malfunctioning aircraft at sufficient altitude for his parachute to open, thereby turning the jet into an unguided missile over a densely populated housing tract, or to remain in the aircraft long enough to guide it into an unpopulated zone. And he must decide this in the matter of a few seconds. The stress of the situation focuses on the decision he must make with respect to risking either his own life or those of others. The anxiety, in this case of imminent death or disaster, stands in sharp relief for this experienced, decorated combat pilot from northern Wisconsin who was newly married, in his mid-20s, with most of life's experiences ahead of him.

Following the algorithm, we ask whether there is any evidence to suggest that Richard Bong's reaction to the stress and its necessary anxiety offer any evidence of Primitive or Immature Domain adaptive mechanisms that might involve either ignoring the situation as though there were nothing at all wrong or blaming it on others and waiting for them to come fix it. Following the same logic applied in the instance of Colonel Olds' violently rolling F-4 in Chapter 17, inaction in this situation, as in that one, meant certain disaster. The evidence suggests that Major Bong did not sit passively in the cockpit waiting for gravity to take its course. Neither Primitive nor Immature Domain adaptive strategies present themselves from the evidence. The accounts cannot provide sufficient detail to allow us to apply the algorithm in assessing the occurrence of the Neurotic Domain mechanisms, other than to say that there is nothing to suggest an angry overcontrolling of the situation, as one might expect in a Reaction Formation.

The evidence suggests the remarkable feat of Richard Bong's having gotten partly out of the cockpit and then climbing back in again above the critical level of about 200 feet. Below that level his parachute would not have opened completely, as all pilots of the era knew. He controlled the aircraft long enough to point it to the unpopulated power line easement into which it crashed, before the aircraft became uncontrollable. Somewhere near this point in the process he left the aircraft for a second time, falling clear of it. Rescue crews found his body and his partially open parachute some distance from the airplane's crash site.

This sequence of events certainly suggests the presence of Suppression, the same Mature Domain mechanism we saw in Colonel Olds' example and probably bred of the same experience of many hours flying aircraft; they were contemporaries and both had flown the P-38 in combat. Practice at gaining control of an uncontrolled airplane is part of the professional preparation and training for everyday flight. But Major Richard Bong's choice of risk—to himself rather than to others—a choice that led to his death, moves well beyond the stoicism of Suppression. To get back into the cockpit of that disabled aircraft at a dangerously low altitude implies that its pilot foresaw the plane coming down in a populated area. His action in returning to the danger, rather than in leaving it to harm others, indicates something of what Schopenhauer referred to as the human compassion that allows us to consider the welfare of others. It allowed Richard Bong to put the lives of others above his own, as both the eyewitness account and the evidence from the crash site suggest.

This defines Altruism as a Mature Domain adaptive mechanism: acting in the best interest of one's own conscious equilibrium when that equilibrium includes the best interests of others. It occurs for the sole purpose of retaining one's sense of psychological well-being. Its importance can be heard in statements like, "If I had done otherwise, I could not have lived with myself." At the same time, true Altruism does not depend on external sources of narcissistic gratification such as those we have discussed as pseudo-altruism in Chapter 16. Like all of the Mature Domain mechanisms, true Altruism both serves and activates human compassion in a dynamic relationship that connects us with others and with the idealism of our existence—with "the better angels of our nature," as Abraham Lincoln phrased it. Richard Bong, a young man who liked to sing and play the clarinet, did not like news reporters calling him the fighter pilot with the most "kills," as we learned in Chapter 16. As General Kenney mentioned there, he did not like others thinking of him as the best killer. When his final flight faced him with being a preserver or a destroyer of human life, he chose the former. He likely could not have done anything else in his last great act of heroism—one that he himself, could he have looked back, would have found admirable.

MEDITATION AS ADAPTATION: ALTRUISM AND THE LIFE OF THE MIND, LIFE OF THE SPIRIT

Teresa of Ávila, whose writings have already served our discussion in Chapter 9, returns here to exemplify the difference between true Altruism, one of the Mature Domain adaptive mechanisms, and its lesser cousin, pseudo-altruism, which we learned to recognize as a form of Reaction Formation in the Neurotic Domain repertoire in Chapter 16. Availing ourselves of her writings for this purpose requires keeping in mind some differences between her experiences in the 16th century and ours in the 21st. Principally, with her own life bracketed by Copernicus (1473–1543) and Galileo (1564–1642), the reader notes that her autobiography contains no reference to the oncoming cultural change in Western Europe that moved explaining the nature of the universe out of metaphor and into science. Rather, Teresa (1515–1582) writes from within the Christian metaphor as she knew it in the Spain of her day and as it had existed in Europe for at least a thousand years before that. In the present day, 500 years later, science rather than theology guides our understanding of the physical setting in which humans live. The major religious traditions—whether biblical (Christian, Judaic, or Islamic), Hindu, or Buddhist, or any of the variations of any of these—survive best as poetic metaphors of human existence rather than as scientific explanations of the contents of space and time or the mechanisms of causality.

Similarly, humans living in the 21st century more likely describe the workings of the mind, the brain, or a combination of both concepts in terms of the scientific models alluded to in Chapter 2, rather than as religious constructs. As a result, where Teresa speaks of God as external to her person but communicating with her, Carl Jung speaks of a common perception that humans carry within them that defines a supreme being through what his model refers to as an archetype of perception.

In translating, therefore, Teresa's external God who comes to her in prayer denotes a phenomenon that people in our era would likely call a poetic metaphor of our own internal perceptions. Twenty-first century diction would formulate this particular notion of communication with an energy or supreme being—depending on one's belief system—as an occurrence that we may notice through meditation. For the purposes of understanding in relation to psychological adaptive mechanisms, Teresa's levels of prayer equal what we might call levels of meditation: levels of the intensity or depth of perceiving—and living in—the mental and physical activity that comes from within oneself. That is, the depth or intensity of internal perceptions that do not result directly from external stimulation.[3] With this translation as background context, however, the present discussion focuses not on the perceptions themselves, but rather on the uses that the same human phenomenon under two different names—Teresa's prayer = 21st-century meditation—bring to the process of human psychological adaptation. In this respect, application of the current model—and especially the recognition algorithm—may prove particularly useful.

To begin our learning from that redoubtable nun and reformer of the 16th-century Spanish Church, a contemporary of other Spanish religious reformers in the persons of Ignatius Loyola (1491–1556) and John of the Cross (1542–1591), consider her concern when discussing with others the experience of prayer. Speaking of the zeal of the newly converted—noting that Teresa's own experience of what she describes as prayer began for her after age 40—she offers a concern that can apply to others new to religious conversion:

> There is another very common temptation; and that is, when one begins to enjoy the common fruit of prayer, to wish everyone else to be very spiritual too. The wish is not wrong; but attempts to bring it about may not be good unless carried out with great discretion and in such a disguised way that one does not appear to be trying to teach. If a person is to do any good in such matters he must be very strong in the virtues, so as not to put temptation in the way of others. This I discovered for myself, and so I understand the danger. For when—as I said before—I persuaded others to practice prayer, on the one hand they heard me say so much about the great blessings that come of it and, on the other, they saw how poor I was in virtues although I prayed.
>
> (Ávila 1957, p. 91)

These words call to mind one of Charlotte Brontë's characters, the Reverend St. John Rivers, whose description appeared in Chapter 16 on Reaction Formation. Reviewed briefly, despite his understanding of having chosen the wrong profession because the ministry served neither his heart nor his mind, he completely reversed his own self regard by transforming into a missionary zealot. He perceived that ministry instead excited him and contained all of those worldly factors, such as renown and the lust for power, that the social and professional pursuits he truly longed for

3. See Immanuel Kant's definition of *a priori* experience in *Critique of Pure Reason* (1929).

would offer him. Add to that, he came to see missionary work as a ticket to Heaven as compared to the humdrum of a daily Hell as a minister. This distant and abstract reward far outweighed even the clear and present love that Miss Oliver offered him. Despite all this, however, Jane Eyre, Charlotte Brontë's narrator, saw in St. John Rivers only a lack of peace in his protestations of idealism. We concluded in Chapter 16 that St. John Rivers' Reaction Formation, an adaptive style in the Neurotic Domain, took the form of a pseudo-altruism designed to prop up his own need to think well of himself. Its purpose was to stave off a profound loss of self-esteem since, as the character says in *Jane Eyre*, without this conversion to missionary zeal his spirit will die in the tedium of his ordinary ministerial occupation. In the model of psychological adaptations, St. John Rivers had not resolved the separation of painful thoughts and painful feelings that might allow him to come to better terms in adapting to his own psychological needs.

Teresa of Ávila in the above quoted passage describes something very similar in first wanting to approach others with the zealousness of her excitement at having discovered prayer—a direct communication with God, in her perception But instead she rejects the zeal rather than embrace it as a new identity. Unlike Charlotte Brontë's character, Teresa has no self-esteem wrapped up in her religious fervor. Nor does she need the love or approval of others to validate her own experience. Rather, she understands that a zealous approach puts people off—as, we recall, St. John Rivers' conversion to missionary had the effect of putting off Jane Eyre. This is not something Teresa wishes to do. Historically, in fact, she was known as a community builder who reformed her own order of nuns in keeping with the prayer she experienced and described for others.

More particularly in regard to the psychological adaptation model, however, Teresa's words recognize that pursuing a pseudo-altruistic zeal as its own cause does not lead to her own peace of mind. She goes on to describe the purpose of her prayer in words that sound familiar in our present 21st-century discussion of responding to stress:

> The security of the soul that applies itself to prayer lies in its ceasing to be anxious for anything or anybody, in its watching itself and pleasing God. This is very important. If I were to tell of the mistakes I have seen people make, through reliance on their own good intentions, I should never be done.
>
> (Ávila 1957, p. 91)

Speaking in the theological terms of her day, she could have as easily been describing the "good intentions" that Charlotte Brontë finds in St. John Rivers 300 years later. In the present adaptation model, we might restate her words as follows: "A person who applies a Mature adaptation strategy ceases to be anxious in coming to know him/her self and their perceptions of the energies of existence. Pursuing good intentions for others instead only distracts from this."

Teresa of Ávila points out this pseudo-altruism as a false start on the road to effective psychological adaptation. An application of the recognition algorithm offers a more detailed look at what she actually does in finding both meaning and adaptation. According to the algorithm, the first task requires definition of the stress that then occasions the anxiety that we have defined as a sense of doom or disaster, resulting in an adaptive response. At first this seems a quandary: what could a nun living in a convent in 16th-century Spain possibly find in life that might be stressful? The answer recalls a Christian metaphor that may seem attenuated to 21st-century ears. The religious metaphor in which Teresa lived—first promulgated in the time of Zoroaster (circa sixth century B.C.) and, and observed in all three of the biblical religious traditions—held that all men and women come into this life as evil beings, owing to a very literal belief in the original sin that cast humans out of the sight of God.[4] Returning to the Garden of Eden—or Heaven, in the theology of Teresa's day—therefore requires a successful redemption of one's innate evil nature. While theological beliefs may show the way, in the metaphor of the Fall from the Garden of Eden, the redemptive process itself is a personal occupation.

In respect to the current model of psychological adaptation, therefore, a first question asks, did Teresa think of herself as evil or, in the language of her day, as sinful? Over and over again throughout the pages of her autobiography, she refers in very specific language to her own sinfulness. To modern ears this may reach the point of tedium, but in the context of her times, she gives us a description of what she perceives as literal reality. The sense of doom or disaster that follows from an essentially evil nature—that is, the anxiety defined in our present model—is likewise a damnation that the Christian beliefs of the time held as eternal exclusion from the sight of God.[5] In the Christian metaphor, this is the punishment of Satan and equates unredeemed humans with the damnation of the Devil himself.

In present 21st-century language, a similar phenomenon may be described as forever having lost touch with one's own vitality, one's own engagement with life that results in the "damnation" of never having lived in an authentic fashion in the root sense of that word, a life in which one "authors" one's own course. The fictional portraits provided by Charlotte Brontë's St. John Rivers or Leo Tolstoy's Ivan Ilyich provide examples in more modern dress of what medieval European religious metaphors meant in respect to the same phenomenon. The stress to which Teresa of Ávila must adapt, put in the language of our present understanding, is one that she shares with all human beings: namely, living a life of personal satisfaction. The opposite, by contrast, is the anxious doom of never having been engaged with human existence from the inside out.

The recognition algorithm next asks, how does she go about this process of adaptation, one that she might think of as redemption? Does she employ Primitive Domain adaptive mechanisms? Recalling the basic stance of the Primitive strategies as a failure to recognize the presence of any stress, Teresa's persistent concern about

4. Those reading these words from the point of view of Western culture and traditions will find a certain familiarity in them. By contrast, those reading the same words from the perspective of Eastern cultures, such as Hindu or Buddhist traditions, will find them very foreign. Neither of the latter two traditions employ any concept of original sin. Humans, viewed as part of nature and emanating from the energies of the universe, come into the world as good, and with no hint of evil. All babies are Buddha babies, as the Zen master and philosopher Daisetz Suzuki commented (see Suzuki, 2007, p. 148).

5. Dante Alighieri, writing his *Inferno* three centuries earlier, takes us inside this aspect of the Christian metaphor in marvelous, concrete detail.

her own "sinfulness"—what today might be construed as being out of touch with one's own nature—argues against the Primitive adaptive strategies in her case. She speaks of the influence of the Devil in very concrete terms, to our sensibilities creating the prospect of a delusion. But in Teresa's time and culture a concrete belief in the Devil was widely held, and consistent with the Christian metaphor for explaining the nature of existence, a belief not at all regarded as contrary to fact.

If she does not ignore her concern for metaphorical redemption, does she locate the responsibility for avoiding the death of her soul outside of herself, in the manner of the Immature Domain adaptive mechanisms? As discussed in Chapter 9, we have already seen her reject the notion that everything wrong with her emanated from what was wrong with her body. She simply stopped considering her illness because, in her view, it led nowhere. Nor do we find Teresa haranguing us with the hellfire and brimstone sermons of the 17th- and 18th-century American fundamentalist preachers, demanding the passive welcome of an external God in order to be "saved." For Teresa, the process of redemption occurs within oneself and does so actively, not passively. The Immature Domain adaptive strategies do not apply in the discovery of what she calls prayer.

Following the recognition algorithm further, assessment of the Neurotic Domain mechanisms requires us to identify the difficult thoughts and the painful feelings that the stress entails and that generate its anxiety. In the terms of Teresa's day, the cognition can be formulated as, "I will live eternally outside the sight of God," and in a 21st-century concept as, "I will never be myself." The affective content does not depend on the terms of the different cognitive formulations of different eras: "I am terrified" works either way. We have already seen that Teresa rejects the option of proceeding in a way that fosters the separation of the painful feeling from its idea: she will not preach the conversion of others to prayer. This distracts her from the necessary work of her own integration of thought and emotion, the task of that she sees as her own redemption. As she argues against Reaction Formation, at the same time we do not hear her arguing only about feeling at the expense of thought, as in Repression, or about thought at the expense of feeling, as in Isolation of Affect. She does not employ the Neurotic Domain psychological adaptive mechanisms but seeks out Mature Domain adaptation.

She does this in a very creative manner of observation, a process akin to what, in our day, we might refer to as research insofar as it aims at understanding a phenomenon that she experiences. For her, this is a process not only of intellectual observation but also one of coming to terms with painful feelings in ways through which thought and emotion inform each other. They then lead her to the resolution of being in close touch with her God, or, as we might say, with herself. For her, resolution is an active process that comes through her life in prayer, or, as we might say in a meditative knowing of oneself, alluding to Socrates' famous dictum "Know thyself." Using the terms of her context, she describes her prayerful life as having occurred in stages, as summarized next.[6] She uses water—a universal symbol of what Schopenhauer, building from the Upanishads, referred to as the will in nature. Western

6. For this, I have used only Teresa of Ávila's own words, although I quote them in abbreviated sections with their titles taken from her writings. Readers may compare these to her original text at their leisure.

religions refer to it as grace—and Teresa uses it to describe her own growth of the spirit, what she might consider the redemptive growth of the soul.

The First Water

We may say that beginners in prayer are those who draw the water up out of the well; which is a great labor, as I have said. For they find it very tiring to keep the senses recollected, when they are used to a life of distraction. Beginners have to accustom themselves to pay no attention to what they see or hear, and to put this exercise into practice during their hours of prayer, when they must remain in solitude, thinking whilst they are alone of their past life.

(Ávila 1957, p. 98)

The Second Water (the prayer of quiet)

Now the soul begins to be recollected, and here comes into touch with the supernatural, to which it could not possibly attain by its own efforts. . . . I mean that the water is closer because grace reveals itself more clearly to the soul. This entailed a gathering of the faculties within oneself so as to derive a greater savor from that pleasure. But they are not lost or asleep.

(p. 98)

The Third Water

The soul does not know what to do; it cannot tell whether to speak or be silent, whether to laugh or weep. It is a glorious bewilderment, a heavenly madness, in which true wisdom is acquired, and to the soul a fulfillment most full of delight.

(p. 112)

The Fourth Water

In this state, the soul still feels that it is not altogether dead, as we may say, though it is entirely dead to the world. But, as I have said, it retains the sense to know that it is still here and to feel its solitude; and it makes use of outer manifestations to show its feelings, at least by signs. . . . So the labor is not felt as such but as bliss.

(p. 122)

. . . [A]nyone who has experienced raptures will, I know, understand me perfectly. To one who has not, however, this must seem nonsense, and it may be so. For one like myself to speak of such a matter, making an attempt to explain something which cannot even begin to be described in words, may very well appear ridiculous.

(p. 124)

Put in modern secular terms, Teresa describes a progression by which one reaches what she describes as a blissful communication with one's own being. Although formulating the stages in different terms, yoga practices of the Eastern religions describe the same phenomenon, for example in the seven stages of the Kundalini system of yoga. The Sanskrit word *ananda*, meaning "bliss," aims at describing the same sense of being fully in tune with even the far reaches of oneself, of what Teresa regards as God. Contrary to Gianlorenzo Bernini's *Saint Teresa in Ecstasy* in the Cornaro Chapel that portrays her in something like a physical orgasm, the bliss, or rapture, that she describes is an active mind/brain effort that occurs, in her description, when the body is essentially quiet and appears so to anyone observing at the time. She goes on to describe the effects of reaching this meditative state, which she calls the highest state of prayer, as a continuous process and one that informs her daily life:

> The mind is now so used to drawing upon real truth, that everything else seems to it childish.... So the soul continues to lead a troubled life, and always has its crosses, but it is a life of continuous growth. Those with whom it has most to do keep on thinking that it has reached the summit, but they soon see it raised even higher, for God is always granting it new favors.
>
> (Ávila, 1957, p. 151)

St. Teresa reaches not a cloistered withdrawal from the experiences of life but a much closer, more exciting, ever-growing engagement with them. Her redemption lies in finding her soul's continuous growth, what those in our day might describe as the continuing growth of the spirit, that unseen part of human nature. An active engagement with the experiences of life brings with it continuing recognition of both the idea of its physical and spiritual nature along with the shared feelings—the compassion—that these entail, ranging from sadness through joy. The active process that includes both idea and feeling defines Mature Domain psychological adaptation in the present model.

But how is this an example of Altruism? Teresa has not given up her life for the lives of others, as in the more dramatic case of Richard Bong's last flight. Referring again to the idea of research, of looking deeper into the nature of things and experiences, Teresa describes what mythological scholars refer to as her own heroine journey: going into unknown and terrifying areas of experience and perception, finding not only a sense of bliss but of personal growth and adaptation in the effort, and then returning to tell others about it. Her adventure at finding her redemption, what we would describe as finding the fullest reaches of herself, shows no indication of her having taken it on solely for the purpose of gaining other peoples' praise and adulation. She does not attempt her adventure of the spirit to please others. To the contrary, she observes that her description of raptures may seem crazy to others and perhaps it is, as she gently makes fun of her own words. She is willing to risk being thought of as crazy, another aspect of her bringing back the knowledge she has gained in the journey and communicating it to others who may wish to take the journey themselves. The risk of adventure in the service of one's own adaptation and the risk of communication in the service of others defines true Altruism whether in a 16th-century convent or a disabled 20th-century fighter jet. The compassion involved allows humans to go places at the risk of their own comfort that they might not otherwise consider and, in so doing, to be of service not only to themselves in respect to living in tune with one's own mind, but also spiritually or materially to others. Consider the last example of this chapter, one of a more everyday nature in being of use to others.

THE INTERN IN PRACTICE: THE REAL DR. WILLIAMS AND ALTRUISM IN ESTABLISHING DIAGNOSIS

Where before the recurring character of the sleepy intern has sprung forth on demand in order to exemplify particular adaptation styles, in this instance, Dr. Williams, who was at one time himself an intern, and possibly a sleepy one, provides us with this chapter's example in a description that occurs well after his internship days. He takes us to Passaic, New Jersey, where he practiced in the 1920s, well before the discovery of antibiotics and their use in treating children with deadly infectious diseases. He examines a child assisted by her parents in their home:

> The child was fairly eating me with her cold, steady eyes, and no expression to her face whatever. She did not move and seemed, inwardly, quiet; an unusually attractive little thing and strong as a heifer in her appearance. But her face was flushed, she was breathing rapidly, and I realized that she had a high fever. She had magnificent blonde hair, in profusion. One of those picture children often reproduced in advertising leaflets and the photogravure sections of the Sunday papers.

The little girl refuses to open her mouth for the doctor:

> If you don't do what the doctor says you'll have to go to the hospital, the mother admonished her severely.
>
> Oh yeah? I had to smile to myself. After all, I had already fallen in love with the savage brat, the parents were contemptible to me. In the ensuing struggle they grew more and more abject, crushed, exhausted while she surely rose to magnificent heights of insane fury of effort bred of her terror of me.

Held down by her father, the doctor maneuvers a tongue depressor between her teeth and pries them open whereupon she bites the stick in half:

> Get me a smooth-handled spoon of some sort, I told the mother. We're going through with this. The child's mouth was already bleeding. Her tongue was cut and she was screaming in wild hysterical shrieks. Perhaps I should have desisted and come back in an hour or more. No doubt it would have been better. But I have seen at least two children lying dead in bed of neglect in such cases, and feeling that I must get a diagnosis now or never I went at it again. But the worst of it was that I too had got beyond reason. I could have torn the child apart in my own fury and enjoyed it. It was a pleasure to attack her. My face was burning with it.

> The damned little brat must be protected against her own idiocy, one says to one's self at such times. Others must be protected against her. It is social necessity. And all these things are true. But a blind fury, a feeling of adult shame, bred of a longing for muscular release are the operatives. One goes on to the end.
>
> (Williams 1957, pp. 131–135)

With recourse to the recognition algorithm, we can identify the stress that the narrator of this passage faces and that ultimately perturbs his conscious sense of well-being. But on the surface it may seem that his own feelings make up the stress in the situation. When I present this passage to psychiatry residents and other trainees, the women in the audience usually notice the sexual overtones in Williams' description: the child's blonde hair in profusion, the narrator's being in love with her while finding the parents contemptible, and his feeling of shame, as examples. The men, by contrast, usually miss this completely and see instead an idealistic physician who must take control of the situation in order to stamp out disease. Put another way, where the women see sex, the men see aggression—both basic energies that we share with the primitive brains of animals where brain-cortex control of them is far less than that which humans have. And while both sets of energies appear in the narrator's description, his interest as a writer lies more in presenting them to us as the ingredients he uses to resolve the stress, rather than to see them as the stress itself.

In the most dispassionate, one might even say cold, phrases in the story, he articulates the stress as the possibility of a dead child if he does not learn what he needs to learn in order to make a diagnosis and begin treatment. He has already seen two cases of other children dead because someone had not thought the matter serious. In addition, to ignore making a diagnosis in this case risks spreading the same deadly disease to others. Preventing the death of this beautiful child makes up true stress that weighs on him. His anxiety lies in preventing the doom of this child who wants no part of him or his medical knowledge and shows it by biting his tongue depressor in half. His duty is to preserve life and her personal disaster will become his professional disaster.

The recognition algorithm next asks whether the narrator ignores the situation and its incipient danger to the child. He does not deny the fact that the child has a high fever and is likely very ill, but the situation is very tense one and difficult for physician and patient alike. He articulates the alternative course that perhaps he could just walk away. But he knows that his anxiety won't allow that. The Primitive Domain mechanisms may be tempting but won't address the child's danger.

The algorithm moves on to the Immature Domain adaptive mechanisms. These too offer the temptation of locating the entire stressful situation somewhere else: the badly behaving little brat deserves whatever she gets. This would be to project the doctor's own anxiety at the situation, and the energy of his own anger that fuels his drive toward the diagnosis, onto the patient. But Neurotic Projection as an adaptive style for the doctor will not work in this situation either. He correctly notes that the child's lack of understanding of any but her most immediate experience of the situation may very likely kill her if her illness is left unchecked. This is her "idiocy" as he describes it. He recognizes that but does not return fire at it, as he might were he using Neurotic Projection.

But he is not completely comfortable with the situation even though he sees her rise "to magnificent heights of insane fury" in her angry behavior. He too has become angry—"a blind fury," as he says. In the recognition algorithm, this description articulates the emotional content of the stress itself, one of the two ingredients needed when considering the Neurotic Domain adaptive mechanisms. It has made the narrator angry. The cognitive content might be formulated as, "Duty requires that I must face this furious little child who makes me so angry that it hurts." While toying briefly with the possibility of a Reaction Formation—defining the child's angry actions in preventing his looking in her mouth at every turn as her rising to "magnificent heights" in her fury—he does not cease the examination and applaud her performance. Similarly, he does not ignore his own feelings, as one might see in an Intellectualization, nor does he ignore the fact of her behavior as causing his anger, as one might see in Repression. The Neurotic Domain defenses have no use to him.

Rather, as the narrator describes, both feeling and idea—anger and the necessity of a professional duty, respectively—work together in this circumstance. His ideal is clear: he is a physician; he is trained to establish diagnoses by looking at and probing into the body. Because of his training he is socially sanctioned, and duty bound, to do so. Referring to one model of human behavior, he will use his critical judgment as a human being in making use of the appropriate cortical brain structures that mediate the socially integrated experiences of this training. Simultaneously, he will harness the energies from the more primitive parts of his brain that the cortex mitigates and shapes into effective action. In this respect, his adaptation to the child's anger and his own response to it occur in service to her health at the cost of his own comfort. He pursues his own Altruism in this course of behavior. In the process he suffers not only her rage but his own as well. In the definition of compassion, anger can be a shared feeling as often as sadness.

Contrasted to the pseudo-altruism of a Reaction Formation, Williams' physician-narrator does not look for applause and admiration from those around him. Nor does he pursue the little girl's diagnosis in order to prop up his own self-confidence (narcissism) or self-esteem (love): as he describes, he would just as soon walk away but he knows that the little girl's life hangs in the balance. As we learn further on in Williams' story, the doctor and the little girl's parents eventually do pry her mouth open, and he gets a brief, if terrifying, look at the membrane that the bacteria has formed at the back of her throat. The child has a case of diphtheria, preventable in our day with a vaccine, but deadly in those years.

Clinical medicine, through supervised repetition, trains physicians and surgeons to look at the horrors of this life. Rather than running from them, it asks that they look with a sense of curiosity as to how those horrors can be understood and made better. Rather than fearing them, it asks that they find a sense of true compassion with those who suffer, even though the immediate emotions may mask the deeper, more troubling ones. Although individual practitioners may be altruistic to greater and lesser degrees, the profession itself serves Altruism: with careful attention to clinical and scientific method, putting the welfare of others above one's own comfort in the sense that Schopenhauer described. Whether in Dr. Williams' practice, Major Bong's flying, St. Teresa's prayer, or the thousands of other activities in which humans engage to better the world for others with no expectation of return for oneself, Altruism is at work. It makes us better people in one model, and connects us with all humanity in another.

EXAMPLES AND USES OF ALTRUISM

Humans may engage in Altruistic behavior frequently in an ordinary day's time. Simple acts, such as holding a door open for another person, deferring one's place in the lunch counter line to someone else, or returning an object that a person has dropped on the sidewalk, and many other such instances, exemplify people going out of their way for others. Is Altruism, the Mature Domain psychological adaptive mechanism, at work in these instances? Or can we simply say that there is no clear stress involved that calls forth anxiety to which people respond with small altruistic actions of this nature? Therefore, as a result, everyday Altruism is a separate phenomenon and not an adaptive behavior. The reader is certainly free to draw the latter conclusion, as may seem a proper one to them. As noted in the Chapter 2, the purpose of this volume is to provide a practical model of psychological adaptive behaviors that perceptive readers may use where it may seem to them appropriately applied.

Viewed through the adaptive model, however, small acts of everyday Altruism may offer another insight. In Chapter 3 and again Chapter 7, we noted that stresses can have positive or negative valences. Potential stresses at work here may include the positive sense of feeling good about oneself, a result of the compassion humans experience in connecting with others. Conversely, missing an opportunity to enjoy that sense of connection with other human beings may, even in small instances, often results in noticeable anxiety, not so much a cataclysmic sense of doom or disaster as one of a discomfort or an unease. Altruism as a Mature Domain mechanism, therefore, may offer us the everyday opportunity of human connection and feeling good, at the sacrifice of human isolation and feeling bad.

This sense of Altruistic connectivity and positive direction may have to do with the universal human self-perception of being on the "right" path or the "wrong" one. Stresses, as we have noted, may come from inside or outside the human person. The positive stress of being in tune with one own energies and perceptions may contrast with the negative stress of being out of touch with them. This implies that oneself, as well as other people, can be the object of Altruism as a Mature Domain psychological adaptive mechanism. Humans value themselves when they "are on the beam," "walking the pollen Path," "doing the Lord's work," finding their "being that is illumination," "knowing thyself," and many other similar formulations from different cultures at different times.[7] Compassion and understanding apply to the self, as well as to others, Altruistically considered in the psychological adaptation model.

It appears also true that the observable behaviors of Altruism may increase in clarity as the stresses we face themselves increase in magnitude or frequency. For

7. Respectively, these formulations come from early aviation, Navajo culture, the Christian metaphor, the Buddhist bodhisattva, and Greek philosophy.

example, one of the most common and yet most profound of Altruistic behaviors in everyday life may come from parenthood. In the interest of their children, who must develop from the most profoundly helpless of beings in infancy to independent, functioning adults, most parents will limit, and even sacrifice, their own comfort for the well-being of their children. The positive stress of catalyzing the growth and development of one's offspring, and the negative stress of failing to do so, may both result from many causes, varying from cultural norms and beliefs through evolutionary biology.

From the observer's point of view, Altruism, considered as a Mature Domain psychological adaptive mechanism, flexibly adapts to many situations, and to their stresses with both positive and negative valence experiences, in the grand opera of human life. It may call for the heroic in the most dramatic cases, but its reach may be far more subtle than the most obvious of examples will provide. Its range includes all of us, every day, in small ways and in large. It allows us to adapt to ourselves as well as to others. Rather than Henry David Thoreau's formulation of lives lived in quiet desperation, Altruism as an adaptive behavior appears to offer the possibility of lives lived in something more akin to personal adventure.

REFERENCES

Ávila, T. (1957). *The Life of Saint Teresa of Ávila, by Herself* (J. M. Cohen, Trans.). London, Penguin.

Bong, C. (1991). *Dear Mom, So We Have a War*. Minneapolis, Burgess.

Kant, I. (1929). Critique of Pure Reason (N. K. Smith, Trans.). New York, Palgrave MacMillan.

Schopenhauer, A. (2005). *Philosophical Writings: Vol. 27. German Library* (Wolfgang Schirmacher, Ed.). New York, Continuum.

Suzuki, D. T. (2007). *Manual of Zen Buddhism*. Charleston, SC, Forgotten Books.

Williams, W. C. (1957). "The Use of Force." *The Farmers' Daughters*. New York, New Directions.

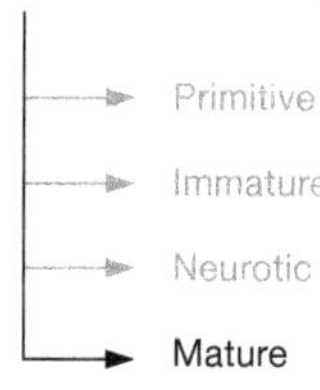

CHAPTER 20

Sublimation

It would be difficult to find a more closely drawn introduction to Sublimation as an adaptive mechanism than that which Dante Alighieri provides in his short book *Vita Nuova* (translated as *New Life*). Written in 1295, at the transition point between Western Europe's medievalism and the oncoming Italian Renaissance, he details an experience that sounds as if it could have been written specifically for the present model of psychological adaptive mechanisms, some 700-plus years later. As if instructed by the recognition algorithm, he describes the stress he experiences, the anxiety that results from it, and then his adaptive responses.

As the passage begins, Dante, in his early 20s, accompanies a friend to a social gathering at which he knows that his beloved (from afar) Beatrice will be present. His arrival at the gathering occasions an anxiety attack:

> So I, thinking to please my friend in so, decided to remain with him in attendance upon the ladies. No sooner had I reached my decision than I seemed to feel a strange throbbing in the left side of my chest which before long spread to all parts of my body. Then, so as not to attract attention, I leaned against a painting that ran along the walls of that house and fearing that people might have become aware of my trembling, I raised my eyes and, gazing at the ladies, I saw among them the most gracious Beatrice. Then my spirits (*senses*) were so disrupted by the strength Love acquired when he saw himself so close to the most gracious lady, that none remained alive except the spirits of sight; and even these remained outside their instruments, because Love usurped their enviable seat to view the marvelous lady.

The ladies, seeing his nearly paralyzed state, ridicule him gently:

> My friend, who in good faith had been deceived, took me by the hand and, leading me out of the sight of these ladies, asked me what was the matter. And I, somewhat restored, feeling my dead spirits come back to life . . . , said these words to my friend, "I have placed my feet on those boundaries of life beyond which no one can go further and hope to return."

In embarrassment, he returns home to his room:

> In the midst of my tears, I decided to write a few words addressed to her, explaining the reason for my transfiguration and saying that I well know that people are not aware of it and that were they aware of it, they would be moved to pity. And I resolved to say these words with the hope that perchance they would reach her ears. Then I composed this sonnet which begins: You join with other ladies.
>
> You join with other ladies to deride me
> and do not think, my lady, for what cause
> I cut so awkward and grotesque a figure
> when I stand gazing at your lovely form.
> Could you but know my soul in charity,
> then yours would melt from its accustomed scorn;
> for Love, when he beholds me near to you,
> takes on a cruel and bold new confidence
> and puts my frightened senses to the sword,
> murdering this one, driving that one out,
> till only he is left to look at you;
> thus, though his changeling, I am not so changed
> but that I still can hear in my own soul
> my outcast senses mourning in their pain.
>
> (Alighieri 1992, pp. 25–26)

Before the figure of Beatrice became the central literary symbol in *The Divine Comedy*, she was a real person. The same age as Dante, they had first met each other at nine, and again at age 18, numbers to which Dante ascribes spiritual significance. Both are divisible by three and are multiples of three squared: three persons make up the Holy Trinity, the triune God of Dante's culture. In discovering his love for her, which he personifies in this book as a god within himself, he discovers love for specific individuals as something to be shared among all humans. He is not describing purely sexual love or its idealized opposite, the traditional Christian love of one's neighbor. As others have noted, neither of these forms require an emotional communication between two discrete individuals. Whether for sex or *agape*,[1] one person is as good as the next. But in Beatrice Dante finds that his emotions overwhelm him to the point of what feels to him like physical death. This universal phenomenon calls to mind Sappho's similar description, quoted in Chapter 7, of being "on the point of death" in the presence of love. Dante's physical sensation of immediate disaster, beginning with the throbbing that starts over his heart and then takes control of the rest of his body, conforms to our definition of anxiety in the current adaptation model. We find its source—the stress, in this case—in Dante's physical proximity to the object of the emotions that overwhelm him. While they

---

1. *Agape* (pronounced ah-gah-pay) is a Greek word that the Christian system of belief uses to refer to the selfless love of all human beings for all other human beings.

include affectionate rapture, they also include pain: as he notes earlier in the book, in Love he has found a god stronger than himself, and now he knows he is going to suffer.[2]

Applying what may seem like the mundane exercise of the recognition algorithm to a setting of such an exalted state of experience, we nevertheless ask whether Dante employs a Primitive Domain mechanism in adapting to this painful situation. It is difficult for him, but there is no indication that he ignores it. He does not deny that Beatrice exists, belittle her importance to him, or construct an illusion that she is inhabited by the Devil. The evidence does not support the presence of any of the Primitive Domain mechanisms.

What about the Immature Domain mechanisms? After all, he seems to blame his suffering on a personification of his feelings that he calls Love as if it were a person, and more than that, as if it were a god. Further, he seems to project his painful emotions into his body. Are we dealing with Neurotic Projection and a Hypochondriasis? To agree with either of these would be to misunderstand both the symbolism that Dante gives to Love's personification as well as the description of the symptoms. We learn in Chapter II of the *Vita Nuova*, for example, that he first beheld Beatrice when both were nine years old. He describes that encounter as the beginning of his spiritual life—his *New Life*—and recognizes Love as a part of himself that he notices both in his brain and in his viscera. The physical reaction he describes above is neither more nor less than the activity of the sympathetic nervous system in the fight-or-flight response to stress that we noted in Chapter 2. Dante's does not locate responsibility outside himself for dealing with the remarkable stress of feeling alive, the stress that Beatrice signifies. Rather, his love for Beatrice guides him to the best aspects of human life. His description takes us well beyond the Immature Domain adaptive mechanisms.

To assess the Neurotic Domain adaptive mechanisms, the observer asks, has he described his rapture and pain as separate from his perception of Beatrice, or do they work together to inform his description and the poem he writes following it? Were Dante to define a cold, emotionless, description of Beatrice's physical and behavioral characteristics on the one hand (intellectualization), or a turgid, and only positive, description of his experience of love in the absence of anyone called Beatrice on the other hand (repression), perhaps a case for the Neurotic Domain adaptive mechanisms might materialize. But neither of these occur.

Instead, Dante transforms all of his distress, all of his rapturous love, and the effect that both have upon him into a sonnet. As suggested at the beginning of this chapter, Sublimation, that creative miracle from the Mature Domain, constitutes his ultimate psychological adaptive mechanism. Reading the version of the sonnet above, or various other translations of it, the same meaning comes through: in her presence, his thought and feeling for her drives all else away from his mind and this changes him. He is grateful for this change that integrates idea and emotion, but it is still painful.

2. "Heu miser, quia frequenter impeditus ero deinceps!" Chapter II. Joseph Campbell translates this as "Now I am going to suffer."

While writing something down may constitute an everyday form of sublimation for any of us, this poem carries the Sublimation process further. Reading it, for example, there is no mention of Beatrice by name. Neither is there mention of Dante. If one copied out the sonnet and handed it to someone else to read who had no idea of its origin in the specific circumstances of Beatrice and Dante, the same meaning and feeling articulated in the poem would still arrive, intact and emotionally moving. This is the mark of Mature Domain Sublimation resulting in a work of art. The creation itself—whether a poem, a painting, a musical performance, or any of the other products born of engagement with the painful, or joyful, feelings and thoughts of human existence—exists independently of its creator. Others, experiencing the work, share in both the thoughts and feelings that inhere in it as their own. They share the experience with the work's creator and feel touched by it. But this occurs from experiencing the work itself, not from its author's direct presence. This kind of creation stands on its own and connects us with the human experience entailed in it, itself.

One need not write poetic verses, sculpt statues out of marble, or compose symphonies to use Sublimation in everyday life. Turning work aggressions into an improved swing at the golf driving range, baking the family's joy into the best apple pie ever, or singing in the choir—however badly—because the music touches something of the fragility of life, all count. Each example creates in its own way and bring us into touch with others, whether the golf foursome, a shared meal, or a momentary levitation into a collective sound. A great Sublimation work, such as Dante's extended treatment of the love for human life that he first knows through his affection for Beatrice—*The Divine Comedy*—requires a special talent. At the same time, however, the most creative Sublimations seem also related to the greatest stresses that in turn call forth exceptional responses. The news of cancer in a beloved relative, for example, calls forth the quest for justice in one person, a jazz solo that moves an audience to extended applause in another, and a painting of variations on the circle in a third.

Nathaniel Fick, the Marine captain quoted in Chapter 16, after consecutive combat tours with his platoon in Afghanistan and Iraq, wrote a description of his experiences that puts his readers in the middle of those conflicts detail by detail, without polemic or gratuitous violence. The meaning of his title *One Bullet Away* does not settle in until the very last chapter. That bullet killed his successor, the next leader of his platoon, well before he wrote the book. His account can be read as a Sublimation of his experiences—including his luck—that puts us in the emotional middle of the action. The narrative and the feelings it evokes work together.

The present model holds that each of these creative efforts serves adaptive purposes. They invite the connection with others that helps resolve the anxiety, if not always removing the stress itself, in the person who is adapting. At the same time the interpersonal connections enliven those who share in them, whether through words, pictures, or a good golf game, among the many examples. Sublimation, like the other Mature Domain adaptive mechanisms, occasions and supports human compassion, even in the most unexpected circumstances, as in the following example from the fighter pilot in the Great War whom we met earlier.

SONG IN THE WIRE, SONG IN THE WOOD: PUTTING STRESS AND ANXIETY INTO MUSIC

At 30, Mick Mannock was older than most fighter pilots when he began flying in 1917. In his first few months at the front, some of the other pilots in his squadron thought he had "the wind up," that is, that he was afraid of combat. In fact, he was more circumspect than most. Prior to the First World War, he had been active in English socialist politics and, had he lived, might have had a successful career in it. Just before hostilities began in 1914, he had taken a job in Turkey and was imprisoned there after war broke out. He nearly starved to death there until he was repatriated in a prisoner exchange. His relative age and his experiences before joining the Royal Flying Corps had given him a circumspection that his colleagues later came to value and to admire. After what today would be considered minimal flight training, Mannock took pains to practice flying armed aircraft, developing the skills he would use in combat. He became expert at it, as we have seen, and reached the point at which flying became second nature. This allowed him to consider the larger challenges of finding effective ways to defeat his opponents in the air. Because he thought about his work, he led his peers in the Flying Corps in developing successful combat tactics against the formidable and equally creative German pilots. Over the months of his wartime deployment, he taught less experienced pilots the skills he had developed in fighting and surviving, and they revered him for this. His quick rise to command of two separate squadrons and promotion to major likewise attested to his ability to think through problems and reach solutions. But he did not enjoy combat operations. Others regularly described him as being ill before flights from the nervous tension, but leading them anyway. This was his duty and he pursued it like the others, for king and country, at least early on.

With experience, however, the reality of the fighting continued to settle on him, as it would in Major Bong's case in World War II.[3] As a squadron commander near the end of his combat days, he instructed his pilots that it was not enough to fight the enemy in the defense of Britannia. His pilots' duty was to kill them. He had no illusions of what they were about. But how different this was from the political socialism that aimed at making life better for the poor and disenfranchised. Here was a man with a sense of idealism about life, who had endured physical starvation at the hands of the enemy. He had become very good at sanctioned killing in aerial combat even though it seemed, literally, to make him sick. Perhaps a small irony exists in the fact that the wood-and-wire contraptions he flew shared at least that much of their construction with Mannock's musical instrument.

Among the grim descriptions of his diary and then those of his fellow pilots who wrote of him, a corner turns and he appears before us in an entirely different light, a dazzlingly bright one against the gray overcast pall of the war. Edward Mannock played the violin. He apparently played it very well from a technical point of view. But against, or perhaps in response to, the massive ongoing stress in flying combat to kill, in machines that could fall apart or catch fire, without the escape of a parachute, and with the continuous loss of good men on both sides above the even

3. See Chapter 16.

worse carnage that filled trenches below, Major Mannock played his violin. He played it, not as frivolous escape, but in a way that touched others. One of his fellow pilots records the following description:

> On Mick's ability as a violinist, MacLenachan said: "Watching Mick's expressive face as he successfully accomplished the difficult double-stopping passages in the *Caprice [Viennois]*,[4] I was amazed at the emotional splendour of his playing. Technique was required, but there was something greater than that, something no other violinist had ever conveyed to me. Mick had the soul of an idealist, one that can endure agonies of mind and body for his ideals, can kill for his beliefs. He told us all this in his playing. Perhaps my appreciation was heightened by my knowledge of his emotions—but I noticed that many of the others were equally spellbound by the tall gaunt figure standing in the half-light at the far corner of the mess. On my telling him of this he refused to play for several days and when we finally persuaded him to do so, he insisted on turning his face to the wall."
>
> (Mannock 1966, pp. 171–172)

This passage calls up the recognition algorithm, but in reverse. The violinist stands off in the corner of the mess hall at evening and after a meal. He draws others into the music by his playing, and the others notice the reactions within themselves. The music touches them, and, for the narrator of this brief passage, it is like no other violin performance he has heard. Major Mannock plays a musical composition that originated on the other side of the front lines, but no one seems to notice. The music itself lifts above the definition of enemy or friend, and at the same time is anchored to it. Idea and feeling coexist in the performance of the composition that seems to ask for peace on behalf of the warriors who must bear the combat. When the other pilots tell Edward Mannock of their reaction to his music and their admiration of it, he refuses to play it for several days. He gives no evidence of a Reaction Formation here: he is not in the center of the hall looking for adulation or applause, nor does not playing it before the others for a few days throw him into an emotional crisis. In the most touching detail of the passage, when he does play the *Caprice* again, he turns his face to the wall. The music he plays has a life of

4. Fritz Kreisler, one of the great violin virtuosos of all time, composed *Caprice Viennois, Opus # 2*, in 1911. Kreisler, an Austrian by birth, fought briefly for his country early in World War I. He was wounded in ground combat and cashiered out of the army. He and his wife migrated to the United States between the two wars, and they eventually became American citizens. While living in America, he converted to Catholicism and enjoyed a career playing concerts and teaching talented youngsters.

Caprice Viennois, a short work, strikes many ears as nostalgic, largely because of the twice repeating sections written in Viennese waltz tempo. It contains these and playful passages as well, but it also contains other brief passages that bring in darker, more suspenseful tones that contrast to a wistful surface. Like a well-written short poem, it contains much in little. For the sophisticated audiences of the day, in an era before recordings when music was more often played than bought, it was in some ways the equivalent of a pop tune of today. This may have been how Edward Mannock came across it and played it a few years later. Kreisler's own recording of it survives today and, at this writing, can be found on the Internet.

its own. It is a Sublimation: it does not depend directly on his personality for others to appreciate it. Yet they can sense the pain in it that he senses, as their own. The same man whose Suppression saved his life when his plane broke apart, and whose regression to Acting Out led him needlessly into dangerous situations and possibly to his death, here in his music reaches others for something like the human ideal, the opposite of the carnage and death—the disaster and doom—around them. If a Sublimation can be called heroic, Major Mannock gives us what that sounds like.

RIGHT HAND AND JOY: TURNING DOWN THE PRIMITIVE AND IMMATURE FOR THE MATURE DOMAIN

One needn't be in the throes of transcendent love or trapped in a war, even one to end all wars, to make use of Sublimation. In ordinary circumstances in the lives of humans, the contrast between the goodness of love and the pain of loss provides one of the most frequent and often one of the most difficult stresses to which all of us must adapt. For us, and all those around us, even love is "time-limited," to use the phrase from modern advertising. Consider this poem from the early 17th century:

On My First Sonne

Farewell, thou child of my right hand, and joy;
My sinne was too much hope of thee, lov'd boy.
Seven yeers tho' wert lent to me, and I thee pay,
Exacted by thy fate, on the just day.
O, could I lose all father now. For why
Will man lament the state he should envie?
To have so soone scap'd worlds and fleshs rage,
And, if no other misery, yet age?
Rest in soft peace, and, ask'd, say here doth lye
Ben. Jonson his best piece of *poetrie*.
For whose sake, hence-forth, all his vowes be such
As what he loves may never like too much.

(Jonson, 1968, p. 20)

Ben Jonson, one of the great poets of the English Renascence era, leaves us in no doubt as to the stress he suffers. It makes up the subject of his poem: the childhood death of his eldest son to whom he gave his own first name, Benjamin. The name can be translated from Hebrew as "one of the right," as in those who sit at the right hand of God on the Day of Judgment in the Judeo-Christian metaphor. This is the compliment he pays to his son in the first line. In the third line he pays his son back to God in the painful description of only having been lent the joy of being the boy's father and that for only a brief period of time. Resulting from this, he suffers that special kind of anxiety that we refer to as grief—a specific sense of doom or disaster at the loss of someone we love. Our purpose, then, is to ask how he adapts to this painful circumstance.

To do this, we apply the recognition algorithm, first asking whether he consciously perceives the existence of the stress and its anxiety. The clarity of his description provides more than enough evidence to say that he does. At the same time, there is no evidence of any Primitive Domain adaptation at work: were he to deny the death of his child, there would be no poem; were he to avoid the stress by distorting it, the poem might assert, in a very literal sense, his son's continuing to live; were he to project it, his son's death might be the work of the Devil as a very literal phenomenon walking about the earth—a physical being of some kind. But none of these or any other expressions of Primitive Domain adaptive styles appear in the poem.

The algorithm asks, does he regard the grief at the death of his son as someone else's problem? That is, does he locate it outside of his conscious self, whether, for example, projecting it into his own body in the form of some unexplained physical illness, or onto someone else as intending him harm delivered through his son's death? Again, none of these or the other Immature Domain adaptive styles appear in the poem. Speaking in the first person, the poet makes it clear that both the pain involved and the grief belong to him as he struggles to find their resolution.

The next step in the hierarchy of recognizing adaptation levels requires first that we describe both the cognitive and emotional contents of the stress. In this example, the poet describes them for us directly: to paraphrase, they include, "My son has died," and "I suffer a sadness that seems incurable." In the Neurotic Domain adaptive styles, in which idea and feeling disjoin, we may ask whether either the emotional content or the thought content have gone missing, suggesting either Intellectualization or Repression, respectively, as the operating adaptive mechanism. Neither has occurred: the poet does not bathe the reader in feeling at the expense of thought, nor does he provide a coldly calculated analysis of the nature of death in childhood. Interestingly, Jonson makes a running attempt at a Reaction Formation when he asks why we lament death when in fact we should welcome it as an escape from the troubles of the world including, if nothing else, old age. In doing so he tries to define good—life—as bad, and bad—death—as good. But in phrasing it as a question, rather than as a statement of fact, he tells us that he himself does not believe it. He follows it with the phrase, "Rest in soft peace," as if to say that somehow a harsh death can be mitigated for his son sake. Though he toys with a Neurotic Domain adaptive strategy, he makes clear that he does not accept it precisely because he has found an integration of thought and feeling, rather than separate, mutually exclusive roles for each.

Ben Jonson's adaptation to his son's death takes us into the Mature Domain psychological adaptive mechanisms. The feeling—a terrible sadness—and the idea—the precipitous death of one's young child—work together to make up both the form and the content of his poem. The verses themselves make up his adaptation. He says farewell to his "best piece of poetry," that is, to the son he has made biologically as he might make a poem in writing, and Jonson again compliments his son, this time in relation to all of the poetry that he has ever written. In the last two lines of the poem, he plays on the difference between the words "love" and "like" in another halfhearted attempt at a Reaction Formation in which some attempt at not liking his children will somehow limit his feelings for them in a way that can prevent the grief of their leaving. But the reader knows, as Jonson himself knows, that this will not work: he will love and like his children, and in so doing accepts both the sadness and the knowledge that they and he will change.

Most readers of this poem will come away with the direct experience of the sadness of the words as well as direct knowledge of the cognitive content of the stress in the child's death. We do not need Ben Jonson present before us to perceive these and be touched by them. The compassion of his experience is at hand solely because the poem exists and we are able to read it. This describes the nature of Sublimation as a Mature Domain psychological adaptive mechanism. The adaptation includes, and at its best approaches, the highest forms of art by establishing a creative work capable of communicating both idea and feeling in a way that draws in the reader/observer and does not require the author's/artist's presence. We perceive these works as touching us in some way, namely allowing us to perceive both idea and feeling in a way that resonates with our own adaptations as we face the chances and events and emotions of living. One of the unique aspects of this poem in particular lies in Jonson's ability to contrast the different ways of ways of adapting to terrible pain. His examples range from the Primitive Domain—as in his wish to be relieved of any sense of fatherhood when he says, "could I leave all father now"—through the two Reaction Formation attempts we have mentioned. He then discards all of them in favor of simply putting in verses his painful ideas and emotions as the most simple, yet the most creative and compassionate, adaptive style accessible to him. Unlike the Neurotic styles that choke off any possibility of sharing the feelings of others, the Mature Domain adaptive mechanisms enhance it, and, of these, Sublimation turns it into the highest forms of human art.

ONE DAY AT A TIME: SUBLIMATION TOWARD RECOVERY

If Dante Alighieri brings us into the light of love, if Edward Mannock's violin touched his comrades with the pathos of human suffering, if Ben Jonson rends our hearts with the loss that rent his, Kenneth Fields extends the reach of Sublimation to include the horrible and the noble in human growth and change. Considering only a portion of his poetic work beginning with the poems in *The Odysseus Manuscripts* and continuing through those in *Classic Rough News*,[5] he presents his readers with a struggle. He uses that remarkable characteristic of verse lines that allows the poet to create a work that conveys emotion and ideas simultaneously. In Fields' work one often finds emotion as the key that opens sequentially deeper levels of thought as the reader settles into the poem with repeated readings over time. Rather than considering the thread of struggle that runs through most of his poems in these two collections—a task far too large for our training manual on adaptive mechanism recognition—we can maintain focus by considering one poem that lives at the center of the struggle. Its subject involves a man named Billy, one of the characters in *Classic Rough News*. It uses the French term *La Pucelle*, which in its lowercase form means

5. Fields (1981, 2005).

"the maid" or "the virgin" and in the capitalized form used here refers to Joan of Arc, who was known as the Maid of Orleans. It also mentions Teresa of Ávila, whom we have met before in this volume. In the eighth line, the narrator mentions "the lash of inwit," that, for ease of reading, we can paraphrase in its medieval meaning as the lash of remorse.

The Interior Castle

Alone, he heard voices, which was not surprising.
Religion did funny things. Did Billy suppose
That La Pucelle and Teresa and those other ladies
Had done it without booze? He did not suppose.
To each his own, his protestant, mystic rule.
And yet he felt hidden from his hidden god,
But did his bidding, loved his narrow cell,
Suffered the lash of inwit, yes, and fasted
To be a worthier vessel for the spirit's light.
In time the voices grew, he came to feel
Somewhat reluctantly, into his own:
"This is my blood, the spirit that hates the world,
Take it, and drink." He prayed in his unbelief,
Then took his humiliation like the cure.

(Fields 2005, p. 16)

On first reading, this poem appears to be about religion: it mentions two saints, refers to the idea of god, and, toward the end, borrows words from the Consecration in the Roman Catholic Mass. But there is also one word that doesn't belong to religion, namely "booze" in line 4. As the reader meditates on that word, the poem transforms into one about drinking: puns on "spirit," for example, include the life within, the life of grace in the Christian metaphor, and alcohol itself as when we referred to distilled spirits. But this is not simply a celebration of drinking. Rather, it is a close description of the kind of drinking that has become Billy's religion. It isolates him, monk-like, in his cell; it takes on the characteristics of a god hidden from sight, a god who deals in remorse and begins to speak to Billy as though in a voice. In lines 12 and 13, the voice speaks but it says the opposite of religion: in its root sense the word *religion* means linking back to others, whereas this god's voice says to sever relations with the world.

But the poem is neither simply about religion nor about drinking. Other words in the poem do not fit either of these themes. A person lives here who begins to recognize the voice of this god as his own voice, who tries to hide from it, in the style of Avoidance from Chapter 5, and finally succumbs to it with the reward only of personal humiliation, having lost control of it once again. The term "humiliation" in the theological sense means that the god is in control and in this instance it means "Once the drinking starts, there is no stopping it." At the same time, however, this charming god creates a sense of simplicity in Billy's narrow cell, as though his god is all he needs. But even Billy himself does not believe this although it is so important to him that he fasts—he gives up food—in order to drink. Recalling Jane Eyre's quote from the Bible mentioned in Chapter 16, there is no god here whose peace passes all understanding. Rather, the idea content that ties this poem together entails the ambivalent, and intense, relationship between Billy and his god. That is between Billy and his booze.

Even this relationship, however, is not static. We have already noted that Billy's Avoidance doesn't serve him. Instead, he is at the point of recognizing that, rather than some external god controlling his fate as in a Neurotic Projection in the present model, the voice of god is only his own voice. In the strategies of psychological adaptation, Billy in this poem starts to move from the Immature Domain into a higher realm as he begins to locate the ambivalence toward his god within himself.

This is all well and good, but what does it have to do with Sublimation? To read the poems in *Classic Rough News* leads us to the knowledge that Kenneth Fields has made public about his own recovery from alcoholism, in scientific language his recovery from alcohol dependence. As a number of researchers, including the present one, have noted in the scientific literature, the same ambivalence makes up the central phenomenon in alcohol dependence. Kenneth Fields himself once commented, "You know it's not good for you. But you don't want to quit."[6] Realizing that he could no longer drink in a predictably controlled fashion—the behavioral result at the center of any substance dependence—constituted his own classic rough news. This, in the model of psychological adaptation mechanisms, makes up the stress with which this poet had to deal himself. Its consequences, viewed as the doom of drinking and the doom of not drinking—creating an ambivalence between them—make up the anxiety component generated from the stress itself. Perhaps in common with other human conditions that involve loss of control of a behavior or of a physical function, the addictive disorders generate anxiety from both aspects simultaneously.

In the face of this, whether Kenneth Fields, like Billy, had to work through the Primitive Domain and then the Immature Domain adaptive mechanisms in order to reach the Mature Domain strategies goes beyond the evidence at hand. The discerning reader, however, will note that the same progression from Primitive through Mature occurs in The Twelve Steps of Alcoholics Anonymous (AA), and published scientific research has established the efficacy of this form of treatment.[7] Be that as it may, the example of Billy above shows us both the horror of alcohol dependence in its loneliness and its loss of self-respect, along with the nobility of the human spirit even in the face of such a two-headed monster. *That* spirit—the true, rather than the false, god in the poem—begins to adapt and to grow. We can sense Billy's pain in drinking, his need to drink, and most importantly the ambivalence that ties them together. As he begins to recognize these, he begins to take on a life of his own, and so does the poem he inhabits. We have both its cognitive content and its emotional

6. Personal communication.
7. Project Match: see Kadden (1996).

ambivalence before us, with the scale beginning to tip towards an affirmation of the world. Kenneth Fields gives us the poem, asking only understanding. And for our purposes, we can locate it as a Sublimation in the most Mature Domain adaptive strategies.

SLEEPY INTERN, OOP-BOP-SH'BAM! WORK SUBLIMATED AS A FORM OF PLAY

The medical chief resident arrives at his office one morning and finds this note on his desk:

> I write this in between medical crises while listening to some Dizzy Gillespie tunes through my earbuds. I feel like calling you Clyde. Would you mind if I called you Clyde? It's so much less common than your real name. And you don't meet too many Clydes these days. Not since Diz and the Bop meisters of the 40s and 50s. Besides, Clyde, I don't know if I'm really between medical crises or not. There've been a few so far, like the woman who reminds me of my grandmother, but with heart failure. Then there was the guy in his early 30s going into DTs, and at such a young age. He must be some kind of genius. Somehow I wanted to call him Mozart but decided against it. And to round things out in the key of Geewhiz, how about that hefty woman my mother's age who brought in her roaring infected gallbladder headed toward a riff on her whole body with a high C fever and everything. She impressed the medical students, those Sears and Roebuck drummers, and scared the hell out of me. But the sweet antibiotics are returning her to her natural state of cool. And they're helping me a whole lot with mine too. In fact I may have more of the Cool than I ever had before. Now I can harmonize with heart failure, shake hands with the DTs—Köchel way up there somewhere, Clyde, as Mozart goes, umlaut and all—and play Prince Valiant to the fat, forty, fertile, and febrile females[8] of America. Ain't it a gas? Or would that be a riff on the flatulent? I used to play the flatulent but gave it up in junior high. True, we'll hand the biliary chick off to the surgeons when she quiets down. All part of the Cool. And I can't say I haven't had my moments, here comes one now—an up-tempo businessman with the wrong triglyceride Clyde and chest pain, another chart from the cats in the ER. Those guys know a chord change when they hear one. I won't call it stage fright, but I'm on in a few minutes and intermission's about over. Besides, you've got to have a little tension in the tune unless you're into soporifics. And I never have been. I dig the fun. And that's what I learn from you and the rest of the band. Catch you later Clyde.

The chief resident writes in the margin of the note, "This intern is chief resident material in another couple years, in the highest possible terms and without reservation whatsoever.—Clyde." He makes a copy to pass on to the department

8. The four Fs of gallbladder disease, plus febrile.

chairman and takes the original home. We leave the well-practiced reader at this point to apply the recognition algorithm to assess sequentially for stress, anxiety, and the Domain of response, leading to the assignment of the appropriate psychological adaptive mechanism in the case of the intern's note. The title of this chapter offers a hint.

REFERENCES

Alighieri, D. (1992). *Vita Nuova*. New York, Oxford University Press.

Fields, K. (1981). *The Odysseus Manuscripts*, Chicago, Elpenor Books.

Fields, K. (2005). *Classic Rough News*. Chicago, University of Chicago Press.

Jonson, B. (1968). *The Complete Poetry of Ben Jonson*. New York, W. W. Norton.

Kadden, R. M. (1996). "Project MATCH: treatment main effects and matching results." *Alcohol Clin Exp Res 20*(8 Suppl): 196A–197A.

Mannock, M. E. (1966). *The Personal Diary of Major Edward Mannock*. London, Neville Spearman.

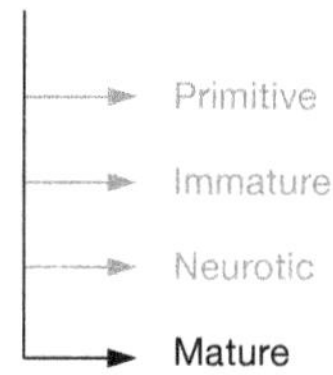

CHAPTER 21

Humor

Humor allows us to bear the unbearable.[1] With it, humans can put into words their most painful thoughts and feelings and do so in a way that draws others to us rather than alienating them. It involves jokes, and the jokes may include others, but not at their expense or demeaning them by way of Displacement as discussed in Chapter 15. This is because in Humor the jokes always include ourselves: in the grammatical sense, the person serves as both the subject and the object of his or her own joke. And as it does not demean others, neither does Humor demean oneself. Self-deprecation does not occur in it, as it may in Passive Aggression, the Immature Domain strategy discussed in Chapter 8. In Humor as an adaptation strategy, we live in the Mature Domain of the psychological adaptive mechanisms. Both in the teller and the tale, we find a sense of freedom in the stories that make us and others laugh. Humor takes us beyond the bounds of our pain—great or small—and out of the range of our preconceptions, whether plainly stated or metaphorical.

Consider Shakespeare's character Jaques,[2] a self-serious courtier bent on finding meaning in external existence. He returns from a walk in the forest, where he has encountered a court Fool. He mentions the experience to his superior, the Duke:

Jaques: When I did hear
The motley fool thus moral on the time,
My lungs began to crow like chanticleer,
That fools should be so deep-contemplative,
And I did laugh sans intermission
An hour by his dial. O noble fool!
A worthy fool! Motley's the only wear.
Duke S: What fool is this?
Jaques: O worthy fool! One that hath been a courtier,
And says, if ladies be but young and fair,
They have the gift to know it; and in his brain,—

1. —even writing books. See also Vaillant (1977, p. 386) on bearing the unbearable.
2. Pronounced JAY-kweez.

Which is as dry as the remainder biscuit
After a voyage,—he hath strange places cramm'd
With observations, the which he vents
In mangled forms. O that I were a fool!
I am ambitious for a motley coat.

Duke S: Thou shalt have one.

Jaques: It is my only suit;
Provided that you weed your better judgments
Of all opinion that grows rank in them
That I am wise. I must have liberty
Withal, as large a charter as the wind....

(Shakespeare, *As You Like It*, Act II, Scene 7)

Poor Jaques. For a brief moment he glimpses paradise and the freedom from his existential[3] shackles. He finds the Fool, wearing "motley"—the coxcomb hat with bells on it and the multicolored doublet and tights. Like professional Fools today—think of standup comedians, for example—this one "morals on the times," that is, he makes jokes on customs, current events, and perhaps on time itself. Jaques wants to imitate the Fool, wear a motley suit, and live in liberty from all that he once thought wise. But he takes the world around him only seriously, looking for meaning in it rather than in himself. He finds no relief from the torments of life, death, and sorrow. As the play ends, he just hasn't the Humor[4] to give them up and retires instead to a monastery, where he will become a monk. Compare this to a later declaration of independence.

LIBERTY BELL: HUMOR IN THE FACE OF PERSONAL RISK

In the summer of 1776, a group of British colonists gathered together in Philadelphia and formally published a document that announced their break with England and their intention to form a new government, one that later became the United States of America. The Battle of Lexington and Concord had occurred in Massachusetts, far to the north, a little over a year before. The English king and Parliament had sent increasing numbers of armed troops to put down the rebellion. The representatives of the 13 colonies, however, had decided to take a stand. They discussed, argued about, and finally wrote the Declaration of Independence. All of them then signed the document, going on record publicly that each individual stood now formally as leaders of the insurrection against the British. Under British law, this was treason. And treason was a capital offense: each of the signers could be hunted down, tried, and put to death.

With over 200 years of hindsight, signing the Declaration of Independence appears of more political or philosophical interest than it does a personal threat to the men who wrote their names on it. But for those of the time, it included the very

3. To use a term from a much later period.
4. Yes, this phrase contains an Elizabethan pun.

specific dimension of personal risk. The oldest of them, Benjamin Franklin of Philadelphia, commented on this to his colleagues in a statement that others attribute to him. "We must all hang together," he said, "or most assuredly we will all hang separately." His punning use of the word *hang* remains with us still.

To apply the recognition algorithm, the stress lay in the threat of death—taking one's own life into one's hands, literally, in picking up a pen and signing a treasonous document. Personal anxiety too came with it: execution is personal disaster. The algorithm asks us then to sort which Domains might apply in this instance of a group of colonials signing what might be melodramatically described as their death warrant. With regard to the Primitive Domain mechanisms, we may safely conclude that all who signed it did not avoid signing it. Nor do we have reports of persons saying that there was no document to sign or that their signature had been put there by persons in league with the Devil. Similarly, considering the Immature Domain mechanisms, none of the leaders of the American rebellion claimed that it was someone else's fault that they had signed the Declaration. If any of them retreated into a fantasy world or suddenly came down with a series of unexplained illnesses, this has not been widely reported. Neither the Primitive nor the Immature Domain responses appear to be at work.

The algorithm next asks whether the emotion, and the cognition, of this act remain separate or whether the two are well integrated in a common effort to tolerate the risk of death. The feeling content may be described as fear and the idea content by the notion of each one risking his life. As to the other signers of the Declaration of Independence, we must depend on historical scholarship to enlighten us as to the specific facts of their responses as individuals. In considering Ben Franklin's adaptation, however, we can focus on the response he gave others, and those of us who come after, in his famous joke.

This returns us to his use of the word *hang*. *Hang together* is an idiom for individuals remaining connected and working toward the same outcome. In this case, were the British to have split the rebellious colonies from one another, new governments loyal to the king would have continued colonial rule. In that case, the treasonous signers would hang separately, which is to say be executed. Both idea and feeling, therefore, manifest themselves in the joke. More elegantly, however, Franklin makes fun of himself as well as his colleagues. All of them have taken a risk and must be able to tolerate the anxiety that results from it. Ben Franklin creates a joke in which they can all participate. In this regard, he uses true Humor, the Mature Domain adaptive mechanism that includes the subject—the one who is making the joke—as the object of the joke. By comparison, laughing at others at their expense while not laughing at ourselves—that is, the Displacement of witty putdowns, as discussed in Chapter 15—exemplify the Neurotic Domain adaptive style of aiming painful thoughts and feelings at others when we have yet to resolve them ourselves. But in his Mature Domain Humor Franklin laughs himself, and invites others to do so as well.

As most U.S. schoolchildren know, the colonists did indeed hang together and instituted the republic in which Americans now live. Five years after the meeting in Philadelphia, they defeated the British at the Battle of Yorktown and made good on the vision of a nation governed by its citizens. Their risk included balancing personal disaster against their personal—and public—gain insofar as setting up a nation dedicated to liberty. But not all such choices necessarily involve personal gain and in these, perhaps, as in no others, Humor might serve us as rescue when no other is at hand.

THE LAST DANCE: HUMOR WHEN THERE IS NO WAY OUT

In Chapter 15 we met the Spartans blocking the pass at Thermopylae, stopping the huge Persian army against overwhelming odds. We saw them just before the battle, preening themselves, much to the perplexity of the Persians, and exercising as though warming up for an athletic contest. Their chronicler, Herodotus, provides a further description of one of their number that reads as freshly now as it did 2500 years ago, when he first set it down in writing.

> Of all the Spartans and Thespians who fought so valiantly the most signal proof of courage was given by the Spartan Dieneces. It is said that before the battle he was told by a native of Trachis that, when the Persians shot their arrows, there were so many of them that they hid the sun. Dieneces, however, quite unmoved by the thought of the strength of the Persian army, merely remarked, "This is pleasant news that the stranger from Trachis brings us: if the Persians hide the sun, we shall have our battle in the shade." He is said to have left on record other sayings, too, of a similar kind, by which he will be remembered.
>
> (Herodotus 1954, p. 519)

As discussed in detail earlier, the stress of the situation emanates from the looming battle, its mortal combat, and the pressing likelihood of death. The anxiety is that of the warriors looking into their doom at the hands of an overwhelming Persian force. Taking the recognition process a step further, however, asks how this particular Spartan adapts to the stress and its coming doom. Another of the Greek fighters, from another town, tells Dieneces that the odds against them are so long and the Persians so many that their arrows hide the sun. That is, he tells a tall tale full of the fear and dread of the Greeks' situation, and we use the recognition algorithm to focus on Dieneces' response to it.

In the first place, does he give any evidence of ignoring the man from Trachis, or avoiding him, or trying to shut up his frightened speech? No description of that occurs in the narrative, revealing evidence that Dieneces responds with a Primitive Domain adaptive strategy: he does not ignore the situation. At the same time, he does not demonize the stranger from Trachis and blame the messenger for his message. That is, Dieneces does not locate his own response to the stress in anyone else, but regards it as his own responsibility. He does not invoke any of the Immature Domain adaptive strategies.

In respect to the next level of the Neurotic Domain adaptive mechanisms, Dieneces shares the same emotional and cognitive contents of the stress that we noticed in his comrades in Chapter 15. The painful feeling is fear of imminent death or disaster, and the painful cognition is something like, "This may be my last day."

Herodotus gives us no evidence that these two components of the adaptive response exist independently, or separately, from each other. Dieneces does not respond with either an emotional outbreak or with an intellectualized description of the relative odds of one of the other parties surviving the battle. One might reasonably ask whether he has not defined good as bad and bad as good, as might occur in a Reaction Formation, in describing the Persians arrows as pleasant news. Looking closer, however, Dieneces does not describe the falling arrows as good news but rather the shade they cast. There is no doubt that, if not by their arrows, then by some other means, the Persians bring certain death.

In response, Dieneces weaves the frightening ideas and feelings into his own tall tale aimed at creating his own psychological shade, or as we would say, his adaptation. He tells a joke and puts himself in it as the source, and the target, of his own humor. The joke is on him, he says in effect. If he looks forward to the many thousands of the Persian arrows that blot out the sun, he will regard it as a pleasant shade. As both the subject—the teller of the joke—and its object or target, he very deftly uses true Humor, often the most subtle of the Mature Domain adaptive mechanisms. Dieneces' joke is both moving and funny at the same time. It could as easily bring tears as laughter, its feelings and thoughts are so well intertwined. We read it 2500 years later and still find it both funny in its intentional exaggeration of the facts and touching in its universal reference to the sad ending of life. Herodotus pays Dieneces' words their ultimate compliment when he says that the Spartan warrior left other sayings of a similar kind by which he would be remembered. That is, Dieneces' Humor connected him with the others of his time, and they with him, in facing the long odds and short span of human life. Had we a time machine, which of us would not like to use it to converse with Dieneces, to talk with him about his Humor and hear more of his tall tales about how to bear the unbearable? But one need not be an ancient Greek warrior on a hot day with the Persian army advancing to engage Humor for the purpose of bearing the difficult moments in life. The lives of the rest of us, that Henry David Thoreau said were lived in "quiet desperation," often find their moments amenable to Humor, as in the next case of a common circumstance.

THE COMMITTEE MEETING: HUMOR IN LIVES OF QUIET DESPERATION

Practical research has defined the leadership characteristics of businesses that work well and those that work superbly well—far above the merely successful.[5] The typical leader of a great business enterprise possesses a characteristic humility that, in the present adaptive model, we have noted before. It lies in the difference between Neurotic Domain pseudo-altruism and true Altruism, the Mature Domain adaptive strategy. The former requires a great show of heroic acts in the service of assuring the actor that he or she is worthwhile, loved, or both. The energies of interacting with others are all directed toward this, and it often precludes trust: how is it possible to trust others if one cannot trust oneself? The latter, by contrast, does not serve

5. See Collins (2001).

either personal narcissistic gratification or personal love needs. It includes trust and therefore delegation of tasks to others. Its heroism is a quiet phenomenon in which the leader derives the most gratification when those for whom he or she is responsible work successfully. It builds an atmosphere of work relationships that fosters the growth of the individuals who work there. The successful leader's role involves articulating a vision and setting goals, delegating responsibility to others and then stepping back to allow them to do their work. It builds, rather than destroys, work and professional relationships. In this context, consider the following vignette.

> A group of accountants in a branch office of a large accounting firm sit in an early afternoon meeting in which they are to review a report for their manager. The report comes from the regional office of their company and it reviews the frequencies of accounting errors throughout the system. The manager requires the review committee to provide him with a brief set of minutes that record as little discussion as possible with no questions or feedback. The manager has a track record of replacing those who report to him every two years, and just such a purge took place about a month prior to meeting. Over the previous two years, about one-third of the employees have found work elsewhere. Unbeknownst to those meeting around the table, the manager himself has now been set on probation by the regional office because of what they see as his inept handling of personnel that has cost them a share of their profit margin.
>
> In the discussion, one of the accountants comments that despite the manager's not wanting any feedback, it may be useful to review the report in the context of improving their operation if possible. Recalling that the manager runs their section "out of his hip pocket" and cannot delegate with any consistency, he jokes that the only way anyone knows that they're doing a bad job is when the manager punches holes in their tires or dents their car doors. Another of the accountants, one of several recently purged by the manager, smiles and irreverently says, "That's what that was!" The first accountant smiles, laughs, and then to the surprise of himself and those around him, breaks out into tears. "That's okay," his colleague says, "I've got another offer. It's a good offer, and I'll be all right."

Inept management, like a slow viral infection, may not be immediately obvious, and especially so to those new to an organization. The result is often the creation of an atmosphere of presumed trust in which, due to the psychological limitations of the person in the leadership position, no trust is possible. Escape from the pathological situation is the only remedy for those who can recognize and respond to it, most often the best and most capable of those who work there. The everyday stress, invoking the adaptive model, is an oppressive, continuing one of working in an environment that neither trusts nor rewards its workers. The anxiety follows in the predictable "doom" of continuing devaluation and demotion.

In this example from mid-level management in the day-to-day marketplace, one of the accountants cracks a joke with the implication that the manager has slashed *his* tires and dented *his* car but that he himself has been too obtuse to ascribe its cause. His colleague first laughs at the joke and then find himself overwhelmed with sadness. By finding a way to laugh at the pathological work atmosphere that their manager has created, they find a way to tolerate the intolerable. And for at least one of them, the laughter makes crying possible. It connects them as human beings in a way in which they find a collegial solace. And Humor may serve to give perspective to the options available to each as they go about their lives. In one option, the accountant who makes the joke at his own expense, using Mature Domain Humor by our definition, moves on to another, better run firm. In another option, let us suppose that the other comes to work at his same firm until he retires, preferring the local town and the community he lives in to all others. In his choice, he finds that that moment of levity helps him tolerate his work. Both find their ways to adapt in a pathological situation of poor leadership.

NATURE'S MIRROR, MY MIRROR: HUMOR AND WHAT I REALLY LOOK LIKE

Sometimes, however, there is no escape from an ongoing stress as there was for one of the accountants. One such stress is simply the passage of time, and the concomitant changes through which we all must proceed over the course of life. Who, for example, would not avoid the worse parts of old age if he or she had the chance to do so and still breathe? We do not have that option and must in some way come to terms with the course of aging. Ben Jonson, the Elizabethan/Jacobean poet and playwright we met in Chapter 20, finds himself face-to-face with this difficulty when he falls in love in a special circumstance: a visit to Scotland. He writes a poem in which he describes the impression he has made on a young woman there.

My Picture Left in Scotland

I Now thinke Love is rather deaf, than blind,
For else it could not be
That she
Whom I adore so much should so slight me,
And cast my love behind:
I'm sure my language to her, was as sweet,
And every close did meet
In sentence, as of subtile feet
As hath the youngest Hee,
That sits in shadow of *Apollo's* tree.
Oh, but my conscious feares
That flie my thoughts betweene,
Tell me that she hath seene
My hundreds of gray haires,
Told seven and fortie years,
Read so much waist, as she cannot imbrace
My mountain belly, and my rockie face,
And all these through her eyes, have stopt her ears.

(Jonson 1968, p. 136)

How may the observer characterize the stress: the tension that Jonson puts in this poem? To begin with, his use of the word "My" in the title tells us that he speaks in his own voice, not through a narrator or a third person. Then he concludes the poem in the first line, when he reverses the old cliché that love is blind, saying that he has found it deaf instead. In the rest of the first stanza, he notes that the lady in question has rejected him despite the elegance of his speech and writing. He deliberately exaggerates his own praise by describing his use of words as sweet, tightly structured, yet subtly rhythmical, and, ultimately, god-like. The reference in the last line of the first stanza recalls the legend of the nymph Daphne, who turns into a laurel tree rather than accept Apollo's sexual advances. Apollo is himself the god of poetry in the Greek pantheon, but here he can only sit in the shade of the wooden Daphne: even the immortals, who are never old, may find themselves rejected by a beautiful woman. "And I write just as well if not better than he does," Jonson claims. "Why should his beautiful language fall on wooden ears? There must be something else at work."

In the second stanza, Jonson gives his readers the picture of himself that is in the mind of the woman he met in Scotland. It is full of waste—in the sense of decrepitude, as well as a pun on his own waist: gray hairs, approaching 50—an old age in that era, followed by that marvelous line "my mountain belly, and my rocky face." She cannot embrace him literally—his girth is too large for her to reach around—nor in the figurative sense of apprehending and valuing the poetry he writes for her.

Recalling the recognition algorithm, Jonson defines the stress as an outright rejection that is based on what he looks like rather than the beauty he can bring to life through his words, an art he has worked at for most of those "seven and fortie years." We know that this spurs a sense of anxiety when we hear of his "conscious fears" that at this point in the algorithm we can hear as a sense of the doom from the rejection. As we address the next step toward adaptive mechanism recognition, Jonson gives us no evidence of his ignoring the lady's rejection. He makes it the subject of his poem, rather than avoid it or claim that it doesn't exist. The Primitive Domain does not apply in the situation. Nor does the Immature Domain: he does not call the woman stupid and tasteless, meaning that the rejection is all her fault. Nor does he retreat into a fantasy or into impulsive action. To the contrary, he locates the difficulty in his own appearance from her point of view.

With this location established, the algorithm asks us to define both the emotional and cognitive meanings conjured up by the stress of the rejection and the sense of doom it entails. In another of those descriptions that seems to have been written for exactly this exercise, like the example from Dante in Chapter 20, Jonson states both feeling and idea plainly: "Oh, but my conscious fears / that fly my thoughts between," he writes. The painful feeling entails a fear of being ignored or avoided, of being thought ugly or unpleasant, of being regarded as a "nonperson" in present-day language. The painful thought might be expressed as "I am being shut out and my love ignored." Very perceptibly, Jonson tells us that this fear is running among his thoughts—that is, that the two of them work together. He does not describe the Neurotic Domain separation of feeling and idea: there is neither emotion present disconnected from his thoughts nor thoughts present disconnected from his feelings.

He does not Displace them on to someone else, Dissociate from them for some brief time, or turn them into a Reaction Formation in which he stalks or pursues her in some unwanted fashion until she finally recognizes his presence.

Instead, the author of *Every Man in His Humor*, one of Johnson's popular verse plays of the time, makes the whole episode into a tender joke. To create a modern pseudo-medical term, he takes credit for having discovered Jonson's Syndrome: a condition whereby the experience of visual unpleasantness renders hearing impossible. But his joke reaches far more subtle depths than that. For one, he includes a sense of compassion with the woman who looks at him and finds him repulsive: he can see himself from her point of view. For another, he tells the joke and yet remains the object of its laughter when he overpraises his own literary prowess and then inventories his physical shortcomings as relatively incidental. He comes to the natural conclusion that the poor woman is clearly deaf to his affection but certainly not blind to his appearance, leading to his conclusion that the two are clearly connected. Her sight of him has stopped her hearing. Worse yet, even Love itself personified—think of Cupid or of Dante's love god from Chapter 20—has gone deaf and refuses to present Jonson's case to the object of his affection.

And, read in another way, we may find one more subtle joke in the poem: if the phenomenon of love is deaf, rather than blind, we may reasonably expect a deaf lover to appear in the verses. But the woman clearly does not love Jonson, as he tells us. Who is the deaf lover? The only alternative is Jonson himself: full of love and not blind to its rejection but, rather, completely deaf to the idea that his love is worthless. In this, perhaps, occur his greatest pathos and his greatest Humor in this poem.

So it is that Humor, perhaps the crowning psychological adaptive mechanism of the Mature Domain group, allows us to tolerate the rejections we find when others judge us as covers rather than as books. Humor alleviates the terrors of feeling and thinking of ourselves as unloved or as undervalued, as in the next example, the last tale of our stalwart, if fictional and shape-shifting, intern.

INTERN, ZERO-ZERO-LOVE: HUMOR IN THE COMPETITIVE ENVIRONMENT

It has been a busy and not particularly restful night in the hospital, and our intern has managed only about 30 minutes of sleep, a catnap between admissions. Seven A.M. has arrived, and it is time for morning report on the medicine service: a review of the night's admissions and crises presented case by case to the chief resident and a senior attending physician, who on this day happens to be the department chairman. "Oh great!" the intern thinks to herself while pouring a cup of coffee in the conference room. "Welcome to the One-Upmanship Derby, ladies and gentlemen. It's a fast track with no rain in sight. Mudders need not apply."

It is a large, busy city hospital, and three teams have been admitting patients during the night. They present in order of the first three consecutive admissions, and our intern is up third: "Batting cleanup," as she says to herself. The chief resident signals to begin, and a senior resident from the first team stands and says, "I am very pleased to report to you that last evening we admitted a 35-year-old man with a high fever. Through diligent diagnostic detective work, we established beyond doubt that his is the first reported case of Tsutsugamushi Fever in our city seen in the last 50 years. It was my honor to assist our team in this effort by recognizing the characteristic black eschars that indicate the disease. Confirmation came from a microscopic identification of this form of typhus. May I have the first slide please? . . ."

"Well done," the chief resident says as the resident concludes the presentation. "Excellent pursuit of a diagnosis that is rare in this geographical area." The department chairman nods in agreement. The intern, sitting off to the side of the room, looks out the window and rolls her eyes to the ceiling and back.

A second senior resident, from the second team, stands and reports. "Doctors, it is not my intent to puff up the expertise or diagnostic prowess of my own admitting team at the expense of my learned colleagues who have presented a most fascinating case. I hope they will not take offense when I report that, as it happens, when admitting a 50-year-old female, we identified a lesion in the brain owing to a remarkably subtle clinical presentation. It could be appreciated only when one considers, as we did, the possibility of transient ischemia in the tortuous artery of Bernasconi and Cassinari that signaled the presence of a meningioma of the tentorium. Because we diagnosed this in its early stages, the neurosurgeons have stated their confidence in using microsurgical techniques to excise the meningioma easily and remove any concern for this patient's health subsequently. Because of this unusual presentation, a search of our hospital's records notes that this is the first such case ever diagnosed within these walls, and a further literature search through the national Library of Medicine database suggests that it is only the fifth such case reported in the history of American medicine."

"Excellently done," the chief resident replies. "Please enlighten us further on the subtleties of the neurological presentation in this case," and he nods to the department chairman, whose eyes have grown wide with wonder as he listens to the history. "Well, golly gee," the intern thinks to herself. "Maybe if we all moved close together, over against one of the walls, we could get a brass band in here."

A few minutes later, the chief resident turns to the intern and says, "Your turn, Doctor." With as much pomp as she can manage, the intern strides to the front of the room, exuding confidence from every pore. She nods to the department chairman, and then to the chief resident, and then addresses the audience. "I realize that you have just heard two cases that presented subtly and, due to the diligence of my colleagues, resulted in the rare and diagnostically gratifying establishment of two illnesses not often seen in these parts. Following suit, I am pleased to report to you that our team as well has set a very high bar in order to maximize the effects of our expertise as diagnosticians and therapeutic interventionists. More specifically, we have made it a policy to admit no one to our service who has not been to a nursing home first."

The department chairman at first smiles and then begins laughing heartily. The chief resident allows himself to do the same, and soon the whole gathering is caught up in the joke. As the laughter eases, the intern goes about presenting the cases of three other patients with common illnesses of whom she has taken good care through the night.

People generally like to feel good about themselves and to find validation of their goodness in the applause of others. Our intern is no exception. But here at morning medical rounds, she finds herself in a serious game of one-upmanship with the cards stacked against her. The other two admitting teams have had astounding luck, in their view, in establishing the diagnoses of not one, but two, very rare conditions. She herself has had the challenges of only very common illnesses that require only a routine knowledge, and yet she has worked long hours with no sleep in providing the best treatment available. She would like some acknowledgment of her work. The stress in this case is that of her feeling undervalued in comparison with the others despite her efforts. Her anxiety takes the form of the sense of doom: of being ignored in the excitement of the other two teams' discoveries. And Ben Jonson has already shown us just how painful it is to be ignored.

To begin the recognition algorithm process, the observer looks for evidence of the Primitive Domain mechanisms. Does she ignore feeling ignored? The vignette gives no evidence of her turning into a wallflower and avoiding the whole irritation, of projecting it out by claiming that the two other teams' patients have come from another galaxy just to torment her, or of denying that the other teams' feats of diagnostic legerdemain ever existed. She does not employ any psychotic adaptive strategies.

Nor, to her credit, does she use the Immature Domain adaptive mechanisms. She does not blame the others for the potential of her work being overlooked and undervalued. She does not regard the chief resident as out to embarrass her for her professional skills (Neurotic Projection), she does not poison the coffee of the other two teams (Acting Out), and she does not drift into a fantasy world (Schizoid Fantasy), come down with unexplained illness (Hypochondriasis), or insist on being first to speak and using all of the time to describe her own patients in minute detail (Passive Aggression). She does not employ the character-level psychological adaptive mechanisms.

In respect to the Neurotic Domain adaptive mechanisms and the task of identifying both the intern's painful feelings and painful thoughts, the observer notes that the first is feeling angry and the second is thinking that she will not get credit for her work while being upstaged by the others. Her thoughts and feelings, however, do not appear to be separate from each other. She does not become inexplicably angry (Repression), nor does she obsessively question the evidence on which the other two teams based their diagnoses (Intellectualization/Isolation of Affect). As well, she does not aim her anger at some lowly medical student (Displacement), pretend she is somewhere else (Dissociation), or institute a wide-ranging chart review of all the hospital's cases in order to find her own case with some other rare diagnosis (Reaction Formation). Hers is not the repetitive Neurotic Domain range of adaptive strategies that make it hard, if not impossible, for her to be a member of the group, and an active contributor to morning rounds.

Rather, she recognizes the stress of being undervalued and the feeling of doom associated with it, regards the painful thoughts and feelings as her own to be dealt with, and integrates the affect and cognition, rather than split them apart. She first makes a series of jokes in her own mind that set the stage for the joke she will tell on herself before the body of medical scholars. She then gets up and makes fun of her bad luck in one-upmanship, gently saying that she specializes in recognizing the common horses while referring the recognition of rare zebras to others. The others reward her with their laughter, even from the department chairman, who inadvertently cues the chief resident. By doing so, she finds herself both valued, the opposite of her sense of doom, and connected to the others in the room who have more often had nights of taking care of routine matters than of demonstrating their medical prowess among the rare conditions. The intern's adaptive mechanism is that of her Humor, her ability to laugh at herself and learn from the process. As readers, we thank her from the heart and thank all of the other interns, for their examples that have instructed us through the course of this volume. Well done, good and faithful servants.

CODA: HUMOR AND LIVING IN TIME

We come to the last of the exercises designed to teach the reader how to use the algorithm in recognizing psychological adaptive mechanisms. It may be useful at this point to consider an instance of perhaps greater subtlety than those seen before. For that, let us use an example of an adaptive response in respect to what people mean when they want to make sense of, think about, or describe the "human condition." Day-to-day Humor itself often presents subtly and does not exist only as a catalyst to obvious belly laughs, uncontrolled giggles, or even pleasant groans. Symbolically speaking, it can simply induce a smile that involves the feeling state of joy. If pity and terror define human tragedy,[6] joy admits us to the human comedy. Consider this sonnet from Kenneth Fields, whom we met in much darker circumstances in Chapter 20.

Poetic

with a line from Basil Bunting
"It might be from a handbook on recorders."

For one thing, it's on the air, you can hear music,
Knowing inflected by the ear. Not *wood*,
Not even *mouthpiece*, but the lovely *fipple*
("Hey, that's like nipple," my little daughter laughs),
And the conveyor of this joy's a player,
Whose breathing tunes the hollow that she fills,
Empties and fills again. I am caught up
In the roll of the hull, this ecstasy of naming,

6. "Pity is the feeling which arrests the mind in the presence of whatsoever is grave and constant in human sufferings and unites it with the human sufferer. Terror is the feeling which arrests the mind in the presence of whatsoever is grave and constant in human sufferings and unites it with the secret cause" (Joyce 1992, p. 368). Practically speaking, Joyce's use of the word *pity* is the same as Schopenhauer's use of the word *compassion*: both denote the concept of sharing feeling with others, whether ours with them or theirs with us, or both simultaneously.

This gathering up of more than fifty years
In a wide harbor, a life made up of words,
All of them here before we finally heard them,
And consolation rolling upon the tide:
As the player's breath warms the fipple the tone clears.
Ardor, attend us as our stars descend.

(Fields 2005, p. 69)

The casual observer will be hard pressed to find any evidence of a psychological stress in this poem. And that is perhaps one of its points. But for the purposes of discussion here, we may recall the Buddhist metaphor: All life is sorrow. One of the properties of time is that it creates both beginnings and endings. And because we live in it, we too begin and end. Endings are full of sorrow. Any of the things that humans can devise—including love—bring sorrow because they end, either by changing shape or by stopping altogether, as in the finality of death. If all life is sorrow, therefore, how can we bear it every day? That is, how can we carry it, and ourselves, forward? How can it be a comedy?

At the beginning of *Paradise Lost*, the blind 17th-century Puritan poet John Milton gives his Satan the following famous lines.

Infernal world, and thou profoundest Hell
Receive thy new Possessor: One who brings
A mind not to be chang'd by Place or Time.
The mind is its own place, and in it self
Can make a Heav'n of Hell, a Hell of Heav'n.

(Book I, lines 251–255)

And a few lines later, the same character utters a marvelous, diabolical Reaction Formation.

To reign is worth ambition though in Hell:
Better to reign in Hell, than serve in Heav'n.

(lines 262–263)

Taken together, Milton says in effect that the mind can adapt to anything. It is important to recall, however, that he was writing from inside the Christian metaphor of human experience and a particularly fundamentalist version of it as a Puritan. That frame of reference, and those of the other biblical religions, as we noted earlier, divide human experience into good and bad, Heaven and Hell. From that point of view, for some, the same division may even inform the present model considered as adaptation (good) and stress (bad). By contrast, however, two major Eastern religions, Hinduism and Buddhism, do not create the same dichotomy.[7] From their

7. Consider the gentle joke of the Buddha saying to the hot dog vendor, "Make me one with everything."

metaphorical constructions of human experience, our model of adaptation would entail a positive communication, not only with life's sorrow but also with its energy, and both of them from a single source. Adaptation, from that point of view, has to do with getting in touch with the common energy that each of us shares with all of existence. We noted a version of it earlier in Schopenhauer's view of the will in nature.

Psychological adaptation in our present model, however, need not restrict itself to one or another of these cultural views exclusively. As we have noticed at different points in this volume, stress can present both positive and negative valences, and anxiety can serve simply as a signal that some threat must be dealt with, in the Western model, or that we are losing touch with our energy toward life, in the Eastern model. Like the Mature Domain mechanisms, the adaptation model itself can be flexible enough to include both Eastern and Western cultural frames of reference just as well as it can the scientific constructs of both mind and brain that we have noted before.

Read with these contexts in mind, Kenneth Fields' blank verse sonnet begins with the title "Poetic," alerting us to watch for something being made or created. The epigraph points out that a recorder—the wind instrument popularized in Renaissance Europe, made of wood and related to the pennywhistle—has something to do with it. The first six and a half lines place the production of music before us as a kind of knowledge coming through the ear. The player creates it literally out of the air that she breathes into the top part of the recorder, known as the fipple. It is a joyful experience to the listener, as well as to the little girl who laughs at the word *fipple* because it rhymes with *nipple*. The process of making music has its own dynamic: the repeated cycles of warm breath help tune the instrument itself. Symbolically speaking, *air* and *breath*, along with other words such as *wind*, frequently refer to the spirit or the life force that humans experience. As an example, in the New Testament, the Holy Spirit can take the shape of a divine wind or inspiration, or that of a dove that flies on the wind. And symbolically, there is a spirit at work in the "Poetic" recorder too, both the musical instrument and, by way of a pun, the poet himself.

Suddenly juxtaposed, the poet sees himself in the hull of a ship that is rolling back and forth, with the wind that pushes it and raises the waves around it, and just as suddenly broadens to include sound waves. This second medium generated through the use of air brings us words, the natural material of the poet who finds music in them. The poem's author has lived with them for 50 years and regards them as an ecstasy[8] that has brought him into a wide harbor, where he can find the music of words from many different sources as he learns to hear them. And even further, there is a consolation—a shared comfort—in the waves of breath through a recorder, of sound to the ear, or of wind on the sea. Line 13 puts it in a quotation: that the repeated active use of breath to make the sound waves warms the recorder's upper chamber, the fipple, and improves the clarity of the recorder's tone. This is true both of the instrument and of the poet as a recorder of words, to voice the pun intended. And the last line shifts again into something like a prayer, beginning with the word *ardor*. That word signifies passion, warmth, and fervor, and recalls the New

8. See St. Teresa of Ávila's definition and use of *ecstasy* in Chapter 19.

Testament vision of the Holy Spirit appearing as tongues of fire. The prayer to Ardor asks that it remain with us even though "our stars descend."

What does all this have to do with recognizing human psychological adaptive strategies? To answer this, we once again bring out the algorithm and ask, what stress occurs in this poem that seems itself a happy celebration of music and words? At first glance, it might seem a comment on middle age and the downturn of life—the stars descending. But it may be better to consider the subject of this poem the course of life itself. Four people appear in the poem: taken in order of age, they are the little girl, the woman who plays the recorder, the poet himself now in middle age, and another poet—Basil Bunting[9]—who is much older, and perhaps deceased, at the time of this poem's writing. Symbolically speaking, all of them course through life, perhaps even considered as waves whether through breath, sound, or the sea. The motion of waves themselves can be stressful, as can their beginning—alluding to the use of nipples—and their end, with reference to self-luminescent stars moving out of sight. This in turn can convey a sense of doom and the feeling of being "locked in" to human existence, not necessarily a pleasant thought in everyday consciousness.

How does this poem handle the sense of doom at being who and what humans are in the lives we experience? Does it split matters into good and bad in the way of the post-Zoroastrian metaphors of original sin and damnation, as in some of the views of Western cultures? More specifically, is there any evidence here of the Primitive Domain adaptive mechanisms at work? The poet does not deny or avoid the facts, either that time continues or that in the course of it humans arrive and depart like stars climbing and setting. Nor does he ascribe this to anything other than the human condition. No Primitive Domain version of Satan walks in the poem.

Is there any evidence here of an Immature Domain Satan instead? We look for a character in the poem that Projects the pain of life outward on to some other person who may then be punished for it, reminiscent of Eudora Welty's murderer in Chapter 11. But none appears. Neither is there an otherworldly Fantasy that seeks escape from this world, nor the distraction either of Acting Out a social conflict or focusing on an unexplained physical illness as the principal source of pain in human existence. Kenneth Fields makes it clear that the pain and sense of doom require adaptation from within, not from without: *we* hear music, and *we* write words. No one foists them upon us.

Isn't this simply making "a Heav'n of Hell and Hell of Heav'n" in the Reaction Formation style of Milton's Satan, generally considered the most interesting figure in that poem? To answer this, the recognition algorithm requires an identification of the cognitive and emotional contents that the stress provides. The painful idea is "I will end," in itself a recognition that only humans, of all living things, find in their awareness, to the best of anyone's knowledge. The painful feeling is terror, that which James Joyce formulated as the grave and constant element that unites our human sufferings with the secret cause (see footnote 6 in this chapter). Joyce's "secret cause" refers to that which humans experience but do not understand, any more than any of us understands, on our own and without benefit of the beliefs of others, why we are here to begin with.

---

9. Bunting was especially interested in the spoken sounds, or the music, of words.

Contrary to a Reaction Formation, neither the poem nor its characters celebrate terror as a desirable part of human life or the certainty of death as happiness. There is no ideal presented of reigning in Hell as better than serving in Heaven; the dichotomy simply does not apply here. Nor do any of the other Neurotic Domain adaptive mechanisms fit: terror and the end of personal existence are not split apart, with one unavailable to the other. Nor are they laughed at derisively—Displaced as if they had nothing to do with us—or Dissociated away, left behind for a time only to return and find them unresolved. The Neurotic Domain psychological adaptive mechanisms do not fit the poem.

What is there to suggest that terror and the transitory nature of life work together in this poem to reach an adaptive resolution of idea and feeling that quells anxiety? What addressed the sense of doom—and allows us to bear the unbearable? "Not *wood*, / Not even *mouthpiece*, but the lovely *fipple*"—how difficult it is to read those lines without smiling or even a gentle laugh. There is something innately funny about the word *fipple* just because of the sound it makes, and perhaps ironically so. The child in the poem finds it funny because of its rhyme. And its meaning in the poem expands as it takes on its character as the part of the musical instrument that changes in contact with the player's breath, the two together clarifying the sound of the music. And even if it sounds funny, *fipple* is still a word, one of the words waiting for us to hear them in that wide harbor of experience. We can hear the delight, the Humor, of being *fipples* ourselves as we interact with the breath that carries oxygen, the source of our own bodily warming as we burn matter into energy every minute. That is, we can take ourselves less seriously and find joy in the music and in the words that our air, our spirit, brings to us. We can become part of the *FIP*ple-ness, the *FIP*ple-osity, the fip*PLE*-itude: Humor allows us to smile and perhaps gently to laugh at ourselves in a way that allows others to laugh with us. We not only bear, but find joy in, that which we might otherwise find unbearable. The last line of the poem prays not to an abstract deity, but to our own ardor, our energy for the music and the words and the breath and the spirit, to give us life in all of those forms as our physical existence descends. It is a prayer that the Mature Domain psychological adaptive mechanisms allow us to answer, each one of us on our own or, as Ben Jonson might say, every man in his Humor.

REFERENCES

Collins, J. (2001). *Good to Great*. New York, Harper Business.
Fields, K. (2005). *Classic Rough News*. Chicago, University of Chicago Press.
Herodotus. (1954). *The Histories*. London, Penguin.
Jonson, B. (1968). *The Complete Poetry of Ben Jonson*. New York, W. W. Norton.
Joyce, J. (1992). *Dubliners and A Portrait of the Artist as a Young Man*. New York, Barnes & Noble Books.
Milton, J. (1957). *John Milton, Complete Poems and Major Prose*. New York, Odyssey Press.
Shakespeare, W. (1955). As You Like It. *The Complete Works of Shakespeare* (W. J. Craig, Ed.). New York, Oxford University Press.
Vaillant, G. E. (1977). *Adaptation to Life*. Cambridge, Harvard University Press.

CHAPTER 22

Clinical and Practical Uses

The first 21 chapters of this book offer the reader a model and a clinical method for recognizing psychological adaptation mechanisms as they appear in everyday life and in many different settings. The stepwise recognition algorithm offers a potentially replicable way of categorizing observable behaviors systematically by first assigning them to the appropriate Domain of psychological adaptive styles and then to the formal mechanisms themselves.

Fulfilling one of the tests of scientific knowledge, the recognition algorithm is potentially repeatable (1) at different points in time by the same observer as well as (2) among different observers who simultaneously assess the same descriptions or recordings of observable behavior. At the time of this writing, the recognition algorithm itself is only theoretically replicable in a systematic manner. Its scientific reliability, in the formal method of test and retest agreement of results, remains to be demonstrated in controlled experiments. For now, it is best regarded in the context of Sir William Osler's injunction to clinical scientists:[1] to see first, that is, to learn to observe clinical phenomenon, and, having done so, then to analyze the phenomena according to the rules of science.

WAYS OF SEEING

As mentioned early on in this volume, considerable empirical evidence supports the existence of psychological adaptive mechanisms—alternately known as ego defense mechanisms in the psychoanalytic model—as independent phenomena. There is no doubt that psychological adaptive mechanisms occur "in nature," as the reliability data of both Vaillant and Perry have established. They each use a similar method of adaptive mechanism recognition in comparing observations of behavior

1. "Medicine is learned by the bedside and not in the classroom. Let not your conceptions of disease come from words heard in the lecture room or read from the book. See, and then reason and compare and control. But see first." Quoted in Thayer (1931, p. 1). See also Belkin and Neelon (1992).

against prearranged criteria for specific mechanisms. Vaillant uses written abstractions of data from transcriptions of independent clinical interviews, and Perry's data follow directly from interviews recorded in video formats. Vaillant then offers the observational power of sequential, prospective, longitudinal observation in three large samples over six to eight decades. Whether in cross-section or over longitudinally repeated measures, this method of "seeing" psychological adaptive mechanisms opens their reality to our understanding. The drawbacks of the vignettes/video method as a clinical procedure lay both in labor intensity, when requiring at least two or more observers providing concurrent observations or conclusions, and reliance on a series of definitions that, in a clinical setting, would require constant attention to accurately repeated application.

Another approach, mentioned in Chapter 2, was pioneered by Bond (2004), resulted in the Defense Style Questionnaire (DSQ), and advanced by Andrews and associates in Australia who revised and validated the DSQ independently; it offers much less intensity of labor. This survey method asks respondents in the here-and-now to endorse, on a 1-to-9 scale, the extent to which they agree or disagree with each of 40 statements that describe behavior in response to a crisis. The statements reflect 20 discrete psychological adaptive mechanisms, with two of the statements dedicated to each respectively, allowing for a crude average between the two. This instrument lumps the Primitive and the Immature Domain adaptive mechanisms together while separating out Neurotic and Mature Domain groups, each for purposes of data analysis. While the DSQ provides a more feasible assessment because of its ease of use, its data contain much greater degrees of inference in leaping from the preset descriptions endorsed on a paper-and-pencil form to the likelihood that they reflect actual behaviors that fit the descriptions of adaptive mechanisms. Its feasibility, however, makes the DSQ useful for some research purposes in describing averages, trends, or associations, as exemplified in a later section of this chapter. But it has little usefulness as a clinical method. No studies validate the inference from questionnaire to specific behaviors in specific persons, and no published DSQ norms or cut points exist that will allow the clinician to pinpoint even the Domain of the adaptive behaviors of the patient who arrives for evaluation.

Nearly 20 years ago, I began developing the clinical approach to the assessment and recognition of psychological adaptive mechanisms that makes up the subject of this book. In developing a clinically useful, systematic, algorithm from theoretical definitions supported by empirical research data, two things became evident. First, both the theory and the stepwise approach could be taught effectively, as demonstrated in test/posttest data comparisons of the material that the residents learned in the seminars (Beresford, 2005). And, second, I found the algorithm useful in my own clinical evaluations of many patients over many years—mainly general hospital inpatients referred by their physicians and surgeons for psychiatric assessment. What follows from this point through the rest of the chapter comes from that experience and contains my belief in, as well as enthusiasm for, the recognition algorithm as a practical and useful evaluative tool, in the medical setting and in other settings as well. It comes with the warning, however, that, as is the case with any enthusiastic author, the innovation must be tested according to the rules of science. In this case, that testing is only in its earliest stages, namely that of individual experience and case examples. With this in mind, the discussion can proceed in the manner Sir William Osler gave us and begin to answer that most telling of all questions, "How do we use it?"

PRECISION IN THE DIFFERENTIAL DIAGNOSIS

In *The Wisdom of the Ego*, Vaillant noted that he retained the term *ego defense mechanism* for descriptive purposes because of his concern that the movement toward what he called the remedicalization of psychiatry in the last three or four decades of the 20th century seemed to be moving away from a focus on individuals and the dynamics of their thoughts and feelings as they went about their lives. More specifically, he responded with concern about the exclusive use of what Leston Havens, one of Vaillant's teachers, described historically as the Objective/Descriptive school of psychiatry.[2] In the late 19th century, Emil Kraepelin and his students pioneered this approach when they began the very difficult work of establishing a reliable symptom and natural history based nosology of the major psychiatric illnesses. That approach to mental illness, active today in the codifications of the *Diagnostic and Statistical Manual of Mental Illness* (DSM) series through its various editions,[3] took on renewed emphasis when the DSM-III was published in 1980. The fourth edition, which focused on syndromes of observable symptoms as diagnoses,[4] incorporated a version of Vaillant's glossary of observable ego defense mechanisms as noted in Chapter 2. Vaillant's concern over remedicalization stood in respect to psychiatrists using *only* the DSM approaches rather than some combination of them and the psychodynamic approaches that consider the patient's painful thoughts and feelings as diagnostically useful.

Although I agree entirely with Vaillant's concern about the dangers of reductionistic rather than complex approaches to psychiatric diagnosis, I take a broader view of the term *medical*. In my view, psychiatric diagnosis requires a parallel series of at least three—and possibly more—approaches that include (1) the DSM model of associated symptoms construed as syndromes, (2) the psychodynamic models that may include intra- and interpersonal approaches as well as existential, mythos-based, cultural, and even evolutionary models, and (3) medical diagnostic models that cover assessments of all of the organ systems of the body including the brain. A working discussion of each of these in relation to the others is not the goal of the

2. See Havens (1973).
3. The first edition was published in 1952, and the fifth is on the horizon at the time of this writing.
4. The diagnoses of psychiatric illnesses and conditions are largely names for collections of symptoms since, as yet, they occur in the absence of definitive biological markers of high validity and reliability. By contrast, medical diagnoses, in the hands of a physician or surgeon, look for proximate causes for symptoms or syndromes (collections of symptoms that occur together with a frequency greater than that explained by chance alone) that can be verified from physical data.

present work. But in day-to-day practice, the techniques of observing a patient's psychiatric symptoms, attending to their painful thoughts and feelings, and investigating proximate medical causes—with specific attention to the differential diagnoses *within each* of these three general areas—leads to a working judgment as to which may be most salient at the time of the evaluation. This constitutes proper psychiatric differential diagnosis in my view. This complex approach mirrors the phenomena themselves and reaches back to a more general *medical* approach—or model—rather than any form of "cookbook medicine" that applies only one model or differential. The model of psychological adaptive mechanisms adds to, and informs, psychiatric diagnosis in each of these three general areas in my clinical experience. Consider the following examples that view psychological adaptation mechanisms over varying lengths of time.

ADAPTIVE GROWTH AND DEPRESSION

A 38-year-old male who has lived most of his adult years as a surfer in Southern California, and never before regarded himself as having a problem, comes to a mental health clinic with a vague sense of feeling blue. The feeling has occurred for six months and makes it hard for him to fall asleep at night. Worse still, his sense of glory and excitement in following the waves seems no longer what it was. In fact, he has begun to sense that he has nothing he can count on—no continuing intimate relationships, no permanent address, and no regular employment in which he finds interest. He has begun to wonder what he can look forward to after living so long in the romantic vision of himself as Man Against the Ocean. Inwardly, he is not even sure that he acts, or looks, or feels "cool" anymore, although the Great Washed Uncool until now have represented all the things he felt he was not.

The clinic health professional he meets finds that the surfer grew up in a very wealthy suburb of Los Angeles, where he was largely ignored by his parents and sent to boarding schools at an early age. He dropped out of university after his freshman year and surfed ever since. Applying the recognition algorithm, the mental health professional concludes that this patient's primary adaptive mechanism for the past 20 years has been his Schizoid Fantasy, one of the Immature Domain mechanisms. Its content is the glorification of his identity as a surfer, ably assisted by Neurotic Projection whereby all else is uncool. The contents of both however, like the Fantasy and Projection mechanisms themselves, are beginning to fade. The professional cannot rule out a DSM diagnosis of major depressive disorder, but this patient does not report a sense of hopelessness and has arrived at the clinic seeking help. Of the hopeless-helpless-worthless triad of the depressive mood disorders, his self-esteem appears to have caused the greatest part of his anxiety, suggesting a stress to his consciousness in that realm. But the anxious surfer does not report any of the classic biological symptoms such as sleep discontinuity with early waking, morning depression, or weight loss that would point more toward a depression diagnosis.

Using only the DSM model, the surfer might nonetheless get a prescription for an antidepressant at this point. Were he to withdraw into a profound sense of hopelessness and the classic biological symptoms of depression as his course unfolded, an antidepressant would be indicated and very likely helpful. But at this point, the best formulation concludes that his presentation of some of the elements of depression may actually indicate the process of psychological growth. His Immature Domain psychological adaptive mechanisms no longer serve him. He has begun the shift to relocating the stress of his existence from his fantasies and his external projections to some part within himself—recognizing the sense of feeling blue as having to do with himself rather than everyone else.[5]

The evaluating professional's working hypothesis, therefore, is that this patient will improve as he constructs new and better adaptive mechanisms, most likely next of the Neurotic Domain variety. He sends the surfer to one of the clinic therapists, who begins helping the patient look at what might be troubling him, but the evaluator retains in mind the possibility that this may be the beginning of a Major Depressive Disorder episode. A few weeks later, the clinician is reassured by the therapist, who reports that the surfer has begun a course at a local community college in order to "try out" his math skills because that was a favorite subject in high school. In the meantime, the patient's continuing jokes about the therapist's "uncool" shoes and other attributes have become the focal point of their conversations. The therapist formulates this as a Displacement, a Neurotic Domain mechanism that allows both patient and therapist to talk about what constitutes "uncool," a displaced way in which the patient can talk about himself and his anxieties.

With respect to using the clinical model and the recognition algorithm, consideration of psychological adaptive mechanisms has here enhanced the DSM diagnostic process, rather than replaced it on the one hand or been ignored by it on the other. Human behavior is complex, and no single model will have all the answers. Differential diagnosis, in this case, involved a working hypothesis that interpreted the facts by using the adaptive model and its recognition algorithm. But it did not give up the possibility that other processes, such as a form of depression that is thought to be based in specific neurochemical actions, may also be at work. The patient's course in this case, as in all others, provides the ultimate test of the clinician's working hypothesis.

The surfer's case further illustrates one very important property of the hierarchy of psychological adaptive mechanisms. Their general momentum, their energy, moves toward growth, toward Maturity. Why this occurs in human nature, and how it occurs, makes up the subject of a good many models of human behavior ranging from religions and cultural psychology to neural structure and molecular physiology.

In the present model of psychological adaptive mechanisms, the first consideration is not why or how growth toward Maturity occurs, but rather that it does occur. The first function of the medical or other professional is to assist the process of growth and, concurrently, not to impede it. *Primum non nocere*—first do no harm, as the ancient medical dictum has it, and then find how best to assist. Active harm in this case might have been to prescribe a benzodiazepine or other sedative that might

5. See the discussion of a similar point of transition in respect to alcoholism, depicted in Kenneth Fields' poem in Chapter 20.

have quelled the surfer's sense of anxiety at no longer being cool without addressing the underlying proximate cause; medications always contain risks as well as benefits. As the patient's course demonstrates, the best assistance in this case was to provide a professional relationship with another human being aimed at assisting in the recognition of the stress and its anxiety, and in finding new ways to adapt to it.

REGRESSION AND THE BRAIN

The surfer's case offers an example of the adaptive mechanism model broadening psychiatric diagnosis through its concurrent use with the DSM symptom syndrome approach. Consider an instance in which psychological adaptation assessment informs a very different model.

A grandfatherly gentleman now in his early 70s, at age 50 had ended a long history of daily heavy smoking when his doctor informed him that his breathing tests indicated irreversible emphysema. In recent years, however, he had begun to suffer lung infections with increasing frequency. These made it even harder for him to breathe and caused him to cough up yellowish, infected sputum. Because of his congenial personality, he had struck up a happy relationship with the medical and nursing staff members of the pulmonary clinic in his local veterans' hospital. He would bring them low-cholesterol oatmeal and raisin cookies, baked from his own recipe, as part of an ongoing informal campaign that he and the clinic staff shared in the effort of "living longer and better." The nurses, attending physicians, and rotating resident staff members, for their part, would joke with him about his campaign. The hospital had even incorporated the phrase "living longer and better" into its antismoking campaigns. Like the members of an extended family, they were always glad to see him, and he them.

One spring morning, a few days after a family gathering in which he was exposed to the cold virus symptoms of his grandchildren, his breathing had become especially labored. His complexion and his nail beds had taken on a bluish cast, suggesting a lack of oxygen, and his family brought him into the clinic. The staff quickly evaluated their favorite patient and admitted him to the ICU to ease the hard work of his breathing, and begin antibiotic treatment for another round of bacterial infection, one that appeared to be superimposed on his cold. His medical team also started him on a course of prednisone—a steroid of the class that manages glucose mobilization—in high doses to control his body's inflammatory response to his lung infection. By evening, he appeared tired but was breathing much more comfortably and had lost the bluish cast in his complexion. His family left after visiting hours, and he spent a quiet night.

When his medical team arrived on rounds early the next morning, however, they were surprised to find him telling them how stupid they were and what terrible doctors they had all turned out to be. In addition, he reported that he had found the nurses completely uncaring and the food terrible. His speech had become rapid, and he had difficulty remaining in one place, alternately sitting on the bed and then pacing back and forth while tethered to his intravenous line. His mood was one of constant irritation. Asked how he felt, he responded by saying, "I'm fine, but this hospital is going to the dogs." Asked whether he saw things out of place or unusual in his hospital room, he replied, "Only the stupidity of doctors like you." Despite this, he had no concerns about others plotting to hurt him or any other kind of delusional belief. He was well aware of time and place and demonstrated no loss of thought process despite his rapid speech and derogatory comments. The medical team harbored a suspicion that their favorite patient had been duplicitous and angry all along and for some reason found it propitious to let them know about it at this time. However, because of the rapid change in his personality, they called in the hospital psychiatrist for a consultation.

That physician, noting the rapid downward shift from the Mature Domain psychological adaptive mechanism of Altruism that consistently and normally characterized this patient's adjustment to his lung illness, to the Immature Domain mechanism of Neurotic Projection that led him to insult his doctors, taken in the context of hyperactivity and rapid speech, made a form of delirum the working diagnosis. This syndrome had most likely occurred as a result of the prednisone treatment. It had not yet reached a severe stage, with greater loss of the ability to think properly or with misperceptions characterized by hallucinations and delusions. Alternatively, the differential diagnosis included delirium due to the infection itself, with the possibility of spread to the brain either in the bacterial or viral form. The patient, however, did not have a fever at this juncture, and this lessened the likelihood of delirium due to an infection. The psychiatrist advised treatment with a very low dose of a dopamine-blocking agent, in this case haloperidol at 0.5 mg, targeting the return of this patient's usual personality along with no irritability or hyperactivity. If this treatment did not to work over the course of the day, the infectious process should be considered again, with the possibility of the need for a lumbar puncture assessment and a magnetic resonance imaging (MRI) scan of the brain. The haloperidol was to be given in a low dose because of the likely heightened sensitivity of the man's brain to any psychoactive agent while in a delirious state.

After an hour, the patient's symptoms had cleared partially, and he was given a second dose. After four hours, he was back to his kindly self, sitting quietly in his bed, speaking logically and in a normal rate and rhythm. When his medical resident asked him about the concerns he had voiced that morning about his doctors' competence, the patient looked at him in a puzzled manner and asked what it was that he had said to them. On hearing the description, he became embarrassed and apologized, saying that he had no memory of his comments and certainly regretted ever having said anything like that, whether he could remember it or not. He continued on the 0.5 mg dose daily for the next five days while receiving the prednisone for his breathing. As he cleared, the prednisone was stopped, as was the haloperidol. The patient's symptoms did not return.

This case illustrates Regression[6]: a phenomenon defined as the downward movement from employing higher Domain psychological adaptive mechanisms to those of a lower Domain. In this case, the grandfatherly darling of the pulmonary clinic,

6. This is alluded to in Chapter 7 in the case of Major Mannock.

who brought them "living longer and better" in his Altruism adaptation to his own lung disease, turned into the snarling ingrate who insulted his doctors when the prednisone entered his brain.[7] As his brain lost its function, his adaptive capability moved down the recognition algorithm. Where before, painful thoughts and emotions combined in adapting to the anxiety of a clear and present illness, now the best the patient's brain could do was to allow an Immature Domain adaptation in which he viewed himself as not all ill and everyone else as stupid. In this instance, the dopamine-blocking agent corrected the brain physiology that had been upset by the prednisone, a medicine the patient needed in order to recover from his acute lung infection. As the brain's neurochemical status corrected with dopamine antagonist treatment, the patient's adaptive state returned to what it was before the insult to the brain occurred. Alternately stated, the Regression ends, and with that the brain returns to the highest level of psychological adaptation that the person had reached before.

Cases of this nature are not at all uncommon and can stem from many different causes. They illustrate the usefulness of noting the observable changes in adaptive behavior as indications of the state of health of the functioning brain. A Regression can travel all the way down the steps of the recognition algorithm to the Primitive Domain adaptive mechanisms in the setting of a failure of brain functioning. At that level, the patient may appear to be suffering from a psychosis. In that case, the clinician often—but not always—finds a concurrent loss in the brain's cognitive functions, such as constructing and retrieving new memories, calculating numbers, responding to standard judgment questions, or failing at bedside tasks that require planning.

In the case of the elderly man with lung disease, the reader will notice that the medical team thought of ascribing their patient's obstreperous behavior to a permanent part of his makeup that had remained hidden to them prior to that time. No one, after all, likes to be called stupid, and the team's human, if not professional, response might have been to become angry and tell the patient that he did not know what he was talking about. In that instance, they might have begun to think of him as characterologically impaired and a very hateful person, rather than the kindly gentleman they had known. The team, however, had sufficient wisdom to consider their patient's unusual behavior professionally, to doubt their own on-the-spot judgment, and to call in an expert for an outside opinion.

Clinically, the key to recognizing the presence of an adaptive mechanism Regression lay in the history of this patient's prior functioning. Recalling the injunction first stated in Chapter 2 and repeated since, that *people use the best adaptive mechanisms available to them at any particular point in time*, this patient's ongoing relationship with his caregivers and their knowledge of him established that his usual adaptive functioning was very high indeed. He engaged others, and they respected him for it. He had even contributed creatively to the prevention or mitigation of lung diseases in other veterans. Without this knowledge, there would be no useful baseline of functioning against which to measure his outburst after receiving the prednisone.

7. The patient regresses from darling to snarling, as it were.

Rather than regarding current behavior as necessarily characteristic of a pattern, the wise clinician will take pains to establish the patient's highest level of adaptive functioning. This generally can be gotten from those who know the patient best over time, such as family members and caregivers.

Table 22.1 lists, in clinical shorthand, comparisons across the domains that the clinician may find useful in understanding the presentation of the patient immediately before him or her in respect to adaptive styles observed in the clinic or at the bedside. The first row recounts the description from the earlier chapters of when specific Domain mechanisms occur normally, regarding this as a clinical behavioral baseline and considered with an allowance for individual variations. The second row recapitulates the characteristic adaptive stances in regard to stress that occurs within each of the Domains and by which they are defined, as we've seen in considerable detail through the course of this volume.

The third row lists very briefly the appearance that the respective Domain mechanisms take on as they appear in adult life to an outside clinical observer using a model of psychiatric descriptive pathology, such as that offered by the DSM series. The term *psychosis* in this row refers to major mental illnesses such as schizophrenia, major depression, or bipolar disorder, and other variants of these that can result in a psychosis as defined by marked impairment of cognition and perception. The next descriptor, *character disorder*, sometimes also referred to as *personality disorder*, obtains when a person's principal adaptive mechanisms lead them to ascribe their own difficulties to persons or factors outside themselves, the common characteristic of all the Immature Domain styles as we have seen.

In the third column, *adjustment disorder*, from the DSM series, refers to the larger phenomenon of repeating dysphoric—meaning painful or uncomfortable—behaviors that characterize the Neurotic Domain mechanisms. And, in the last column, the Mature Domain psychological adaptive mechanisms make no appearance because they are defined specifically as healthy in adult life.

Table 22.1 PSYCHOLOGICAL ADAPTIVE MECHANISM DOMAINS IN DIFFERENTIAL DIAGNOSIS

	Primitive	Immature	Neurotic	Mature
Age appropriate	Early childhood	Adolescence	Adulthood	Adulthood
Response to stress	Does not exist	Someone else's problem	Affective/cognitive disjunction	Affective/cognitive integration
Adult pathology	Psychosis	Character disorder	Adjustment disorder	None
Environmental response	Hospitalization, social isolation	Ostracism, crisis, incarceration	Advise help	Social connection, integration
Regression differential	Systemic/brain illness	Systemic/brain illness	Generally none, possible brain syndromes	Health

The fourth row in Table 22.1 provides brief characterizations of the response of the environment to persons using the respective Domain adaptive styles in adulthood. Stated very briefly, those using Primitive Domain mechanisms are generally not difficult to identify because of their bizarre behavior and are often either ignored or brought into hospitals or other social agencies out of concern for their safety or that of others. Immature Domain adaptive styles, by contrast, generally serve to irritate the other persons in the social network who surround those deploying them. Characteristically, those who function in this range of adaptive styles do not seek help but may be actively extruded from their social setting into the therapist's office or the ER when the environmental network can no longer tolerate this level of adaptive behavior. By contrast, those in the Neurotic Domain range find themselves in pain or discomfort, and communicate it to their trusted social contacts, who will often respond by suggesting they seek professional help. Persons functioning in this Domain generally come to the clinic on their own initiative seeking professional assistance with their dysphoria, as we noted in the case of the surfer earlier in this chapter. And last, in contrast to the other Domains, the Mature Domain psychological adaptive mechanisms link persons with those in their environment in productive and satisfying ways. Psychological adaptation at this level includes forming satisfying relationships, as for example the relationship between our elderly emphysemic patient and his clinic.

The last row of Table 22.1 lists the general areas for which a medical disease model must account when faced with the patient in any of the respective adaptive Domains. As noted, both brain diseases and those of the body's other physical systems can result in impairments that are then expressed as the Regression from higher to lower Domain adaptive mechanisms.

Both the Primitive and Immature Domain adaptive mechanisms presenting in adult life—especially in settings of acute change or as part of a less striking, downhill course from higher adaptive Domain functioning—call forth the clinician's attention to the medical differential diagnosis that may identify an underlying cause amenable to treatment. Proper treatment of a proximate cause of this nature, as we noticed in the case of our elderly lung patient exposed to the steroid anti-inflammatory agent, can resolve the Regression with the return to health.

Last, in considering the Mature Domain mechanisms, no differential diagnostic efforts need occur on their account. Medical illnesses may be present, but not of the sort that result in an adaptive Regression. Rather, and I often find myself recommending this to colleagues and house officers, it is entirely permissible in the medical setting to admire those who come to terms, often heroically, with a medical illness and its circumstances. Consider, for example, the case of a man with very few economic resources who arrives at a public hospital on a mid-October day with terrible pain in one of his feet. He learns that the disease in the blood vessels of that foot has progressed to a point requiring amputation. Admitted for that purpose, he appears somewhat depressed and withdrawn over the first day as he considers how he might live without being able to walk properly. He begins to trust the treatment team, who not only begin preparing him for his surgery and the work needed to make use of a new prosthesis, but help him to find a place to live during and after his rehabilitation. On the third day and prior to his amputation, he says to the surgical team, "Well, this way I can dress up as the Peg Leg Pirate every Halloween." He, and they, find laughter helpful as a way to adjust to this difficult situation. One can only stand in awe at the elegance of which humans find themselves capable.

REGRESSION AND STRESS

An impairment of brain function is not the only cause of Regression in the present model of psychological adaptation. Stress itself can do so, especially when delivered either in a heavy dose in a short period of time—connected with anxiety defined as an impending sense of disaster—or in a continuing, relentless assault over a period of time with no respite—consistent with anxiety defined as an ongoing sense of doom. The second of these recalls Edward Mannock's dangerous behavior examined in Chapter 7, and, to illustrate the first definition with regard to disaster, consider the following incident.

An intelligent and well-educated woman in her early 40s has suffered epilepsy since childhood. For the previous 10 years, however, she has not had any seizures whatsoever. With her neurologist's consent and direction, she weans herself off of her anticonvulsant medications. All goes well for another 10 months until early on a summer evening when she drives along a coastal highway in California. The sun is low over the sea as she passes a long row of palm trees. She flashes through the alternating light and shadow as the trees create a strobe effect with the sun, triggering a seizure. She loses control of her car, veers across the highway into an oncoming lane and crashes into another vehicle. She suffers a broken hip and ankle, but the crash kills the driver of the other car. Her next memory after the flashing sunlight occurs some hours later, when she wakes in the ICU of a large medical center to which she has been airlifted. She does not suffer pain but knows that she is in a hospital and has been injured. She closes her eyes, pulls her sheet up over her head, and refuses to talk with her surgeons. They order a psychiatric consultation for the next morning.

When the psychiatrist arrives, the patient continues to lie still in her bed with her hands at her side and the bedsheet pulled up over her head in the manner of a corpse. In gentle tones, the psychiatrist introduces herself and waits for a few moments. With no response from the patient, she asks the patient's name and again gets no response. The psychiatrist then gently pulls the edge of the sheet down from the patient's head to below her chin, exposing her face. The woman holds her eyes tightly shut and, in a quick motion, with a hint of violence, pulls the sheet back up over her head and holds it there. The psychiatrist, again gently, says she will come back to talk with the patient later and leaves the room. She concludes from her interview that this patient has likely regressed from a higher functioning state to one in which Primitive Domain Avoidance is now the last best adaptive mechanism available to her.

The doctor advises the nurses and the medical team that she is very concerned about this patient, who appears to be in a very dangerous situation that may lead to thoughts of self destruction. They agree to keep a close eye on her, and to notify the psychiatric on-call team immediately of any change in the woman's condition.

Over the course of the day, the psychiatrist talks by phone with the patient's sister and learns that the patient's husband has been on the opposite coast for business and is due back late that evening. At the same time, she learns that the patient herself is a very high functioning freelance editor and writer who is much in demand by the advertising firms based in Los Angeles. She has not suffered any mental illness, in the sister's awareness, and her only physical illness is her epilepsy. Her sister describes her as an outgoing person who has many friends, whose relationship with her husband is close and affectionate, and whose two children are both in college and doing well.

The next morning when the psychiatrist returns to the ICU, she meets the patient's husband, a tired-looking man of middle age who greets her appropriately and then asks about his wife's health. They converse outside the patient's room, where the husband says that he has heard the details of the auto accident but has not spoken with his wife about them for fear of saying something inappropriate. "I just don't know what I should say or even what she knows already," he says. In response to the doctor's questions, he adds that his wife recognizes him and will look at him while holding the sheet down below her eyes, but she will not speak to him. She closes her eyes tightly and looks away or pulls the sheet over her face once again. The doctor points out that this is an improvement over yesterday and that the two of them should go in and talk with her now.

In the room, the psychiatrist stands on one side of the bed and the husband on the other; the patient lies flat with the sheet in place as before. The psychiatrist introduces herself again and adds that she is one of the doctors in the hospital and would like to ask the patient some questions. She adds that the patient's husband is here too and can stay for the interview. After a few moments, the patient pulls the sheet down below her face and stares to the side, looking at her husband with her eyes partially closed as if squinting. A few moments later, she opens them wide and says to her husband in an angry accusatory voice, "You're not telling me the truth. There's something you're not telling me!" The husband looks nervously at the psychiatrist, who responds to his glance with an affirmative nod back at him. The husband looks back to his wife and tells her that she has been in a road accident in which a person in an oncoming car was killed. Her doctors think she may have had a seizure immediately before the accident, and they're treating her for some broken bones. Before he can get the last part of the sentence out, his wife startles the entire ICU with a howl of anguish that, he later says to the psychiatrist, reminds him of what he has heard about the howl of the Banshee, the harbinger of death in Irish mythology. After some sedation, the woman no longer howls, but neither does she speak. She does not attempt to move again and lies quietly, this time without pulling the sheet over her head. The psychiatrist lets her know that her husband will remain with her, that the patient's realization of the tragedy has come with a great deal of effort, and that she is safe here in the hospital. The nurses will be in frequent contact, and the psychiatrist herself will return to see the patient the next day.

On the third morning, the psychiatrist returns to see the patient sitting up in the ICU bed and making eye contact. Her husband sits in a chair near the bed. The patient's facial expression is one of disgust, if not repulsion, when she looks up. As the doctor introduces herself again, the patient immediately tells her, "I should have died in that accident rather than that other person. I must die myself in order for it all to be fair. Life is bad and worthless. I must die to make it fair." The psychiatrist acknowledges the woman's words, adding that many other patients in her experience have mentioned concerns about death in this way, sometimes thinking of it as a last relief. "If you're alive, I can be of use to you," she says to the woman. "If you're dead, there is nothing I can do for you. It might be better for us to look at other options in handling a difficult situation." The patient looks unmoved, but quietly seems to accept the possibility of looking into the matter further with the doctor. The three of them discuss the matter for a few minutes, going over what the patient knows of the facts of the accident and of her own injuries and their prognosis. The doctor ends the interview after asking the woman whether she is having any further suicidal thoughts, especially any that might have turned into plans about how to kill herself. The woman answers negatively, and the doctor asks whether she will notify the nurses and her husband if any suicidal thoughts return. The patient responds that she will do so.

The psychiatrist continues to meet with the patient and her husband over the next several days, including her transition out of the ICU and on to an orthopedic floor on the fifth day. At that time, the psychiatrist asks whether the patient feels safe without the presence of another in-room person around the clock. The patient, who speaks with greater ease, although not back in the lilting rhythms of her regular conversation style according to her husband, states that she continues to feel safe, though she is still puzzled about how to "make up" for the death of the other person in the accident. The psychiatrist senses a good therapeutic alliance with the patient as well as the realistic perception of the sense of helplessness—in this case the inability to turn time back and change the fact of the accident—that sometimes forms the beginning of positive steps forward in resolving stress.

A week later, the patient returns to her hometown to begin rehabilitation from her injuries as well as work with a therapist in her locale in coming to terms with the accident. A few months later, the psychiatrist receives a phone call from the patient, thanking her for her concerns and saying she is back at work and both she and her husband are doing well. She adds, "Although I'll never feel right about this whole thing, I've started an organization that looks into how best to take care of people after a car accident, including the families of those injured or killed."

This extended vignette illustrates Regression in response to a particularly devastating acute stress, namely an auto accident that causes the death of another person. The woman's medical condition—the seizure she suffered—in this case likely plays a role, namely her postseizure state of unconsciousness, her returning cognitive faculties, and her lack of memory for the event itself. A seizure with no accident following would not cause an extreme regression. However, a small piece of her memory of the incident had survived, enough to allow her to sense early on that something terrible had happened.

As the course of the Regression unfolded however, the psychiatrist saw that this patient's first adaptive recourse was to the Primitive Domain mechanism of Avoidance. In a very concrete style, she pulled the sheet up over her head and would not interact with the world around her. Her surgeons correctly called in the psychiatrist.

Recognizing this as a Primitive Domain adaptation in an otherwise previously psychologically healthy woman as corroborated by her family, the psychiatrist immediately sensed the danger coming from this patient's own anxiety: being cornered with no other way out in the face of overwhelming disaster. A Regression of this magnitude is not the stuff of normal, everyday functioning, and its presence indicates clinical danger.

As the patient began to recover from the stress of the accident, she next engaged the Immature Domain mechanism of Neurotic Projection: blaming her husband and those around her for not telling her the truth, for hiding something from her. Her husband's words triggered an emotional expression that contained all of the terror and sadness that she herself felt. She expressed it in a way that all those around her could sense as well. This was so overwhelming as to require the external support of the ICU staff and the brief, time-limited use of a sedative agent.

The next step in her adaptive mechanism reconstitution led her to engage a Reaction Formation, one of the Neurotic Domain mechanisms: she herself should die in the name of atonement, viewing her own death as good and her life as bad. The psychiatrist's approach at this point was to look at this with her and help her doubt that her Reaction Formation was the best option. The woman was able to make use of the alliance with the psychiatrist in the effort to move back to her prior level of healthy functioning. This made itself evident in her last step, namely engaging the Mature Domain mechanism Altruism in finding a way to share her experience with other people in a way that might make the world a little better off.

Clinically, it is useful to note two points in this case that may possibly occur in a generalized fashion in other instances of a similar nature. First, the acute stress could drive psychological adaptation all the way down from the Mature Domain in the recognition algorithm to the Primitive Domain at its bottom, and do so in a very short period of time. This portends that all of us can suffer Regression when the stress is bad enough.

Second, although the Regression occurred quickly, so too did the reconstitution, in this case taking several days instead of several years. In healthy individuals, such as the woman in the accident, the process of reconstitution contains its own power to return the person back to Mature Domain functioning. In most cases, theory suggests that the same energy toward reconstitution will return them to the highest level at which they were capable of functioning before the stress. This may be to any of the Domains above the Regression in the recognition algorithm, whether Immature, Neurotic, or Mature. This psychological resiliency of motion toward the highest level of previous functioning allows the present model to offer some insight into why it is that some persons respond quickly from Regression after a traumatic event while others appear to respond very slowly or not at all. Much has to do with the pretrauma starting point of psychological adaptation mechanism maturity, the model would suggest.

The woman with the auto accident, for example, regressed dramatically from the Mature Domain adaptive mechanisms that she had developed through the normal course of her life. By contrast, the retired carpenter introduced in Chapter 12 had managed only the Neurotic Domain mechanisms, at his best, in his developmental course through life. He had never been able to trust others, either in intimate relationships or at work, being instead locked in Immature Domain Neurotic Projection and the notion that others would always let him down. His Schizoid Fantasy of the same Domain led to his using all of his resources to move to Costa Rica, where he would live like a king and find a young wife to take care of him. Contrasted to the woman with the auto accident, a Regression in the carpenter's case might mean moving from a tenuous Neurotic Domain Repression mechanism to Primitive Domain Avoidance when faced with the task of locating a place to live. Reconstitution in his case would return him to a combination of the Immature and Neurotic Domain psychological adaptive mechanisms. From our points of view as outside observers, he may appear as intransigent and perhaps as regressed as before. This judgment, however, may have more to do with our perception of intransigence: he appears to us unable to reconstitute because that process, like his Regression, covered much less ground, when viewed in the Domain hierarchy, than in the case of the woman with the auto accident. Understanding a patient's optimal level of adaptive functioning—his or her baseline before a Regression—is crucial in formulating an understanding of Regression and in charting a clinical reconstitution.

FURTHER EXAMPLES OF POSSIBLE USES

To sum up, since beginning this book, both author and reader will have spent considerable time and effort in moving from a theoretical model of psychological adaptive mechanism assessment, based in observable behaviors, through an algorithm-guided process of adaptive mechanism recognition that can be used clinically. With this, the present chapter has so far brought the realization that this method affords a systematic way of seeing a patient's adaptive abilities in a clinical setting. In that setting, the clinical hypotheses that derive from this recognition approach must be further tested in respect to accuracy in repeated assessments. In addition to on-the-spot recognition, this chapter has also added the dimension of time, noting that the phenomenon of positive growth allows people to move toward measurable maturity of psychological adaptation. At the same time, factors such as medical illness and either acute severe or chronic unrelenting stress can drive a Regression from the higher to the lower domains of adaptive functioning described in the recognition algorithm. When this occurs, however, the factors that make up human psychological resiliency can often energize the processes of psychological adaptation and allow for reconstitution of the highest psychological adaptive mechanisms that an individual reached before a Regression. In the last section of this chapter, we will explore some examples in which this recognition process of adaptive mechanisms might be used in other settings.

As we have seen in specific examples throughout this work, the spectrum of ways in which people adapt to the circumstances of their lives has fascinated writers, historians, and creative artists through the course of human existence. In offering a systematized version of observation, we may now hypothesize how to put it to practical use. The number of ways in which to apply this way of seeing is limited only by our imaginative abilities. We have already noted that it has particular use as (1) a model for measuring personal change in the setting of psychological treatment, as in our example of the surfer. Similarly, as in the man with emphysema, it can serve as (2) an indicator of subtle and often early loss of brain or bodily function, triggering medical evaluative processes that include those of psychiatry. And, as in the case of the woman with the seizure disorder, it can (3) serve as treatment guide to the reconstitution of optimal adaptive functioning following both acutely and chronically delivered stresses to the person. In what follows, the reader may consider some heavily disguised samples from further clinical experience that might allow consideration of these and other settings in which this recognition method may be used.

ADAPTATION VERSUS DEPRESSION IN THE SETTING OF CANCER

In working with medical and surgical services, one ongoing concern among cancer specialists is whether and when to offer their patients antidepressant medication. Some years ago, widely publicized studies noted increased survival rates among cancer patients who underwent psychotherapeutic treatment. But a subsequent multicenter study failed to replicate improved survival after behavioral treatment, and other studies found similarly conflicting results. Separately published reports from noncancer treatment studies suggested that the patients most likely to benefit from psychotherapies are generally those with the most psychological adaptive maturity. This led our research group to an alternative explanation: the suggestion that the underlying maturity of psychological adaptive mechanisms may themselves be related to cancer survival. No studies to that time had considered adaptive mechanisms as potential mediating variables in the conflicting results reported in both psychotherapy treatment studies and, remarkably, in trials of antidepressants in cancer patients. Our group therefore applied measures of both depression symptom frequency and psychological adaptive mechanism maturity, in this case the DSQ, to assess the relation each bore on survival probability in a sample of cancer patients. We hypothesized that (1) increased depression symptom frequency and (2) Immature Domain adaptive mechanism endorsement would, independently, predict lower cumulative survival probability at five years. To test this, we collected data from a series of patients undergoing cancer chemotherapy who were not in extreme pain or experiencing delirium symptoms, and then followed them for five years.

To our surprise, as seen in Figure 22.1, the frequency of depression symptoms had no relationship with cancer survival in the Most versus the Least depressed extreme cases in the sample. By contrast, the Mature and Immature case extremes in adaptive Domain styles differed widely and well beyond the expectations of chance alone. After five years, 50% of the Mature adaptors remained alive while 50% of the Immature adaptors had not lived beyond 18 months.[8] The study suggested to us the necessity of understanding the characteristics of the Immature Domain group as a way of better defining how addressing psychological adaptive styles themselves might

8. Beresford (2006).

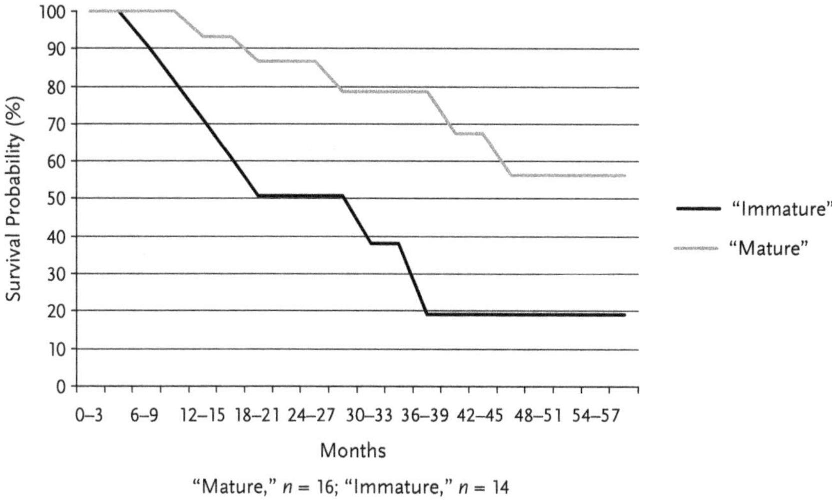

Figure 22.1
Five-Year Cumulative Cancer Survival Probability by Maturity of Adaptive Styles

be helpful in the face of a very serious, often frightening illness. It further pointed out that future studies of antidepressant medication in this group would require measures of psychological adaptive mechanism along with measures of symptoms of depression or psychosis. The adaptive model presented in this volume, in short, presents profound implications in respect not only to diagnosis but also to treatment outcome in illness-related behavioral disorders.

TO TRANSPLANT OR NOT TO TRANSPLANT: LIVING DONATION

Because the availability of suitable organs for donation limits the capacity of liver transplantation to save lives, methods of donating one of the two lobes of the liver taken from a willing, living donor have been developed as a method of increasing organ availability. To both recipients and transplant surgery teams, preserving the life of an organ recipient constitutes a final good. Without the donation, the recipient must either receive a scarce cadaveric donation or die. One difficulty inheres in the word *willing*, however. No surgical team will take a donated organ from a person who does not wish to give it. But how a person reaches the decision to donate an organ, as in kidney donation, or a part of one, as in liver lobe donation, remains to be explored in respect to psychological adaptive mechanisms. Consider the following case examples.

Case 1: Twelve months after a closed head injury in an auto accident, a 37-year-old male sought Good Samaritan status as an anonymous liver lobe donor. His family agreed. At interview, his cognitive examination, however, revealed deficits in both short-term memory and frontal lobe executive functions. An assessment of his psychological adaptive mechanisms identified Primitive Domain Avoidance/Distortion in his belief that the public notoriety from his liver donation would restore his business that had failed after his accident. The psychiatrist and the transplant team agreed on pursuing his candidacy no further.

Case 2: A 33-year-old, three times divorced, male presented for live donation of a liver lobe to a married but childless woman in her late 20s. The recipient happened to be an alumna of his mother's college sorority whom he had met at a social gathering. During the psychiatrist's evaluation, he described an incident at age 10 when he had discovered his mother's exsanguinated corpse, dressed in her sorority sweater, on their living room floor. He presented a clear cognitive state but became vehemently upset and argumentative at the suggestion that the donation might be related to his mother's death. He said his donation was only so the recipient would be healthy enough to have children and it made him sad to think that she could not.

In the psychiatrist's judgment, his highest level of psychological adaptation was a very brittle Reaction Formation, one of the Neurotic Domain mechanisms. Below that lay a Neurotic Projection, one of the Immature Domain mechanisms, in which the donor ascribed his own anger to the psychiatrist. And further down appeared his attempt at undoing his mother's own unfortunate suicide in the style of Primitive Domain Avoidance/Distortion. This constellation suggested that he would not do well when he found that his live organ donation did not resolve his own psychological trauma, consistent with the properties of pseudo-altruism, discussed in Chapter 16.

The psychiatrist advised the transplant team against accepting this patient's lobe donation for transplant. The team disagreed, however, and successfully removed his lobe and grafted it into the recipient. Three months after the procedure, the team began receiving phone messages from the donor saying that his life was worthless. He refused further psychiatric contact, saying, "They don't know what I'm going through." He was not heard from again.

Case 3: A 26-year-old, married father of a six-month-old son presented for lobe donation assessment with his wife. A jet pilot himself, he wished to donate to his uncle, a former astronaut whose heavy drinking had resulted in terminal cirrhosis. At interview, he described growing up in a chaotic household with two drug-abusing parents and looking up to his uncle as the guiding star of his life. He readily acknowledged that he hoped to extend his uncle's life because the man's example had meant so much to him. His wife, age 23, said she doubted the uncle's continued sobriety and that she did not like her husband taking unnecessary health risks with an infant son at home and their plans to have more children. The psychiatrist reviewed the likely consequences of the procedure—including the potential loss of his flying career due to health status—and assessed whether the man understood the alternative of cadaveric donation for his uncle. In the setting of the patient's clear cognitive examination, the psychiatrist noted to himself that the potential donor's adaptive mechanism qualified as a Neurotic Domain Reaction Formation—a pseudo-altruism in which the donor put his own well-being, career, and family at risk to save his uncle. Two weeks later, after further discussion between husband and wife, the man withdrew his request and asked for a referral to "talk to someone about feeling sad."

Case 4: A 32-year-old married teacher and mother of two junior high schoolers learned that her best and longest childhood friend, her first cousin and "other sister," needed a transplant because of nonalcoholic liver disease. At interview, she and her husband described their concern on hearing the news six months earlier and then together began learning about liver disease, transplantation, and donation through online searches and reading. They began discussing it with her physician two months before interview and then with their extended family. Several family members mentioned concern for her health and also applauded her willingness to consider donation; none had tried to influence her toward a decision to donate. At interview, her cognitive state was clear. Asked how tissue mismatch or other medical concerns precluding donation might affect her, she said she would rest comfortably knowing she had "done all I could for my sister." She and her husband described their plans for child care and economic adjustment during her operative recovery. The psychiatrist recorded true Altruism, a Mature Domain mechanism, as her primary adaptive strategy, along with "a healthy dose of Anticipation." Both the psychiatrist and the transplant team agreed with her proceeding to lobe donation.

As illustrated, potential donors follow many paths to the transplant team's door. Careful clinical evaluation can assess their mental capacities as well as motivation and states of mind. In the first case, assessment of the donor candidate's cognitive state led to the differential that revealed the brain trauma history. Both his history and cognitive state fit with his Primitive Domain adaptive mechanism, recalling that the Maturity spectrum of adaptive mechanism functioning is related to the health of the brain. The brain's cognitive state can be measured clinically as part of a comprehensive evaluation.[9]

The remaining three cases, all with normal cognition as tested during the interview, present much greater clinical challenges and controversy. The second patient, for example, when at his best presented a pseudo-altruism, as noted above. Its confirmation came subsequently when his apparent altruism crumbled after finding that his heroic act had no effect on his own, unintegrated painful thoughts and feelings. Consistent with the Neurotic Domain adaptive mechanisms that only repeat painful affect and cognition rather than resolve them, his heroic act left him only more desperate than before. Further, in contrast to the third case, the second donor candidate had no ability to consider alternatives, including reviewing his own sources of motivation. He projected both his need and his anger outward instead.

By contrast, the jet pilot in the third case, who also used a Reaction Formation in risking his own health and his family's well-being to save an idealized uncle, evidenced the flexibility to weigh alternatives and to experience the sadness needed to give up this Neurotic Domain adaptive mechanism. The contrast between Cases 2 and 3 suggests that assessing the ability to consider alternative actions is empirically useful as a measure of the potential for growth in individual cases. Case 2 could not

9. For wide application, a combination of the Mini-Mental State Examination or similar exams and the Frontal Assessment Battery provide effective cognitive screens; the MMSE does not address the complex cognitive processes mediated by the fronto-subcortical tracks. See our neuropsychiatry textbook for further description (Arciniegas and Beresford 2001).

move from his hard-won Reaction Formation, whereas Case 3 used the interaction with the lobe donation process itself as an occasion for growth.

In the fourth case, a careful decision process became evident and included (1) unimpaired cognition, (2) an independent examination of the pros and cons of the procedure itself, (3) a review with others who were not part of the transplant team, (4) no evidence of family coercion, and (5) empirical assessment of psychological adaptive mechanisms. In this case, the patient employed Mature Domain adaptive mechanisms: for example, being asked about not donating elicited a sense of comfort in having exhausted all of the alternatives. Contrast this to the projection of the painful emotions of subjective anger and sadness in Case 2, or in ultimately choosing the present over the past in Case 3.

While most will agree with use of the first four of the assessment factors listed in the last paragraph in addition to the standard history and physical examination, the psychological adaptive mechanism evaluation may seem foreign. The present model and its recognition algorithm, however, provide a systematic approach to that clinical evaluation. In so doing, it aims to mobilize the large empirical literature that supports the observable occurrence of psychological adaptive mechanisms "in nature" and to make appropriate use of them in clinical decision making.

The practical need for psychological adaptive mechanism assessment highlights the disagreement between the psychiatrist and the transplant team in Case 2. Practically speaking, the recipient remained alive and was better off. One can argue that the donor was worse off, however, and that evidence existed to predict this beforehand. Did the team's decision honor the medical dictum *primum non nocere*—first, to do no harm—in the second donor's case? Did extending the life of the recipient because of the liver lobe graft outweigh clinical importance of the donor's psychological state postdonation? No clear or simple answers appear.

The greater clinical precision afforded by psychological adaptive mechanism recognition does, however, offer a new and useful method of weighing psychological harm against physical benefit. This may lead to better clinical definitions of psychological harm. In the meantime, systematic attention to psychological adaptive mechanisms through the use of the recognition algorithm offers the likelihood of improving assessment and care of those who come to us, whether to grow, to heal, to reconstitute, or to put their own health at risk in the service of others. All of them deserve our best efforts in understanding their heroism, their vulnerability, and our own practice.

REFERENCES

Arciniegas, D. B., and Beresford, T. P. (2001). *Neuropsychiatry: An Introductory Approach.* Cambridge, Cambridge University Press.

Belkin, B, and Neelon, F. (1992). "The art of observation: William Osler and the method of Zadig." *Ann Int Med 116*: 863–866.

Beresford T. P. (2005). "Learning to recognize ego defense mechanisms: results of a structured teaching experience for psychiatric residents. *Academic Psychiatry 29*(5):474–478.

Beresford, T., et al. (2006). "Cancer survival as a function of psychological adaptation mechanisms versus depressive symptoms." *Psychosomatics* 47: 247–253.
Bond, M. (2004). "Empirical studies of defense style: relationships with psychopathology and change." *Harvard Review of Psychiatry* 12(5): 263–278.
Havens, L. (1973). *Approaches to the Mind*. Boston, Little Brown.
Thayer, W. S. (1931). Osler the Teacher. In *Osler and Other Papers*. Baltimore, Johns Hopkins Press.

INDEX

Note: Page numbers followed by "*f* " and "*t*" refer to figures and tables, respectively.

www.ingramcontent.com/pod-product-compliance
Lightning Source LLC
Chambersburg PA
CBHW072008020126
37647CB00003B/331
9780199794492